Guides to Clinical
Aspiration Biopsy

Retroperitoneum
and Intestine 2nd Ed.

Guides to Clinical Aspiration Biopsy

Series Editor: Tilde S. Kline, M.D.

Prostate
Tilde S. Kline, M.D.

Thyroid
Sudha R. Kini, M.D.

Retroperitoneum and Intestine 2nd Ed.
Kenneth C. Suen, M.B., B.S., F.R.C.P.(C)

Lung, Pleura and Mediastinum
Liang-Che Tao, M.D., F.C.A.P., F.R.C.P.(C)

Head and Neck
Ali H. Qizilbash, M.B., B.S., F.R.C.P.(C)
J. Edward M. Young, M.D., F.R.C.S. (C)

Liver and Pancreas
Denise Frias-Hidvegi, M.D., F.I.A.C.

Breast
Tilde S. Kline, M.D.
Irwin K. Kline, M.D.

Flow Cytometry
Philippe Vielh, M.D.

**Infectious and Inflammatory Diseases and
Other Nonneoplastic Disorders**
Jan F. Silverman, M.D.

Diagnostic Immunocytochemistry and Electron Microscopy
Hossein M. Yazdi, M.D., F.R.C.P.C.
Irving Dardick, M.D., M.Sc., F.R.C.P.C.

Pediatrics
Philippe Vielh, M.D., Ph.D.
Lydia Pleotis Howell, M.D.

Guides to Clinical Aspiration Biopsy

Retroperitoneum and Intestine 2nd Ed.

Kenneth C. Suen, M.B., B.S., F.R.C.P.(C)

Pathologist
Vancouver Hospital and Health Sciences Centre

Consulting Pathologist
British Columbia Cancer Agency

Clinical Professor of Pathology
University of British Columbia
Vancouver, British Columbia, Canada

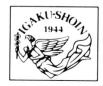

IGAKU-SHOIN   New York   •   Tokyo

Published and distributed by

IGAKU-SHOIN Medical Publishers, Inc.
One Madison Avenue, New York, New York 10010

IGAKU-SHOIN Ltd.,
5-24-3 Hongo, Bunkyo-ku, Tokyo 113-91.

Library of Congress Cataloging-in-Publication Data

Suen, Kenneth C.
    Retroperitoneum and intestine / Kenneth C. Suen. — 2nd ed.
       p.   cm. — (Guides to clinical aspiration biopsy)
    Includes bibliographical references and index.
    1. Retroperitoneum—Cancer—Cytodiagnosis.   I. Title.
  II. Series.
    [DNLM: 1. Retroperitoneal Neoplasms—diagnosis. 2. Biopsy,
Needle. 3. Intestinal Neoplasms. WI 575 S944r 1994]
  RC280.I5S84 1994
  616.99'49507582—dc20
  DNLM/DLC
  for Library of Congress   94-4776
                                             CIP

ISBN: 0-89640-256-8 (New York)
ISBN: 4-260-14256-9 (Tokyo)

Printed and bound in the U.S.A.

10 9 8 7 6 5 4 3 2 1

Preface

It has been over seven years since the publication of the first edition of this monograph. This new edition, like the first, is written primarily for practicing pathologists, pathology residents, and cytotechnologists.

Each chapter in this new edition is headed by a "Key Facts" section which identifies the key points and sets the theme for the text that follows. The chapter entitled "Retroperitoneum" in the first edition is now divided into four chapters: Overview, Lymphoproliferative Disorders, Soft Tissue Tumors, and Metastatic and Germ Cell Tumors. We have seen many more extragonadal germ cell tumors and peritoneal mesotheliomas since the publication of the first edition. (I suspect many of these cases had been classified as poorly differentiated adenocarcinoma, primary site undetermined). In this edition, I have discussed these two interesting entities in more detail. An entirely new chapter on mesothelioma has been added. Other chapters have been revised and updated. More charts and tables for easy reading as well as an updated bibliography have been included.

One of the goals of the first edition was to describe sites that were little-known. Though this certainly is still true, diagnostic problems in connection with these sites now affect many more cytopathologists due to increasing utility of fine needle aspiration. In the new edition, I have expanded considerably the "Diagnostic Pitfalls" sections of the important disease entities.

The last few years have witnessed many technological advances in the field of diagnostic cytopathology. Undoubtedly, intelligent differential diagnosis with the light microscope is still the mainstay of our daily practice, but flow cytometry and molecular genetics, in addition to immunocytochemistry and electron microscopy, have also found their roles in diagnostic cytology. It is now well established that many malignant tumors have DNA ploidy and genetic abnormalities. The clinical applications of all these modern techniques are generously incorporated into the discussions of difficult lesions.

Considerable changes have taken place in the practice of cytopathology due to both government regulations and the development of new technology. All these changes will not displace us from our role as diagnosticians and teachers. With the help of new technology, we are able to make accurate diagnoses with increasingly smaller amounts of tissue. Cytopathology has a vital opportunity to assume an even greater leadership role in medical diagnosis, and we must seize this opportunity.

Kenneth C. Suen, M.B., B.S., F.R.C.P.(C)

Contributors

Peter L. Cooperberg, M.D., F.R.C.P.(C)
Head, Department of Radiology
St. Paul's Hospital
and
Professor of Radiology
University of British Columbia
Vancouver, British Columbia

V. Allen Rowley, M.D., F.R.C.P.(C)
Director of Abdominal Imaging
Department of Radiology
Vancouver Hospital and Health Sciences Centre
and
Assistant Professor of Radiology
University of British Columbia
Vancouver, British Columbia

Contents

Preface   **v**

1. **Introduction and General Considerations**   **1**

2. **Abdominal Imaging Techniques**   **27**
    V. Allen Rowley, M.D., F.R.C.P.(C)
    Peter L. Cooperberg, M.D., F.R.C.P.(C)

3. **Retroperitoneum I: Overview**   **39**

4. **Retroperitoneum II: Lymphoproliferative Disorders**   **49**

5. **Retroperitoneum III: Soft Tissue Tumors**   **85**

6. **Retroperitoneum IV: Metastatic and Germ Cell Tumors**   **135**

7. **Stomach and Intestine**   **169**

8. **Peritoneal Mesothelioma**   **199**

9. **Adrenals**   **213**

10. **Kidneys and Urinary Tract**   **247**

    Index   **287**

Key to Abbreviations

ABC	Aspiration biopsy cytology
CEA	Carcinoembryonic antigen
EMA	Epithelial membrane antigen
FCM	Flow cytometry
HCG	Human chorionic gonadotropin
HD	Hodgkin's disease
LCA	Leukocyte common antigen
MRI	Magnetic resonance imaging
NAB	Needle aspiration biopsy
NHL	Non-Hodgkin's lymphoma
PLAP	Placental alkaline phosphatase
R-S	Reed-Sternberg

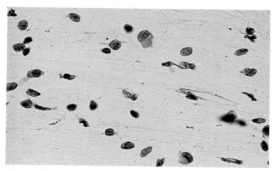

Plate 5.1. Embryonal rhabdomyosarcoma in the retroperitoneum, ABC. **A.** Note scattered small cells with atypical nuclei. Some cells have eosinophilic cytoplasm, consistent with rhabdomyogenic differentiation. (H & E preparation; ×500).

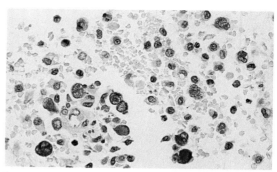

Plate 5.1. B. Cell block, prepared from the same aspirate, immunostained with antidesmin. Note some of the tumor cells showing strong cytoplasmic positivity. (Immunoperoxidase technique; ×500).

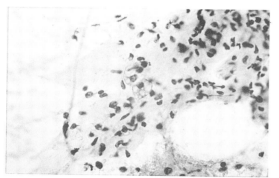

Plate 5.2. Retroperitoneal myxoid liposarcoma, ABC. Note many atypical spindle cells and two lipoblasts (*center*) in a myxoid background. (Papanicolaou preparation: ×500).

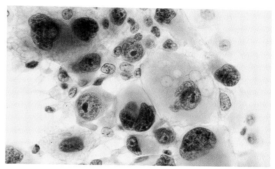

Plate 5.3. Retroperitoneal malignant fibrous histiocytoma, ABC. Note many large pleomorphic cells with macronucleoli. Multiple vacuoles are seen in the cytoplasm of a large tumor cell, but they do not indent the nucleus as in lipoblasts. (H & E preparation; ×500).

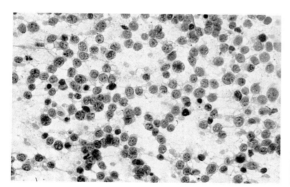

Plate 5.4. Extraosseous Ewing's sarcoma in the pelvis, ABC. **A.** Note many uniform, small, round cells with scant cytoplasm. (H & E preparation; ×500).

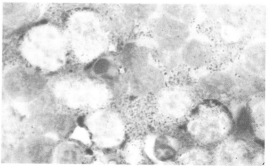

Plate 5.4. B. Periodic acid-Schiff staining of tumor cells showing purplish-pink cytoplasmic granules, indicative of glycogen. The reaction is abolished by diastase digestion (not shown). (Periodic acid-Schiff stain; ×1,200).

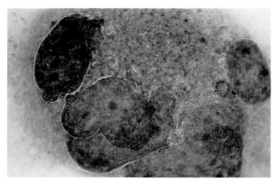

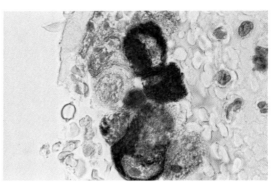

Plate 6.1. Extragonadal retroperitoneal choriocarcinoma, ABC. **A.** Note a syncytiotrophoblast cell with multiple bizarre nuclei and abundant granular cytoplasm. (May-Grünwald Giemsa preparation; ×1,000).

Plate 6.1. B. Cell block preparation showing a strong immunoreaction for beta-HCG. (Immunoperoxidase technique; ×1,000).

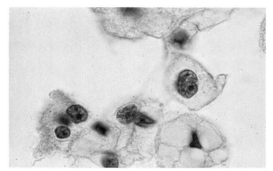

Plate 10.1. Renal cell carcinoma, ABC. Note a group of tumor cells with abundant clear cytoplasm. There is only minimal pleomorphism, but the nucleoli are prominent and the nuclear membranes are thickened. (H & E preparation; ×500).

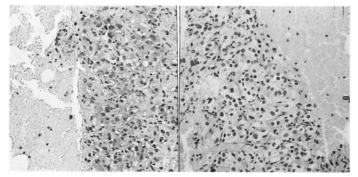

Plate 10.2. Cell block sections prepared from a fine needle aspirate of a renal cell carcinoma. *Left panel:* The tumor cells show a positive periodic acid-Schiff reaction (magenta), prior to diastase digestion. *Right panel:* Tumor cells show a negative reaction after diastase digestion. These findings are indicative of presence of cytoplasmic glycogen in the tumor cells, which is a feature characteristic of renal cell carcinoma rather than adrenocortical neoplasm. (Periodic acid-Schiff stain with and without diastase; ×310).

1

Introduction and General Considerations

KEY FACTS

► Fine needle aspiration biopsy is an outpatient procedure.

► In interpreting aspiration biopsy cytology, evaluation of cellular morphology and evaluation of architectural pattern are equally important.

► Cytologic diagnosis should never be based on a single criterion; multiple criteria should always be sought.

► Any cytologic diagnosis must be rendered with full knowledge of the clinical context. Close communication between the clinician, radiologist, and pathologist (team approach) is crucial.

► False-positive reports are usually caused by inexperience of the interpreter.

► False-negative reports are caused by a number of factors, some of which are beyond the control of the pathologist. Hence, a negative report for malignancy does not necessarily exclude a malignancy. An immediate microscopic examination of the aspirate specimen reduces the number of false-negative reports.

► In a modern diagnostic cytology laboratory, the pathologist utilizes a number of adjuvant special techniques to aid cytologic interpretation. These include immunocytochemistry, electron microscopy, flow cytometry, image cytometry, and molecular biology. However, these modern techniques are labor-intensive and costly and they should not be used indiscriminately.

Since the publication of the last edition of this monograph in 1987, aspiration biopsy cytology (ABC) has attained a prominent status in diagnostic pathology. This prominence results from several factors. Perhaps the most important is the recognition that ABC is a powerful diagnostic tool, widely accepted by both pathologists and clinicians. Secondly, modern advances in imaging techniques have enabled lesions that formerly could have been sampled only at surgery to be visualized and studied by percutaneous needle aspiration biopsy (NAB). This is particularly true in abdominal and retroperitoneal diseases. Thirdly, the current climate of medical cost containment has

1

encouraged the wider use of NAB, which can be performed in the outpatient setting, to save time and expense while allowing better planning of patient care.

SOURCES OF MATERIAL

Fine needle aspiration biopsy was introduced in British Columbia in 1978 by the author, who set up the province's first NAB service at the Vancouver General Hospital.[1] At about the same time, Dr. Hugh Pontifex was organizing a similar service at the British Columbia Cancer Agency. Since then, NAB has been a diagnostic technique widely practiced in the province, accepted by both physicians and patients. About 90% of the material in this book came from these two medical centers. The remainder was contributed by other hospitals, most of which are in British Columbia. This collection of material is rather unique. Vancouver General Hospital is a 900-bed acute-care general hospital where NABs are routinely used as an initial investigation rather than at the end of a long sequence of other diagnostic procedures. Currently, about 1,000 to 1,500 NABs are performed annually. In contrast, the British Columbia Cancer Agency is the cancer referral center for the whole of the Province of British Columbia, where NABs are done chiefly for cancer recurrence, staging, and follow-up in patients who already have a diagnosed cancer. About 2,000 NABs are performed annually. All types of malignancy are seen, follow-up information is readily available, and opportunities for cytohistologic correlation are superb. In addition to the above, there are about 1,000 cases performed annually off-site by physicians in their offices (mostly breast and head and neck masses).

TECHNIQUE OF ASPIRATION

Intraabdominal NABs are performed by radiologists under imaging guidance, using 22-gauge fine needles. The imaging and aspiration techniques are discussed in detail in Chapter 2. A cytotechnologist is always present to receive the needle and syringe directly from the radiologist immediately after the needle has been withdrawn from the lesion. The needle is then detached from the syringe, and the plunger is retracted to allow air to fill the syringe. The needle is reattached and the content is expelled onto properly labeled, clean glass slides by pushing down the plunger. If a smear is too thick, the material can be spread gently with the needle tip. The prepared smears are immediately fixed in 95% ethyl alcohol for 3–4 minutes. To prevent air-drying artifacts, it has been suggested that slides be precoated with 2% Carbowax preservative.[2] After the preparation of smears, the needle and syringe are rinsed with physiologic saline, and the rinse is used for preparation of cytocentrifugation (Cytospin) specimens. Should small tissue fragments be found in the syringe or in the rinse, they are gently removed with forceps and transferred to formalin fixative for cell block preparation as needed. Immunoperoxidase stains can be conveniently performed on cytocentrifuge smears or on cell block sections.

To circumvent the necessity of having a cytotechnologist prepare smears on the spot, many workers[3-5] have advocated collection of the aspirate sample in a fixative, e.g., Saccomanno's Carbowax solution. This collection method is particularly useful when aspiration procedure is done outside the hospital and by many individuals. It permits transportation, at the convenience of the operator, to a laboratory where smears can be prepared by trained personnel according to the preferred method of the laboratory.

FIXATION AND STAINING

The individual's familiarity with a stain is more important in achieving the desired result than the particular qualities claimed for any given stain. Like many others,[6,7] we prefer hematoxylin and eosin stain or Papanicolaou stain and use May–Grünwald Giemsa stain only if a lymphoproliferative lesion is suspected. Immediate fixation of smears for 1 to 2 minutes is crucial if hematoxylin and eosin stain or Papanicolaou stain is used. One of the following fixatives is recommended for routine use: 95% ethyl alcohol or Clarke's solution (75 ml of 100% alcohol and 25 ml of glacial acetic acid). The glacial acetic acid in Clarke's solution lyses the red blood cells, thus providing a cleaner background in case of a bloody aspirate. Both hematoxylin and eosin stain and Papanicolaou stain have similar staining qualities, using hematoxylin as a nuclear stain. They permit a better visualization of the nucleus and, hence, a more detailed evaluation of its structure than is possible with May–Grünwald Giemsa stain. Hematoxylin and eosin stain and Papanicolaou stain, particularly the former, are familiar to tissue pathologists and permit easy comparison between the morphologies of the cells in aspirates and those in tissue sections.[6,7] Moreover, the architectural pattern of cell groups can be appreciated even in thick smears. The conventional Mayer's or Harris's hematoxylin tends to overstain the nuclei. We recommend use of Carazzi's hematoxylin, which gives excellent and crisp nuclear detail when used as a double-strength solution with a shortened staining time. The shortened staining time is an advantage when speed and accuracy are essential, as in immediate reporting of NAB results. The preparation of Carazzi's hematoxylin and the hematoxylin and eosin staining procedure are given in **Table 1.1.**

Smears are air-dried if a Romanowsky stain, such as May–Grünwald Giemsa, is to be used. May–Grünwald Giemsa stains both the nucleus and cytoplasm intensely. Background materials such as mucus, colloid, and secretions are readily stained. It also has the merit of staining lymphoid and hematopoietic cells in a manner familiar to hematologists.

If electron microscopy is planned, a portion of the aspirate specimen should be fixed in 2% glutaraldehyde. Alternatively, a separate aspiration may be performed for electron microscopy.

PREREQUISITES FOR SUCCESSFUL NEEDLE ASPIRATION BIOPSY

Optimal interpretation of ABC depends on many factors. **Figure 1.1** lists the key requirements needed for successful NAB. Some of these factors are discussed below in greater detail.

TABLE 1.1. Preparation of Carazzi's Hematoxylin and Rapid Hematoxylin and Eosin Staining Procedure

Preparation of Carazzi's Hematoxylin*
Hematoxylin	2 gm
Glycerol	200 ml
Potassium alum	50 gm
Distilled water	800 ml
Potassium iodate	0.4 gm
	(1,000 ml)

1. Dissolve the hematoxylin in the glycerol.
2. Dissolve the alum in 700 ml of water.
3. Allow to stand overnight.
4. Add the alum solution to the hematoxylin solution, mixing thoroughly.
5. Dissolve the iodate in the remaining 100 ml of water. Avoid heating if possible.
6. Add the iodate solution to the hematoxylin mixture, mixing constantly.
7. Filter into Coplin jar for use. Solution is ready for use immediately. It has a reliable storage life of 6 months at room temperature, and it will remain usable for longer if stored at 4°C.

Rapid Hematoxylin and Eosin Staining Procedure
1.	Fix smears promptly in 95% ethyl alcohol or Clarke's solution	2 minutes
2.	Tap water	10 dips
3.	Carazzi's hematoxylin	$^3/_4$–1 minute
4.	Tap water	10 dips
5.	Lithium carbonate (bluing solution)	10 seconds
6.	Tap water	10 dips
7.	Eosin	20 seconds
8.	95% ethyl alcohol	10 dips
9.	95% ethyl alcohol	10 dips
10.	100% ethyl alcohol	10 dips
11.	100% ethyl alcohol	10 dips
12.	Xylene	10 dips
13.	Xylene	10 dips

*This double-strength modification of Carazzi's original formula is intended to be used as a progressive stain; it works well on cytologic material and frozen sections.

Pathologist's Experience

It is not unusual for a more experienced pathologist to render a diagnostically useful report on a smear which a less experienced colleague may regard as unsatisfactory. The same can be said about almost any other branch of anatomic pathology in which subjective morphologic recognition, based on past experience, plays a crucial role in correct diagnosis. For example, a frozen section that presents an interpretative problem to a novice may be diagnosed with ease by an experienced pathologist.

Two attributes are essential for a cytopathologist to be proficient in NAB interpretation. First, he or she must be motivated and have an interest in cytopathology. It is absolutely necessary to spend time correlating the aspiration biopsy cytology with histologic sections and obtaining clinical follow-up information for quality assurance

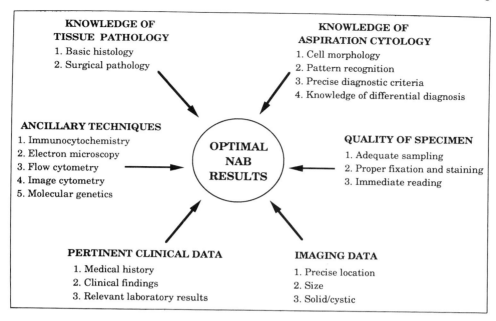

Fig. 1.1. Prerequisites for successful NAB.

and continuing education. The learning process must be augmented by studying imprints and aspiration smears prepared directly from routine autopsy and surgical specimens.[8,9] This method of study is more effective and intellectually more stimulating than reading an atlas of aspiration cytology. Second, one must be well-versed in histopathology because cytologic alterations reflect the histopathologic changes of the underlying disease. The ABC criteria of malignancy are often type-specific rather than general; each organ may have its own set of morphologic criteria with many variables. For example, alterations in individual cell morphology may be more dramatic than architectural pattern in one diseased condition and the reverse may be the case in another condition (see section on "What to Look for in a Needle Aspiration Specimen"). A thorough understanding of the histopathology of various disease processes is therefore essential.

Quality of the Specimens

The quality of the specimen depends on the skill with which the aspiration is performed and the way the smear is prepared. An experienced aspirator capable of obtaining adequate diagnostic material is crucial for a successful biopsy. Superficial, palpable lesions are aspirated by a variety of physicians, who must be familiar with the aspiration technique and fix the aspirate in the manner preferred by the laboratory concerned. In many centers, especially in Scandinavian countries, the aspiration procedures are done by pathologists. This has the advantages of minimizing the numbers of improperly prepared smears and at the same time providing an opportunity for the pathologist to examine the patient, thus facilitating subsequent cytologic intepretation. In cases of deep-seated lesions, aspirations are done by radiologists under radiological guidance (see Chapter 2). The radiologist must be familiar with the technique and smear preparation. Ideally, a cytotechnologist is in attendance to prepare the smears and wet-fix them promptly, if they are to be stained by the Papanicolaou technique or hematoxylin and eosin. Rapid fixation enables the fixative to penetrate the cytoplasm and nucleus quickly; it prevents cell distortion, shrinkage, and swelling. In our laboratory we routinely stain smears using a rapid hematoxylin and eosin method **(Table 1.1).** This is the stain familiar to all surgical pathologists, and the stained smears are ready for examination within 5 minutes of procurement of the specimen. We strongly recommend immediate microscopic assessment of the aspirate specimen so that if it is found to be inadequate, aspiration can be immediately repeated. This reduces the number of unsatisfactory and false-negative reports, and eliminates the need for recalling the patient for a second aspiration.

Consultation Among Pathologist, Radiologist, and Clinician (Team Approach)

The proper evaluation of a biopsy specimen does not begin with the pathologist; it begins with the clinician. The pathologist does not work in a clinical vacuum. His or her interpretation of disease depends on the information and tissue provided by the clinician. Many avoidable mistakes are made because of insufficient or total lack of clinical data. In our laboratory, a special NAB requisition form is used and the cytotechnologist in attendance requires that the form be filled out properly. Clinical data should always include the patient's age and sex, location and character of lesion (solid or cystic), duration of disease, patient's symptoms, and clinical diagnosis. Previous therapeutic procedures such as chemotherapy and radiation may elicit cytologic changes simulating malignancy; hence, it is essential that the cytologist be informed of these procedures. If the patient has a history of malignancy this important information should also be included because comparison of the histology of the previous malignancy with the results of the current NAB will greatly facilitate cytologic interpretation. Special stains, bacterial culture, electron microscopy, or any combination of these procedures may be necessary at times to establish the diagnosis. Many of these special techniques require special handling, and a discussion about the suspected nature of the lesion between the clinician and cytopathologist prior to the biopsy will help the latter to decide how the specimen should be handled.

On the part of the cytopathologist, poor wording of the reports can impede effective communication. The use of a numerical classification, such as class I–V, is best avoided; one should use clearly understood, acceptable diagnostic terms so that the clinician who receives the report will have clear guidance for appropriate action.

WHAT TO LOOK FOR IN A NEEDLE ASPIRATION SPECIMEN

The following aspects of a NAB smear must be assessed carefully by the cytologist.

Cellularity of the Smear

Generally, aspirates from malignant lesions are more cellular than those from benign lesions. This is because cellular cohesion is decreased among malignant cells (thus, cells can be more easily dislodged and aspirated), and also because the number of cells per unit volume is increased in actively proliferating lesions such as malignant tumors. An exception occurs, of course, when a malignant lesion is densely fibrotic, in which case the aspirate may be hypocellular.

Morphology of the Individual Cells

In general, the conventional cytologic criteria of malignancy are applicable to most cases. These include increased nuclear–cytoplasmic ratio, irregular chromatin distribution, irregular nuclear contour, uneven nuclear membrane thickness, prominent or angular nucleoli, and variation in cell and nuclear size. It must be emphasized that there is no single morphologic criterion that is absolutely diagnostic of malignancy. Rather, a combination of criteria, evaluated on the basis of previous experience, is required for the final interpretation.

What makes ABC so interesting and challenging is that the general cytologic criteria described above are not applicable to all cases, because some tumors may have unique morphologic features that are type-specific. There are some malignant tumors that do not always display the usual cytologic features of malignancy. For example, cells derived from a well-differentiated renal cell carcinoma may exhibit only minimal features of malignancy and may mimic benign histiocytes (see Chapter 10). Aspirates from pseudomyxoma peritonei may show cytologically innocuous mucinous cells, and yet the lesion exhibits invasive behavior (see Chapter 7). Similarly, neoplastic cells of a well-differentiated hepatocellular carcinoma may mimic reactive hepatocytes.[10] Conversely, there are some benign lesions in which the cells may exhibit features of malignancy. A pheochromocytoma, because of its pleomorphic cellular features, may be misinterpreted as malignant (see Chapter 9), and cellular schwannoma may show cytologic atypia to a degree that simulates sarcoma (see Chapter 5). Furthermore, reactive or irritated cells and even normal cellular components may be confused with malignancy, e.g., megakaryocytes inadvertently aspirated from bone marrow[11] and smooth muscle fragments from bowel wall (see Chapter 5, section on Leiomyosarcoma). These are only a few examples demonstrating the need for careful evaluation of all the clinical and cytologic parameters, based on a sound knowledge of surgical pathology, in order to arrive at the correct diagnosis. **Table 1.2** summarizes the cytologic appearance of the different cell types commonly encountered in ABC.

Architectural Pattern

Specimens produced by NAB lie on the border between exfoliative cytology and histopathology. The cytologist who studies only the morphologic features of the individual cells is not doing justice to the technique because valuable additional information can often be elicited by assessing the architectural patterns formed by the cells. The term "architectural patterns" refers to the tendency of cell aggregates to form structures that result in an organoid arrangement, which may be well developed, moderately developed, or poorly developed. Not uncommonly, patterns overlap among several diseases. For novices, pattern recognition in ABC is often difficult because the process is either not emphasized or is poorly defined. **Table 1.3** lists some of the common cellular patterns seen in ABC, most of which will be discussed in later chapters.

TABLE 1.2. Cell Morphology with Suggested Cellular Origins*

Malignant columnar or cuboidal cells (see Figs. 6.6, 6.7, 7.1, and 7.7)
   Adenocarcinoma, particularly of the gastrointestinal tract, pancreaticobiliary tract, lung, and uterus

Keratinized cells (see Figs. 6.1, 6.2, and 10.19)
   Squamous cell tumors

Vacuolated cells without compressed nuclei (see Figs. 5.8B, 5.16, 6.5, 9.6, 10.6, 10.28, and 10.29)
   Adenocarcinoma, adrenal cortical tumors, renal cell carcinoma, liposarcoma, malignant fibrous histiocytoma, chordoma, and histiocytes

Vacuolated cells with compressed nuclei (signet ring cells) (see Figs. 5.5C, 5.10B and 7.4)
   Adenocarcinoma, particularly of the gastrointestinal tract and breast, and lipoblasts in liposarcoma

Cells with abundant, granular, eosinophilic cytoplasm and central nuclei (see Figs. 10.8B and 10.23)
   Renal cell carcinoma of the granular cell type, renal oncocytoma, adrenal cortical tumors, and primary hepatic tumors

Small round cells (see Figs. 4.5–4.7, 5.12, 5.13, 6.13, 9.13, and 10.13)
   Small cell anaplastic carcinoma (oat cell carcinoma), Wilms' tumor, neuroblastoma, lymphoma, embryonal rhabdomyosarcoma, and Ewing's sarcoma

Plasmacytoid cells (see Figs. 4.6, 4.10, 6.16, and 10.18)
   Plasmacytoma, immunoblastic lymphoma, melanoma, transitional cell carcinoma, and carcinoid tumor

Spindle or elongate cells (see Figs. 5.3, 5.4, 5.19, 6.4, 6.17, 8.10, and 9.11)
   Mesenchymal neoplasms, melanoma, pheochromocytoma, mesothelioma, and spindle cell carcinomas.

Multinucleated giant cells (see Figs. 4.14, 4.16, 5.8, 5.10, 6.8, 6.24C, and 9.10)
   Pleomorphic sarcomas, giant cell carcinoma, adrenal cortical carcinoma, choriocarcinoma, Hodgkin's disease, and histiocytes

Cells with macronucleoli (see Figs. 4.10, 4.16, 5.8, 6.5, 6.14, and 6.21)
   Pleomorphic sarcomas, giant cell carcinoma, adenocarcinoma, melanoma, seminoma, Reed-Sternberg cells, and immunoblastic lymphoma

Pigmented cells (see Figs. 3.1E and 6.14)
   Melanoma, hepatic cells with lipofuscin or bile, and macrophages with hemosiderin

Cells with intracytoplasmic spherical hyaline bodies (see Figs. 6.22 and 6.23)
   Yolk sac tumor, embryonal carcinoma, malignant fibrous histiocytoma, and hepatocarcinoma

*Tinctorial characteristics described are based on hematoxylin and eosin stain. This table excludes supradiaphragmatic neoplasms not discussed in the text.

Noncellular Background Material

The smear background may provide important clues as to the nature of a lesion. A mucinous background suggests a mucin-producing tumor. A myxofibrillary background suggests myxoma, schwannoma, myxoid liposarcoma, or myxoid variant of malignant fibrous histiocytoma in the case of a soft tissue mass, pleomorphic adenoma in the case of a salivary lesion, and hamartoma in the case of a lung nodule. Amyloid material can accumulate in medullary thyroid carcinoma, renal cell carcinoma, or amyloidoma, whereas colloid material may be seen in association with thyroid tumors.

TABLE 1.3. Summary of Cytologic Patterns Discussed in the Text

Glandular pattern with glands containing large, irregular lumina (Figs. 6.6, 7.2, and 7.7)
   Many adenocarcinomas, particularly those from the gastrointestinal tract, pancreaticobiliary tract, lung, uterus, and ovary
Acinar pattern with small glands containing tiny lumina (see Figs. 6.9, 7.3, 7.13, and 7.15)
   Prostatic carcinoma, carcinoid tumor, breast carcinoma, and, less frequently, adenocarcinomas of the gastrointestinal system and pancreas
Papillary pattern (see Figs. 6.11, 6.12, 7.8, and 10.8)
   Adenocarcinomas of ovary, gastrointestinal tract, pancreaticobiliary tract, and kidney; transitional cell carcinoma of urothelium
Rosette pattern (differs from acinar pattern in that the central area of a rosette is not occupied by a lumen, but contains fibrils or granular material) (see Figs. 6.19 and 9.13)
   Neuroblastoma, Ewing's sarcoma, granulosa cell tumor
Thin trabecular pattern (see Fig. 7.15)
   Carcinoid tumor
Fascicular pattern (see Figs. 5.3, 5.4, and 6.4)
   Spindle cell sarcoma and spindle cell carcinoma
Isolated cell pattern (see Figs. 4.5–4.15, 5.8, 5.10, 6.8, and 6.14)
   Lymphoma, pleomorphic sarcomas, some anaplastic carcinoma, and melanoma
Mixed patterns (see Figs. 6.18, 7.21, 8.10, and 10.15)
   1. Mixed epithelial and spindle cells, e.g., carcinosarcoma, mesothelioma, malignant mixed mesodermal tumor, Wilms' tumor, epithelioid smooth muscle tumor, pseudosarcomatous carcinoma, and synovial sarcoma.
   2. Mixed squamous and glandular cells, e.g., mucoepidermoid carcinoma, adenosquamous carcinoma, and adenoacanthoma
   3. Mixed epithelial cells and lymphocytes, e.g., thymoma and seminoma

A hemorrhagic background may be seen in hematoma, vascular tumors, and choriocarcinoma. Necrosis in the background may be due to tuberculoma, abscess, or tumor necrosis. Psammoma bodies, characterized by basophilic, laminated calcific spherules, are seen in papillary carcinomas (e.g., ovary, thyroid, and lung carcinomas).

REASONS FOR FALSE-POSITIVE AND FALSE-NEGATIVE REPORTS

False-positive reports are in large part due to interpretative errors attributable to the cytopathologist's inexperience. One should not try to diagnose malignancy unless one is familiar with the histologic and cytologic alterations peculiar to that organ. Criteria of malignancy vary from organ to organ; criteria that are useful for the diagnosis of thyroid neoplasms, for example, cannot be applied to the diagnosis of gastric carcinoma. It is always unwise to diagnose malignancy on the basis of a single criterion; multiple criteria should always be sought. With experience and caution in interpretation, the occurrence of false-positive diagnoses can be minimized or eliminated.

False-negative or unsatisfactory reports are caused by a number of factors.

1. Faulty technique, such as misplacement of the needle, inadequate suction, or poor smear preparation.
2. Intrinsic properties of the lesion, such as dense fibrosis or extensive necrosis.
3. Interpretative problems, encountered in well-differentiated malignancies in which the cellular changes may be subtle and mimic benign disease.
4. The clinical information (or lack thereof) provided: e.g., even though it is hypocellular, a pancreatic aspirate sample containing the appropriate cellular components can be reported to be consistent with cystic pancreatic neoplasm rather than unsatisfactory,[12] if the pathologist is given the information that the lesion is cystic or, better still, if he or she has the opportunity to review the radiographs with the radiologist who has given assurance that the needle was correctly placed within the lesion.

Since false-negative or unsatisfactory reports are caused by a number of factors, some of which are beyond the control of the pathologist, it is impossible to totally eliminate them. Hence, the clinician must be made aware that a negative cytologic report does not necessarily exclude malignancy and can only be used as an adjunct to the clinical and radiological investigations. By repeating the aspiration biopsy from different parts of the lesion to obtain representative samples, the operator enhances the diagnostic significance of a negative finding. Moreover, the judicious use of modern ancillary diagnostic techniques, discussed below, can substantially reduce the numbers of nondiagnostic reports.

MULTIPARAMETER APPROACH TO INTERPRETATION

Although light microscopic examination remains the mainstay of cytologic diagnosis, today's cytopathologists must enlist a variety of technological advances to answer specific questions that often cannot be answered by light microscopy. Such modern adjuvant diagnostic techniques include immunocytochemistry, flow cytometry, image analysis, electron microscopy, and molecular analysis **(Table 1.4)**. However, it is important to remember that these special techniques are costly and labor-intensive and they should not be used indiscriminately.

Immunocytochemistry

Only a brief discussion on immunocytochemistry is possible in this volume. The reader is referred to the volume *Diagnostic Immunocytochemistry and Electron Microscopy*[13] in this *Guides Series* for more detailed discussion. The principle of immunocytochemical methodology is based on the fact that an antibody will bind specifically with the antigen that stimulated its production. Tagging an antibody permits localizing the corresponding antigen. Immunocytochemical stains may be performed on direct smears, cell block sections, or cytocentrifuge (Cytospin) smears. The Cytospin smears are readily prepared using equipment, Shandon Cytospin II, which is available in most cytology laboratories. The prepared smears are fixed in cold acetone

TABLE 1.4. Modern Adjuvant Diagnostic Techniques

Adjuvant Diagnostic Technique	Applications to Aspiration Biopsy Cytology
Immunocytochemistry	1. To classify poorly differentiated tumors 2. To determine the site of origin of metastatic tumors 3. To distinguish between some malignant and benign lesions, e.g., lymphoma vs. lymphoid hyperplasia 4. To identify pathogenic organisms
Flow cytometry	1. DNA ploidy and S-phase fraction determination for diagnosis and grading of certain malignancies 2. Immunologic marker analysis of lymphoma/leukemia for diagnosis and lineage assignment
Electron microscopy	1. To differentiate between carcinoma, lymphoma, and sarcoma 2. To classify poorly differentiated tumors
Molecular genetic analysis	1. To detect antigen-receptor gene rearrangements (as clonal markers) in lymphomas 2. To detect specific chromosomal translocations, e.g., t(8;14) in Burkitt's lymphoma, and t(11;22) in Ewing's sarcoma 3. To detect viral genomes and mutations in cellular genes (including oncogenes) in some solid tumors, e.g., EBV, HPV, *ras* gene.

EBV = Epstein-Barr virus; HPV = human papillomavirus.

for 5–6 minutes, and stored in a refrigerator until they are stained. In our experience and those of others,[13] cell block and Cytospin preparations are preferable to direct smears because there are fewer artifacts and less background staining, thus rendering interpretation easier. Furthermore, multiple slides can be prepared from cell block or Cytospin preparations, enabling one to perform a panel of immunostains.

Immunoperoxidase techniques are the most popular procedures used today in the immunodiagnosis of cytologic and histologic materials. The antigens in the cells are detected by virtue of the specific antigen–antibody interactions. In the direct immunoperoxidase method, antigenic sites are recognized by application of a primary antibody, which is labeled with horseradish peroxidase. In the indirect method, a primary unlabeled antibody binds to a corresponding antigen under investigation. To localize this attachment, a second peroxidase-labeled antibody is used to bind to the first antibody. This technique is more versatile than the direct method because a variety of primary antibodies made in the same animal species can be used with one conjugated secondary antibody. As a rule, the sensitivity for antigen detection is amplified by using sequential antibodies directed against the previously applied antibody preparation. Visual detection of these reactions is accomplished by labeling one of the secondary antibodies with an enzyme (horseradish peroxidase). The interaction of the enzyme with its substrate (hydrogen peroxidase) and a chromagen produces a colored end-product that can be seen with the conventional light microscope.

Although many laboratories can now perform these procedures, the need for careful monitoring of techniques with appropriate positive and negative controls cannot be overemphasized. Attention must be paid to the quality (specificity) of the reagent

TABLE 1.5. Panel of Simple Antibodies Used in Differentiating Carcinoma, Sarcoma, and Lymphoma

Results		*Preliminary Conclusion**
Cytokeratin	+	Carcinoma
Vimentin	−	
LCA	−	
Cytokeratin	−	Sarcoma, melanoma
Vimentin	+	
LCA	−	
Cytokeratin	−	Lymphoma
Vimentin	±	
LCA	+	

*See also Table 1.7 for aberrant immunoreactions.

LCA = leukocyte common antigen; + = positive immunoreaction; − = negative immunoreaction.

antibodies in that they represent the "recognition" limb of the method. Fortunately, refinements in monoclonal techniques are progressing rapidly; hopefully they will make recognition more specific than was possible with the earlier polyclonal antibodies.

Clinical Applications

The choice of antibodies must be dictated by the morphologic appearance of the lesion and the differential diagnostic considerations. In daily practice, the most common diagnostic problem is in differentiating anaplastic carcinoma, lymphoma, and sarcoma. The use of relatively simple panels of antibodies is generally sufficient (**Table 1.5**). When indicated, further classification of the tumors can then proceed using more lineage-restricted (but not necessarily lineage-specific) antibodies (**Fig. 1.2**). Antibodies against the following antigens are most widely used and found to be diagnostically useful: cytokeratin, vimentin, leukocyte common antigen, carcinoembryonic antigen, S100 protein, HMB45, and chromogranin (**Table 1.6**).[14] Lymphoid tissue can be studied for evidence of monoclonality by using anti-κ and anti-λ antibodies, thereby improving evaluation and differentiation of reactive lymphoid lesions from malignant lymphoma. Since cancer is a clonal disease and all the neoplastic cells of a B-cell lymphoma originate from a single B-cell ancestor, only a single immunoglobulin light chain (κ or λ) is expressed. The demonstration of light chain restriction (monoclonality) is therefore strongly suggestive of B-cell lymphoma.

Although tumor diagnosis can now be fine-tuned with the use of antibodies by virtue of their specificity, it is crucial that the pathologist be familiar with the "aberrant" expressions of some of these antigen–antibody interactions (**Table 1.7**). For example, epithelial membrane antigen is expressed not only by epithelial tumors but also by anaplastic Ki-1 lymphoma.[15] Cytokeratin has been found sporadically in mesenchymal tumors,[16,17] conversely some anaplastic spindle and giant cell carcinomas express vimentin and/or muscle-specific actin.[18] Some tumors are, in fact, characterized by their abilities to express more than one tissue-restricted markers, e.g., coexpression

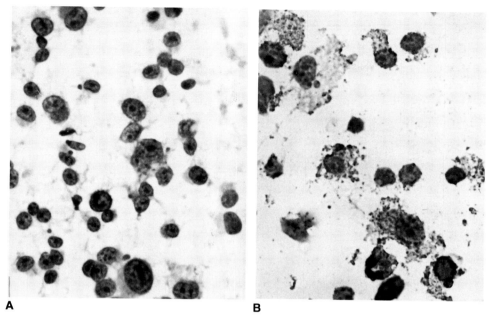

A   **B**

Fig. 1.2. Aspirate of lymph node with metastatic melanoma. **A.** Note dispersed tumor cells with round nuclei and prominent nucleoli. (H & E preparation; ×500). **B.** Tumor cells, immunostained with antimelanoma monoclonal antibody (HMB45), show strong cytoplasmic reactivity. Tumor cells do not show reactivity for cytokeratin (not depicted). (Indirect immunoperoxidase technique, ×500).

TABLE 1.6. Commonly Used Immunologic Markers

Immunologic Marker	Target(s)
Cytokeratin	Epithelial neoplasms, mesothelioma, synovial sarcoma
Epithelial membrane antigen (EMA)	Epithelial neoplasms, mesothelioma, synovial sarcoma, anaplastic (Ki-1) lymphoma
Vimentin	Mesenchymal tumors
Leukocyte common antigen	Lymphoid tumors
Kappa and lambda light chains	B-cell lymphoma
Lymphocyte subsets	Phenotyping lymphoma
Carcinoembryonic antigen (CEA)	Many adenocarcinomas (mesothelioma is generally negative)
Alpha-fetoprotein	Hepatocellular carcinoma, germ cell tumor
Prostate-specific antigen	Prostatic carcinoma
S100 protein	Melanoma, neural tumors
HMB45	Melanoma
Chromogranin	Neuroendocrine tumors
Desmin	Muscle tumors, some lymphomas
Muscle-specific actin	Muscle tumors
Myoglobin	Rhabdomyosarcoma
Leu M-1	Epithelial tumors (mesothelioma is negative), Reed-Sternberg cells

TABLE 1.7. "Atypical" Immunoreactions Observed in Some Selected Neoplasms

A. "Nonepithelial" neoplasms expressing cytokeratin/EMA:
    1. Synovial sarcoma
    2. Epithelioid sarcoma
    3. Chordoma
    4. Some leiomyosarcomas (focal positivity)
    5. Some anaplastic (Ki-1) lymphomas (express EMA)
B. Noncarcinomatous neoplasms expressing CEA
    1. Chordoma
    2. Granulocytic sarcoma
    3. Epithelioid and synovial sarcomas
    4. Some leiomyosarcomas and malignant nerve sheath tumors (focal positivity only).
C. "Nonmesenchymal" neoplasms expressing vimentin
    1. Renal cell carcinoma
    2. Mesothelioma
    3. Melanoma
    4. Some anaplastic giant cell carcinoma
    5. Papillary carcinoma of thyroid
D. Nonneuroectodermal or nonmelanotic neoplasms expressing S100 protein
    1. Cartilaginous tumors
    2. Liposarcoma
    3. Pleomorphic adenoma of salivary gland
    4. Some mammary carcinomas
    5. Papillary carcinoma of thyroid
E. Nonmyogenic neoplasms expressing desmin/muscle specific actin
    1. Malignant fibrous histiocytoma
    2. Anaplastic giant cell carcinoma
F. Hematolymphoid neoplasms nonreactive for LCA
    1. Some Ki-1 lymphomas and histiocytic lymphomas
    2. Some plasmacytomas
G. Carcinomas nonreactive for EMA
    1. Adrenocortical carcinoma
    2. Hepatocellular carcinoma
    3. Germ cell neoplasms

EMA = epithelial membrane antigen; CEA = carcinoembryonic antigen; LCA = leukocyte common antigen.

of cytokeratin and vimentin in renal cell carcinoma, mesothelioma, synovial sarcoma, and epithelioid sarcoma.[19] It is important that the cytopathologist always correlate the immunocytochemical data with morphology before making a diagnosis.

Flow Cytometry

Material obtained by fine needle aspiration provides an important source for flow cytometric analysis. For a detailed discussion of flow cytometry (FCM), the reader is referred to a specialized volume, *Flow Cytometry*,[20] in this *Guides Series*. In addition, many excellent recent reviews of the applications of flow cytometry to cytopathology have been published.[21–23]

The basis of flow cytometry is the principle of fluorescence. Substances possessing this property upon excitation give off a secondary emission that has a longer wavelength than the exciting light. Flow cytometers are machines that measure the fluorescence of objects (cells), flowing in single file across a source of light, usually a laser beam. By tagging cells with suitable fluorescent dyes, various characteristics of the cells can be assessed. The cellular component to be assessed may be a nucleic acid (binding to propidium iodide) or cell-surface antigens (which bind to fluorogen-tagged antibodies). The fluorescence and optical signals are converted to electrical pulses, which are in turn converted to digital form for acceptance by a computer. The advantages of FCM include objectivity, greater sensitivity than immunocytochemical techniques, and high speed. The disadvantages are the high cost of the equipment, the inability to visualize cell morphology microscopically, and the need for skilled, dedicated personnel.

Clinical Applications

The two aspects of flow cytometric analysis most relevant to diagnostic cytopathology are:

1. DNA ploidy and cell proliferative activity;
2. Analysis of various immunologic characteristics of cell populations (immunophenotyping).

DNA PLOIDY AND CELL PROLIFERATIVE ACTIVITY. Abnormal DNA content, recognizable by conventional stains as nuclear hypo- or hyperchromasia, has long been regarded as an important feature exhibited by a variety of human malignancies. For FCM analysis, the cell nuclei are stained with a DNA-specific fluorescent dye, usually propidium iodide, which intercalates into the DNA molecule, such that the amount of emitted fluorescence of the dye–DNA complex is proportional to the DNA content. The emitted fluorescence can be displayed as a histogram, where the X-axis (abscissa) represents fluorescence intensity (DNA content) and the Y-axis (ordinate) represents the number of cells or nuclei. Normal lymphocytes, with DNA diploid content, are added to the test sample as standard. A histogram of DNA diploid cells **(Fig. 1.3)** exhibits a predominant peak in the diploid (2c) region, corresponding to cells in the presynthetic phase (G0/G1) of the cell cycle. A smaller fluorescence peak with twice the intensity of the G0/G1 peak usually occurs in the tetraploid (4c) region, corresponding to the cells in the postsynthetic and mitotic growth phases (G2/M). The relative percentage of cells undergoing DNA replication, i.e., in the synthetic (S) phase, is represented by the number of cells above the baseline that lie between the major diploid and tetraploid peaks. Computer algorithms can estimate percentages of G0/G1, S, and G2/M from the histogram. Flow cytometric detection of abnormal DNA content is based on detection of an abnormal "stemline" relative to internal (or external) diploid reference G0/G1 cells. The degree of aneuploidy is defined by the DNA index, which is the ratio of the DNA content of the G0/G1 aneuploid peak of the cells under analysis relative to the G0/G1 diploid peak of the reference cells.

Recent literature has shown that approximately three-fourths of all primary human carcinomas have flow-detectable DNA abnormalities.[21] For many tumors, therefore, the presence of DNA aneuploidy **(Fig. 1.4)** is strongly suggestive of malignancy. However, it is important to remember that DNA aneuploidy can also be observed in

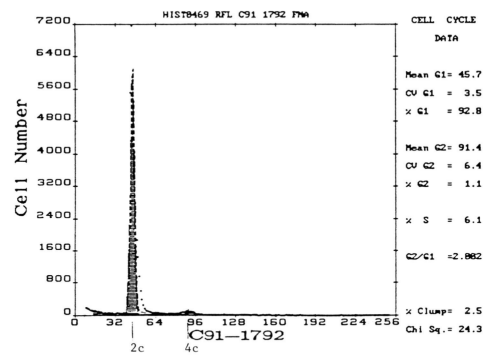

Fig. 1.3. DNA histogram of a reactive lymph node. No DNA abnormality is detected. The channel number (X-axis) indicates the relative DNA content of each cell. The left peak represents diploid G1 cells at 2c and the right peak represents tetraploid G2 cells at 4c.

some benign neoplasms, e.g., thyroid adenoma and colon adenoma.[24,25] Similarly, the absence of DNA aneuploidy does not rule out cancer. A major use of DNA measurements is in grading and prognosticating certain types of cancer. DNA grading of cancer is tissue-specific. For example, breast or prostatic carcinomas with DNA aneuploidy are always high-grade and have a poor prognosis.[26–28] Although this may also be true for many other tumors, exceptions exist, especially in some pediatric tumors such as neuroblastoma and childhood acute lymphoblastic leukemia, in which aneuploidy may be a favorable prognostic marker.[29,30]

In light microscopy, the proliferative activity of a tumor is traditionally evaluated by counting the number of mitoses present on the section. Cell cycle analysis by FCM gives a measure of the growth rate of the tumor. (What is actually measured is the percentage of cells in the S phase of the cell cycle). The tumor types whose biological aggressiveness have been shown to be most predictable by cell-cycle analysis include breast carcinoma, particularly the node-negative cases, and the non-Hodgkin's lymphoma. In these cases, cell cycle analysis may be of value in that rapid proliferation (elevated %S-phase value) may indicate unfavorable prognosis even in the absence of DNA aneuploidy.[31]

IMMUNOPHENOTYPING. Another application of flow cytometry is in the immunophenotypic analysis of cell populations, particularly in the evaluation of lymphomas and

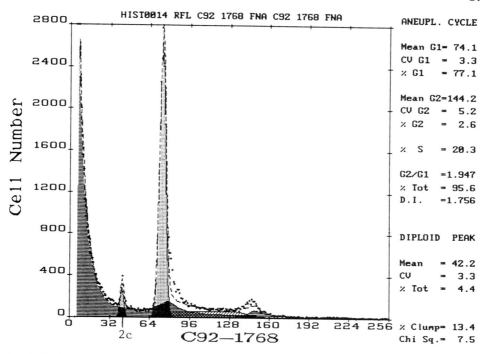

Fig. 1.4. DNA histogram of an aneuploid carcinoma of the pancreas. The specimen contains an abnormal cell population (DNA index is 1.75). The replication rate is high, S + G2/M = 23%.

leukemias.[21,23,32] By labeling surface structures, such as immunoglobulins or related structural proteins, a particular population of cells can be sorted and characterized. This is best illustrated in the B-cell lymphomas, where anti-κ and anti-λ reactivities may be used as a highly sensitive, rapid technique for identifying the monoclonality of a suspected B-cell lymphoma **(Fig. 1.5).**

Furthermore, the development of monoclonal antibodies that can recognize specific subsets of B and T cells has aided in further subclassification of the non-Hodgkin's lymphomas. For example, CD5, an antigen found on normal T cells, is also expressed frequently by B-cell small lymphocytic lymphoma/CLL and intermediate lymphocytic lymphoma. This fact has made CD5 a useful marker for identifying these particular lymphoma types **(Fig. 1.6).**

Electron Microscopy

Many reviews of the techniques of electron microscopy applicable to fine needle aspiration specimens have been published.[33–36] Aspiration samples, containing single cells, small cell clusters, or small tissue fragments, can be optimally fixed in glutaraldehyde. Kindblom reported that the morphologic preservation of small tissue fragments (<0.6 mm) found in fine needle aspirates was superior to that obtained from large postoperative specimens.[37] There are three basic approaches to retrieve material from fine needle aspirates for ultrastructural studies: (1) particle separation by filtration

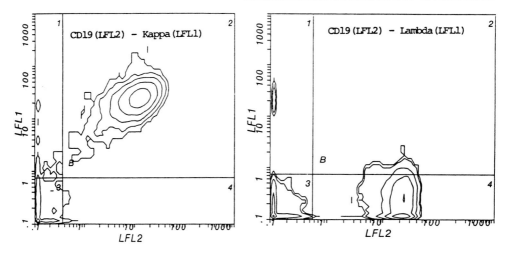

Fig. 1.5. Two-color flow cytometric analysis illustrating light chain restriction in a B-cell lymphoma. The antibodies used are anti-CD19 (LFL2), which is a pan-B cell marker, anti-kappa (LFL1, *left panel*), and anti-lambda (LFL1, *right panel*). The results show that the B cells are monoclonal kappa-bearing lymphoid cells. (Courtesy of Dr. B. Dalal, Division of Hematopathology, Vancouver General Hospital).

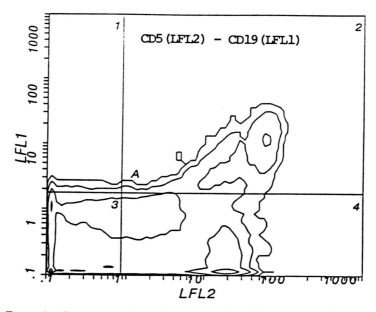

Fig. 1.6. Two-color flow cytometric analysis using a B-cell marker, anti-CD19 (LFL1, ordinate) and a T-cell marker, anti-CD5 (LFL2, abscissa). In addition to a population of reactive T cells (quadrant 4), there is an abnormal population of cells coexpressing CD19 and CD5 (quadrant 2) suggestive of a B-lymphoproliferative neoplasm, i.e., small lymphocytic lymphoma/CLL or intermediate lymphocytic lymphoma. (Courtesy of Dr. B. Dalal, Division of Hematopathology, Vancouver General Hospital).

TABLE 1.8. Ultrastructural Diagnosis of Tumors

Ultrastructural Features	Associated Tumor Type
Desmosomes and tonofilaments	Carcinomas (most abundant in squamous tumors)
Microvilli, luminal borders, cell junctions	Adenocarcinomas
Dense-core neurosecretory granules	Neuroendocrine tumors, peripheral neuroectodermal tumors, and small cell anaplastic carcinoma
Premelanosomes and melanosomes	Melanoma
Myofilaments with dense bodies, basal lamina	Leiomyogenic tumors
Thick and thin myofilaments, Z bands	Rhabdomyogenic tumors
Long interdigitating cytoplasmic processes with replicated basal lamina; microtubules	Neurogenic tumors
Abundant rough endoplasmic reticulum	Fibroblastic tumors
Ruffled cell border with filopodia, lysosomal bodies, lipid	Histiocytic tumors
Long brushy microvilli, perinuclear tonofilaments	Mesothelioma
Paucity of cytoplasmic organelles, lack of cell junctions	Lymphoma

techniques or removal of visible fragments by forceps, (2) centrifugation to pellet the cells from fixative, and (3) reprocessing method using light microscopy to identify cells of interest, followed by plastic embedding of the selected cells. For full detail of these preparatory techniques, interested readers should consult the report by Davidson and Goheen.[38]

Clinical Applications

It should be noted that the majority of neoplasms presented on NAB can be diagnosed and classified on routine light microscopy, and electron microscopic studies are therefore superfluous. On the other hand, electron microscopy is very rewarding in classifying poorly differentiated tumors which may otherwise be unclassifiable and enabling the pathologist to make more specific diagnoses. This is particularly true in poorly differentiated tumors with equivocal antigenic expression and in soft tissue sarcomas with overlapping morphologic features. Helpful ultrastructural characteristics in the diagnosis of tumors are summarized in **Table 1.8.**

The presence of desmosomes associated with tonofilaments is diagnostic of squamous cell carcinoma **(Fig. 1.7).** Surface microvilli, intercellular lumina, and juxtaluminal tight junctions are features of adenocarcinoma regardless of the site of origin. In some cases of adenocarcinoma **(Fig. 1.8)** intracytoplasmic lumina lined with microvilli can be observed. Certain tumors can be identified by their cytoplasmic products, such as melanosomes **(Fig. 1.9)** and neurosecretory granules **(Fig. 1.10).** Rhabdomyogenic tumors **(Fig. 5.1)** show Z-band material with attached myofilaments (about 10 nm in diameter). Smooth muscle tumors **(Fig. 5.2)** possess pinocytic vesicles and

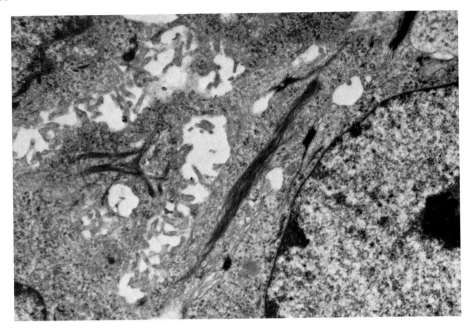

Fig. 1.7. Electron micrograph of a squamous cell carcinoma showing desmosomes and bundles of tonofilaments. (Uranyl acetate and lead citrate preparation; ×11,400).

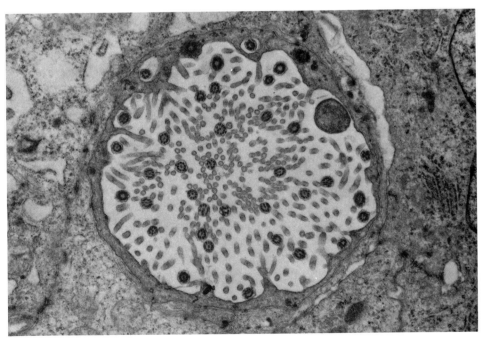

Fig. 1.8. Electron micrograph of an adenocarcinoma showing an intracytoplasmic lumen. Note microvilli and cilia projecting into the lumen. (Uranyl acetate and lead citrate preparation; ×13,300).

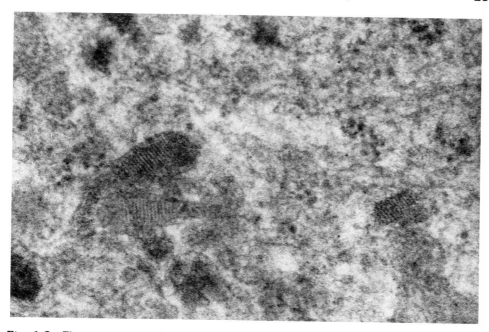

Fig. 1.9. Electron micrograph of a melanoma. Note premelanosomes with diagnostic cross-striations. (Uranyl acetate and lead citrate preparation; ×107,000).

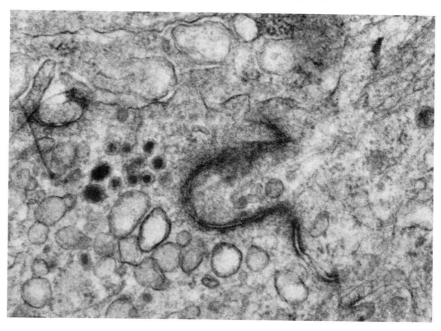

Fig. 1.10. Electron micrograph of a small round cell tumor (lymphoma vs. small cell anaplastic carcinoma). The presence of membrane-bound, dense-core granules and cell junctions identifies the tumor as small cell anaplastic carcinoma. (Uranyl acetate and lead citrate preparation; ×41,900).

fine cytoplasmic actin filaments (about 5 nm in diameter) with condensations into characteristic dense bodies. Tumors of Schwann cell origin show extensive branching of thin cytoplasmic processes, surrounded by basal lamina. Lymphomas are characterized by absence of cell junctions and paucity of cytoplasmic organelles.

Molecular Genetic Studies

Recombinant DNA technologies for the purpose of detecting nucleotide sequences of clinical importance are now being utilized in many fields of diagnostic pathology. DNA is double-stranded, and if the strands are separated by heating, they can accurately rematch. If a specific probe is present, it can recombine with matching DNA, replacing the normal opposite strand. A DNA probe is a small piece of synthetic, single-stranded DNA that binds specifically to complementary DNA. The coding sequence in the probe is known, permitting detection of any DNA with the same nucleotide sequence. The probe is labeled with either a radioactive or chromogenic marker, so that binding can be detected. The unreacted, labeled probe and single-stranded DNA are removed, leaving the hybrids which can be detected by reagents that recognize the label on the probe.

Southern blotting is the current standard technique used in the detection of DNA.[39] The technique utilizes restriction enzymes (nucleases) that cleave the DNA into many fragments at specific locations. The fragments are separated by size on a gel, blotted to filter paper, and then hybridized with probe. If the probe is radioactive, it is detected by x-ray film placed on the filter paper. If it is chemically tagged, it is detected enzymatically to give a colored reaction. While Southern blotting is regarded as the gold standard in detecting DNA, the technique is tedious, the turnaround time is about 10 days or more, and radioactive substances are usually employed.

The recent development of the polymerase chain reaction (PCR) technique[40] obviates some of these drawbacks, enabling rapid cyclic amplifications of a discrete region of genomic DNA, enhancing markedly the sensitivity in DNA detection, and eliminating the use of radioactive substances. By providing two primers, one flanking each end of a segment of DNA, the DNA in the middle will be copied by a heat-stable enzyme (DNA polymerase). With the aid of a computer-programmed thermal cycler, denaturation separates the two complementary strands of the target DNA at a high temperature and then allows annealing of the primers to the target at a much lower temperature. Finally, elongation of the primers by the action of polymerase occurs at an intermediate temperature. The cycle is usually repeated 30–40 times to obtain the desired amplification. The increase in the number of copies of DNA segment is exponential because both the original DNA and the new copies can be used as templates for the next cycle.

Clinical Applications

Recombinant DNA technologies can be applied to fine needle aspirates and have a number of clinical uses.[39–43] They are most frequently used in the diagnosis of lymphoproliferative disorders, by providing information on the alterations of gene structure, such as antigen-receptor gene rearrangements in lymphocytes and oncogene activation characterized by specific chromosomal translocations in neoplastic cells.[41–43] Cancer is a clonal process, in which every cell within a tumor descends

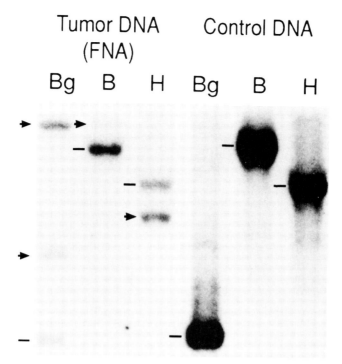

Fig. 1.11. Southern analysis of B-cell lymphoma DNA obtained from a fine needle aspirate (FNA) and hybridized with an immunoglobulin heavy chain gene (J_H) probe, showing germline (−) and rearranged (→) DNA fragments in each of the tumor DNA restriction enzyme digests, compared to germline fragments only in control (placenta) DNA. Bg = BglII; B = BamHI; H = HindIII. (Courtesy of Dr. Doug Horsesman, British Columbia Cancer Agency, Vancouver, B.C.).

from a single progenitor malignant cell. Detection of clonal B or T cells is based on the fact that during their development B and T cells undergo rearrangement of the immunoglobulin genes and T-cell receptor (TCR) genes respectively. In a lymphoid malignancy, clonal proliferation of the neoplastic cell results in identical receptor-gene rearrangements for all cells of the clone. A gene rearrangement of the same type (clonal) is represented by a discrete, nongermline band of hybridization on Southern blotting **(Fig. 1.11).** In a reactive lymphoid hyperplasia containing a polymorphous population of lymphocytes responding to many different antigenic epitopes, numerous rearrangements will occur, giving a mixture of so many different-sized fragments on the Southern blot that the hybridization pattern will appear as a diffuse smear along the lane. Although not always diagnostic, monoclonality of a cell population strongly suggests the presence of malignancy. Immunoglobulin (Ig) probes used for the establishment of a clonal population of B cells are the joining segment of Ig heavy chain (J_H) and constant regions of lambda (C_λ) and kappa (C_κ) light chains. The TCR β and α genes are the most reliable probes for the detection of clonal populations of T cells.

Detection of chromosome abnormalities using conventional karyotyping and band-ing methods is technically tedious. Chromosomal translocations and deletions involving DNA rearrangements can now be detected by Southern blotting or polymerase chain reaction using radiolabeled or biotinylated commercially available DNA probes covering the specific genes. It is now well established that certain chromosomal translocations or alterations resulting in oncogene activation are characteristic of certain tumors and may be regarded as genetic tumor markers. For example, a number of studies have emphasized the importance of the t(14;18) translocation (*bcl-2* oncogene rearrangement) in follicular lymphomas and some diffuse large cell lymphomas, t(8;14) translocation (*c-myc* oncogene activation) in Burkitt's lymphoma, and t(11;22) translocation in Ewing's sarcoma.[44–47]

The presence of certain oncogene mutations and viral genomes can be detected by molecular DNA technology in fine needle aspirate specimens of tumors or diseased tissues. Tada and colleagues,[48] using polymerase chain reaction and direct sequencing technique, were able to detect *k-ras* gene (oncogene) mutation in specimens obtained by needle aspiration of pancreatic adenocarcinomas, a finding that can be used as supporting evidence for the diagnosis of pancreatic malignancy. Feinmesser and colleagues[49] detected viral genomes of Epstein-Barr virus in the aspirates obtained from metastases of nasopharyngeal carcinoma. Shibata and associates[50] identified genomes of human papillomavirus type-16 in metastatic squamous cell carcinoma of the uterine cervix. Detection of these viral genomes (as tumor markers) by DNA probes is a sensitive and powerful tool for the identification of the tissue of origin of these metastatic carcinomas.

Molecular genetic methods, while now labor-intensive, will likely be automated in the near future. Progress in automation will, in turn, facilitate the technology transfer from the research to the clinical laboratory.

References

1. Hicken P: Editorial: Percutaneous biopsy procedures. *Brit Col Med J* 23:525, 1981.
2. Nathan NA: Improved alcohol-fixed smears of fine needle aspirates for cytology of breast and other palpable lesions. *Am J Clin Pathol* 99:721–725, 1993.
3. Atkinson BF: Carbowax fixation of needle aspirates. *Diagn Cytopathol* 2:231–232, 1986.
4. Young GP: Enabling more physicians to do aspiration biopsy. *Diagn Cytopathol* 2:229–230, 1986.
5. Crystal BS, Wang HH, Ducatman BS: Comparison of different preparation techniques for fine needle aspiration specimens. *Acta Cytol* 37:24–28, 1993.
6. Gublin N: Hematoxylin-and-eosin staining of fine needle aspirate smears. *Acta Cytol* 29:648–650, 1985.
7. Pak HY, Yokata SB, Teplitz RL: Rapid staining techniques employed in fine needle aspiration. *Acta Cytol* 27:81–82, 1983.
8. Suen KC, Yermakov V, Raudales O: The use of imprint technic for rapid diagnosis in postmortem examinations. *Am J Clin Pathol* 65:291–300, 1976.
9. Suen KC, Wood WS, Syed AA, et al: Role of imprint cytology in intraoperative diagnosis; value and limitations. *J Clin Pathol* 31:328–337, 1978.
10. Suen KC: Diagnosis of primary hepatic neoplasms by fine needle aspiration cytology. *Diagn Cytopathol* 2:99–109, 1986.

11. Chen KTK, Tschang TP: Megakaryocytes in fine-needle aspiration biopsy of breast. *Diagn Cytopathol* 7:433–435, 1991.

12. Suen KC: Seeing, not just looking (editorial). *Diagn Cytopathol* 7:335–336, 1991.

13. Yazdi HM, Dardick I: *Diagnostic Immunocytochemistry and Electron Microscopy.* Guides to Clinical Aspiration Biopsy. New York, Igaku-Shoin, 1992.

14. Gatter KC, Mason DY, Heyderman E, et al: Which antibodies for diagnostic pathology? *Histopathol* 11:661–664, 1987.

15. Chott A, Kasesrer K, Augustin I, et al: Ki-1-positive large cell lymphoma: A clinicopathologic study of 41 cases. *Am J Surg Pathol* 14:439–448, 1990.

16. Miettinen M: Immunoreactivity for cytokeratin and epithelial membrane antigen in leiomyosarcoma. *Arch Pathol Lab Med* 112:637–640, 1988.

17. Litzky LA, Brooks JJ: Cytokeratin immunoreactivity in malignant fibrous histiocytoma and spindle cell tumors. *Mod Pathol* 5:30–34, 1992.

18. Nakhleh RE, Zarbo RJ, Ewing S, et al: Myogenic differentiation in spindle cell (sarcomatoid) carcinoma of the upper aerodigestive tract. *Appl Immunohistochem* 1:58–68, 1993.

19. Domagala W, Weber K, Osborn M: Diagnostic significance of coexpression of intermediate filaments in fine needle aspirates of human tumors. *Acta Cytol* 32:49–59, 1988.

20. Vielh P: *Flow Cytometry.* Guides to Clinical Aspiration Biopsy. New York, Igaku-Shoin, 1992.

21. Johnson TS, Katz RL, Perhouse M: Flow cytometric applications in cytopathology. *Anal Quant Cytol Histol* 10:423–458, 1988.

22. Klemi PJ, Joensuu H: Comparison of DNA ploidy in routine fine needle aspiration biopsy samples and paraffin-embedded tissue samples. *Anal Quant Cytol Histol* 10:195–199, 1988.

23. Moriarty AT, Wiersema L, Snyder W, et al: Immunophenotyping of cytologic specimens by flow cytometry. *Diagn Cytopathol* 9:252–258, 1993.

24. Harlow SP, Duda RB, Bauer KD: Diagnostic utility of DNA content flow cytometry in follicular neoplasms of the thyroid. *J Surg Oncol* 50:1–6, 1992.

25. Goh HS, Jass JR: DNA content and the adenoma-carcinoma sequence in colorectum. *J Clin Pathol* 39:387–392, 1986.

26. Zetterberg A, Esposti PL: Prognostic significance of nuclear DNA levels in prostatic carcinoma. *Scand J Urol Nephrol* 55(Suppl):53–58, 1980.

27. Ronstrom L, Tribukait B, Esposti P: DNA pattern and cytological findings in fine needle aspirates of untreated prostatic tumors. A flow-cytofluorometric study. *Prostate* 2:79–88, 1981.

28. Palmer JO, McDivitt RW, Stone KR, et al: Flow cytometric analysis of breast needle aspirates. *Cancer* 62:2387–2391, 1988.

29. Oppedal BR, Storm-Mathisen I, Lie SO, et al: Prognostic factors in neuroblastoma. *Cancer* 62:772–780, 1988.

30. Pui CH, Williams DL, Raimondi SC, et al: Hypodiploidy is associated with a poor prognosis in childhood acute lymphoblastic leukemia. *Blood* 70:247–253, 1987.

31. Diamond LW, Braylan RC: Flow analysis of DNA content and cell size in non-Hodgkin's lymphoma. *Cancer Res* 40:703–712, 1980.

32. Johnson A, Akerman M, Cavallin-Stahl E: Flow cytometric detection of B-clonal excess in fine needle aspirates for enhanced diagnostic accuracy in non-Hodgkin's lymphoma in adults. *Histopathol* 11:581–590, 1987.

33. Akhtar M, Bakry M, Nash EJ: An improved technic for processing aspiration biopsy for electron microscopy. *Am J Clin Pathol* 85:57–60, 1986.

34. Mackay B, Fanning T, Bruner JM, et al: Diagnostic electron microscopy using fine needle aspiration biopsies. *Ultrastruct Pathol* 11:659–672, 1987.

35. Kindblom L, Walaas L, Widehn S: Ultrastructural studies in the preoperative cytologic diagnosis of soft tissue tumors. *Semin Diagn Pathol* 3:317–344, 1986.

36. Strausbauch P, Neill J, Dabbs DJ, et al: The impact of fine-needle aspiration biopsy on a diagnostic electron microscopy laboratory. *Arch Pathol Lab Med* 113:1354–1356, 1989.

37. Kindblom LG: Light and electron microscopic examination of embedded fine-needle aspiration biopsy specimens in the preoperative diagnosis of soft tissue and bone tumors. *Cancer* 51:2264–2277, 1983.

38. Davidson DD, Goheen MP: Preparation of fine needle aspiration biopsies for electron microscopy. In: Schmidt WA, Miller TR, Katz RL, et al. (eds): *Cytopathology Annual.* Baltimore, Williams & Wilkins, 1993, pp 255–264.

39. Lubinski J, Chosia M, Kotanska K, et al: Genotypic analysis of DNA isolated from fine needle aspiration biopsies. *Anal Quant Cytol Histol* 10:383–390, 1988.

40. Greiner TC: Polymerase chain reaction: Uses and potential applications in cytology. *Diagn Cytopathol* 8:61–65, 1992.

41. Cartagena N Jr, Katz RL, Hirsch-Ginsberg C, et al: Accuracy of diagnosis of malignant lymphoma by combining fine needle aspiration cytomorphology with immunocytochemistry and in selected cases, Southern blotting of aspirated cells. *Diagn Cytol* 8:456–464, 1992.

42. Hu E, Horning S, Fynn S, et al: Diagnosis of B-cell lymphoma by analysis of immunoglobulin gene rearrangement in biopsy speicmens obtained by fine needle aspiration. *J Clin Oncol* 4:278–283, 1986.

43. Lubinski J, Chosia M, Huebner K: Molecular genetic analysis in the diagnosis of lymphoma in fine needle aspiration biopsies. I. Lymphomas versus benign lymphoproliferative disorders. *Anal Quant Cytol Histol* 10:391–398, 1988.

44. Weiss LM, Warnke R, Sklar J, et al: Molecular analysis of the t(14;18) chromosomal translocation in malignant lymphomas. *N Engl J Med* 317:1185–1189, 1987.

45. Williams ME, Frierson HF, Tabrarah S, et al: Fine needle aspiration of non-Hodgkin's lymphoma: Southern blot analysis for antigen receptor, Bcl-2, and c-myc gene rearrangement. *Am J Clin Pathol* 92:754–759, 1990.

46. Turc-Carel C, Aurias A, Mugneret F, et al: Chromosomes in Ewing's sarcoma. I. An evaluation of 85 cases and remarkable consistency of t(11;22)(q24;q12). *Cancer Genet Cytogenet* 32:229–238, 1988.

47. Jacobson JO, Wilkes BM, Kwiatkowski DJ, et al: Bcl-2 rearrangements in de novo diffuse large cell lymphoma. *Cancer* 72:231–236, 1933.

48. Tada M, Omata M, Ohto M: Clinical application of ras gene mutation for diagnosis of pancreatic adenocarcinoma. *Gastroenterol* 100:233–238, 1991.

49. Feinmesser R, Miyazaki I, Cheung R, et al: Diagnosis of nasopharyngeal carcinoma by DNA amplification of tissue obtained by fine needle aspiration. *N Engl J Med* 326:17–21, 1992.

50. Shibata D, Cosgrove M, Arnheim A, et al: Detection of human papillomavirus DNA in fine-needle aspirations of metastatic squamous cell carcinoma of the uterine cervix using the polymerase chain reaction. *Diagn Cytopathol* 5:40–43, 1989.

2

Abdominal Imaging Techniques

V. Allen Rowley
Peter L. Cooperberg

KEY POINTS

▶ Imaging techniques, such as ultrasound, computed tomography, and magnetic resonance, are of value for both detection and staging of retroperitoneal lesions.

▶ The specific diagnosis of a retroperitoneal mass is generally dependent on biopsy, which can be accomplished in most cases by percutaneous aspiration techniques using sonography or computed tomography for localization.

▶ The combined use of the modern imaging techniques and percutaneous NAB has dramatically diminished the time required to arrive at a diagnosis, which in turn has reduced patient hospitalization.

▶ The success of needle aspiration biopsy depends on an interdisciplinary team approach between the radiologist and cytopathologist. In situations where a cytopathologist or cytotechnologist is not available in the radiology department, the procedure is much less likely to be successful, except for rather large and relatively superficial lesions.

▶ Our cytopathologists are well versed in interpreting fine needle cytology. Large core needle biopsy increases the likelihood of complications and is reserved for selected cases only when cytology is nondiagnostic.

The field of radiology has experienced great technological advances in the last few years. The newer imaging techniques of ultrasound, computed tomography (CT), and, most recently, magnetic resonance imaging (MRI) use powerful computers and allow us to produce sectional images. By avoiding the superimposition of structures that was inherent in more traditional radiologic techniques, soft tissue structures throughout the body, particularly in the abdomen, can be easily identified. There has been considerable hope that all of these physical modalities would in some way yield a "tissue signature" that would clearly differentiate different lesion types. In most cases, cysts can be differentiated from solid lesions by ultrasound or computed tomography. Fatty lesions can be differentiated from water-density lesions by computed tomography. However, differentiation of benign from malignant lesions, or greater specificity about benign or malignant lesions, is still beyond the technological capability of current equipment in the vast majority of cases. There is considerable work underway using the physical parameters of sound or magnetic spectra in different types of lesions. Nonetheless, it will be a long time before clinicians will accept a diagnosis based on a measurement of some physical parameter or a probability based on radiologic interpretation instead of the finality of a pathologist's report. The combined use of modern sophisticated imaging techniques and percutaneous needle aspiration biopsy (NAB) has dramatically reduced the time required to arrive at a diagnosis, which in turn has reduced patient hospitalization.

Modern imaging techniques are exceptionally suitable not only for identifying lesions and determining their size, but also for localizing them within the body.[1-8] Furthermore, convenient external landmarks can easily be determined to direct fine needle aspiration biopsy to yield material for cytologic examination. These imaging techniques allow exquisite determination not only of the position of the lesion and the point on the skin for access, but also the direction in both planes and the depth that the needle must be inserted. Especially with real-time ultrasound, the respiratory motion of the structures, if any, can easily be seen and allowed for.

Although there is a trend toward automated core biopsy procedures using 16- to 20-gauge devices such as the Biopty gun (CR Bard, Covington, GA)[9,10] which routinely obtain larger core tissues that are more easily interpreted by less experienced pathologists, we limit this device to selected cases requiring histologic diagnosis such as the liver (e.g., hepatitis and cirrhosis), kidneys (e.g., glomerular disease), or prostate, or when a fine needle aspirate is nondiagnostic and a safe approach is possible. The use of cutting needles, however, significantly increases the likelihood of complications, and is not generally appropriate for a retroperitoneal lesion, especially if bowel must be traversed on the way to the lesion. We have had no complications of perforation, leakage, or infection by traversing bowel (or for that matter, the pleura, or even the bladder or gallbladder) using a 22-gauge needle. We believe that the necessity for larger gauge needles is more dependent on the capability of the cytopathologist than on the technique of guided-needle biopsy.

LOCALIZATION OF MASSES FOR NEEDLE ASPIRATION BIOPSY

Abdominal masses can be localized by either palpation, fluoroscopy, ultrasound, computed tomography, or magnetic resonance imaging, but these diagnostic modalities are not equal in utility for guiding fine needle aspiration biopsy. **Table 2.1** summarizes their relative strengths and weaknesses.

Palpation

The simplest way to localize a mass for a percutaneous fine needle aspiration biopsy is, of course, by palpation.[11] However, palpation for guidance of biopsy of abdominal masses has two major problems. First, one must know what the palpated structure

TABLE 2.1. Comparison of Localization Modalities

	Advantages	Disadvantages
Palpation	Real-time (fast). Inexpensive. Widely available.	Superficial or large lesions only. No visualization of needle tip. Rarely useful in the retroperitoneum.
Fluoroscopy	Real-time (fast). Widely available. Inexpensive. Needle tip easy to see. Used in high-contrast areas such as bone and chest.	Radiation. No depth perception.
Ultrasound	Real-time (fast). Widely available and portable. No radiation. Relatively inexpensive. Needle path and tip fairly easy to visualize. Good soft tissue differentiation. Used for majority of neck, kidney, liver, and some pancreas biopsies.	Limited by overlying gas, bone and generally by obesity. Somewhat operator-dependent.
Computed tomography	Precise identification of needle tip possible. Not limited by gas, bone, or obesity. Less operator-dependent. Good soft tissue differentiation. Used for pancreas, general, retroperitoneal, adrenal, and pelvic biopsies.	Not real-time (slow). Limited availability. Radiation. Expensive.
Magnetic resonance imaging	No radiation. Good soft tissue differentiation.	Not real-time (very slow). Limited access to patient while scanning for monitoring, etc. Needle visualized only as signal void. Concern about magnetic interaction ferrous needles and magnetic field. Most expensive. Rarely, if ever, indicated at present.

is. Occasionally, a normal structure such as the liver, kidney, spleen, or even gallbladder can be displaced into a palpable position by an abnormal underlying structure. Second, and most common, is that most abdominal lesions are not palpable and, therefore, some guidance technique is needed to locate them.

Fluoroscopy

Fluoroscopy can be used to guide fine needle aspiration.[5] It is particularly useful in the lungs, where the surrounding intrapulmonary air provides natural contrast. Fluoroscopy is not as useful in the abdomen, with the exception of occasional fine needle aspiration biopsies for biliary lesions in patients who have had direct cholangiography, or aspiration biopsies of lymph nodes in patients who have had lymphangiograms.[8] The disadvantages of fluoroscopy are that opacification techniques are generally time-consuming and technically difficult, and both the patient and radiologist are exposed to radiation. Assessment of depth is difficult as well unless biplane fluoroscopy is used, and this is rarely available.

Ultrasound

Ultrasound can be used to guide NAB in several ways. The easiest way is for the operator to localize a big lesion with ultrasound and then memorize its position relative to surface landmarks. If the angles and depth are also memorized (taking into account the compression of subcutaneous tissues by the transducer, which does not occur with the needle), the fine needle aspiration biopsy is usually straightforward. The biopsy is easiest to perform if one is attempting to aspirate a fluid collection, and the "pop" will be felt as the needle enters the fluid. Furthermore, it is easy to confirm the fluid entering the syringe. Most solid tumors are hard enough so as to give a tactile sensation when the needle is in the lesion; this can be helpful as well.

If the lesion is small, one can use ultrasound to visualize the needle traversing the tissue and to guide its passage toward, and subsequently into, the lesion **(Figs. 2.1 and 2.2)**. This can be done with a two-person technique: one person holds the transducer and watches the imaging screen while the second person stands on the other side of the patient, aiming the needle for the appropriate place as determined by the transducer. This, of course, requires good coordination and communication between the two people performing the biopsy; it is much easier for a single operator to achieve the hand–eye coordination necessary. It is important that the point of needle insertion and the transducer's position on the skin for visualization of the lesion both be appropriately chosen. Sometimes, one must compromise on the best pathway for the needle in order to have good sonographic visualization. Optimal visualization is achieved by using a linear transducer, if possible, and selecting the most appropriate focal zone. Orienting the intersection of the needle path and the ultrasound beam to as close to 90° as possible also optimizes the visualization of the needle. The difficulty here is in keeping the needle within the plane of section. The benefit is that the ability to move the needle is entirely flexible and, if the needle misses the lesion, it is easy to change direction and advance again.

Various devices have been developed that fit over the end of the transducer and keep the needle within the appropriate plane of section **(Fig. 2.3)**. Although this technique does keep the needle within the plane of section, it is totally inflexible. The

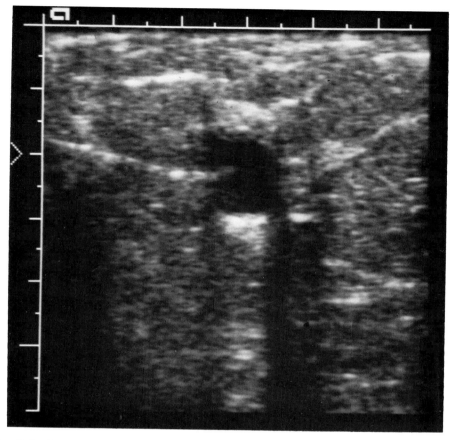

Fig. 2.1. Linear-array real-time ultrasound scan showing the needle entering a small cyst.

angle of the needle is fixed by the device and, once the needle passes through the device, one cannot change the orientation without completely removing the needle. The more flexible free-hand technique is preferred by most experienced radiologists.

We also prefer to use a control syringe (available from Becton, Dickinson & Co., Rutherford, NJ) for biopsy that allows the procedure to be performed with one hand **(Fig. 2.3).** This also prevents inadvertent advancement of the needle and syringe instead of retraction of the plunger, as can happen with the usual two-handed syringe.

Computed Tomography

Although ultrasound is the most useful technique for the majority of cases, computed tomography can be used, especially for lesions in which there is overlying bowel gas or when a posterior approach is necessary. Commonly, retroperitoneal lesions require computed tomography for aspiration biopsy because there is considerable overlying bowel gas, especially in relatively small lesions.[6] Computed tomography is time-consuming, the equipment is expensive, and most computed tomography scanners are heavily used and may not always be available when needed. Even if the scanner

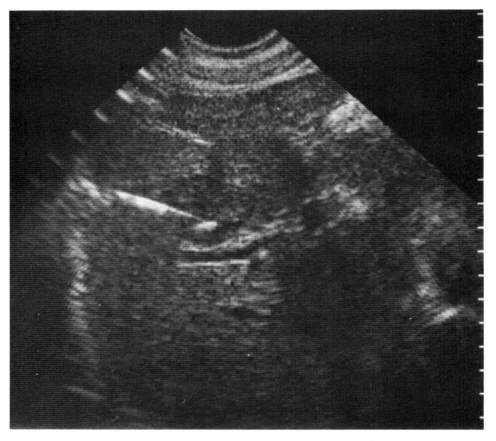

Fig. 2.2. Real-time sector scan showing a needle with tip in solid lesion of the liver.

is available for an adequate time, it is still a cumbersome technique. The lesion has to be identified on the scan, the patient moved back into the gantry to the appropriate level, and a repeat scan performed. A marker is then placed on the patient, the patient removed from the gantry, and the needle is inserted using the correct position, angle, and depth. This usually works satisfactorily on the first pass only if the needle is in an axial plane and the lesion is fairly superficial. With the needle in place, the patient is moved back into the gantry and an AP or lateral scout image taken. A single axial slice at the level of the tip of the needle is then done to show its orientation to the lesion targeted **(Fig. 2.4).** If the needle tip is seen to be outside the lesion, the patient must be removed from the gantry, the needle repositioned, and the patient rescanned. This entire process has to be repeated for each subsequent aspiration. Although computed tomography is the best technique if ultrasound cannot be used, and is the best technique to confirm that the tip of the needle is in the lesion, we usually reserve its use for difficult cases. Even smaller lesions are not necessarily easier to handle with computed tomography. In determining whether or not to use computed tomography, the location of the lesion, rather than its size, is more important.

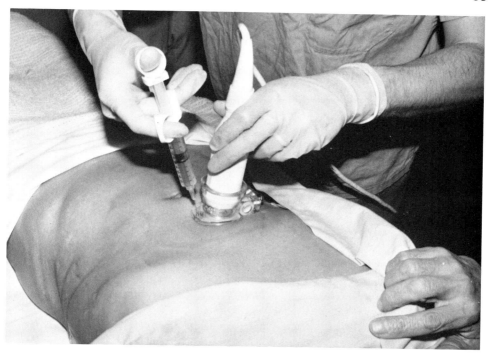

Fig. 2.3. A lucite biopsy guide is attached to the real-time sector scanner in the operator's left hand. The needle attached to the control syringe is passing through one of the holes in the biopsy guide.

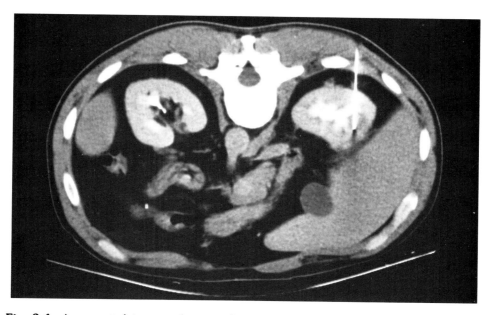

Fig. 2.4. A computed tomography scan showing a posterior approach with the tip of the needle in a small renal cancer.

Magnetic Resonance Imaging

Currently, the closed-bore (cylindrical) nature of MRI scanners, their relatively slow (not real-time) scanning capabilities, and the danger of ferrous biopsy needles becoming projectiles near the strong magnetic field prohibits MRI-directed aspirations. Over the next decade, open-bore scanners capable of scanning one image per second (virtually real-time) and the use of titanium (nonferrous) needles may make MRI-guided aspirations possible. However, they will likely remain relatively expensive and of limited availability for the foreseeable future.

TEAM APPROACH

The success of NAB depends on an interdisciplinary team approach between the radiologist and cytopathologist. At the time of aspiration biopsy, a cytotechnologist familiar with the aspiration technique is present to receive the needle and syringe directly from the radiologist. This ensures optimal specimen fixation and smear preparation. The endpoint of a successful aspiration is easy to determine if fluid is obtained. If solid material is sought, it is important to have the aspirate examined quickly to determine if the appropriate cells are seen. Although in rare occasions we have gone as high as 8 or 9 needle passes at one session, we prefer to do one or two passes and check the material. In our experience, this is diagnostic in greater than 90% of cases. We only continue if no appropriate material has been aspirated. If the lesion is small and the patient tachypneic, we may stop after just a few passes, knowing that it will be a difficult procedure. Also if the likelihood of the lesion being malignant is slim, we may stop after just a few passes. If it is important to prove that the lesion is benign, it is sometimes necessary to do nine or ten passes to increase the likelihood that malignant cells would have been obtained if the lesion was malignant. However, it is usually the temperament of the radiologist and patient that determines when an unsuccessful attempt will be accepted and the procedure terminated. If necessary, the patient can be brought back another day or another physician can continue the attempt. Local anesthesia is utilized only if more than one pass is anticipated or the biopsy is likely to be difficult as we have found the injection of local anesthetic causes as much discomfort as a single aspirate (analogous to the situation when one receives an immunization).

Most of our aspiration biopsies are not scheduled in advance. In most cases, a lesion is found at ultrasound (or computed tomography) and the referring clinician is contracted. The only relative contraindications to fine needle aspiration biopsy are uncontrollable bleeding disorder, lack of a safe biopsy approach, and an uncooperative patient. We only perform a coagulation screen if there is reason to clinically suspect a bleeding problem or if we anticipate having to go to a larger core biopsy needle. Because it is most efficacious for the patient to have the biopsy done during the same visit, we try to do so even though this makes scheduling difficult. Nonetheless, with good cooperation between the departments of radiology and pathology, both the patient and the referring physician can receive the best service. In situations where a cytopathologist or cytology technician is not available in the radiology department, the procedure is much less likely to be successful, except for rather large and relatively superficial lesions.

SPECIFIC SITES

Retroperitoneum

With modern imaging techniques, it is now possible to perform biopsies on even small para-aortic lesions and retroperitoneal lesions in both flanks. Using 22-gauge fine needles, there is no danger in traversing small blood vessels or bowel in aspirating retroperitoneal lesions; however, guidance does help avoid these structures. Although retroperitoneal masses can frequently be identified and biopsied sonographically, there is a higher percentage yield of positive diagnoses with computed tomography.[12] This is due to the inability of ultrasound to traverse bowel gas thus obscuring deeper lesions. However, if the lesion is large enough, it usually displaces the bowel gas so that it becomes visible on ultrasound, especially if any compression is applied to the transducer. We have found that the size of the spleen often provides important information regarding the nature of retroperitoneal masses. If the spleen is large, the retroperitoneal lesion is likely to be a lymphoma. Whenever possible, we try to refrain from using fine needle aspirations as the sole basis for an initial diagnosis of lymphoma. However, when the lymphoma is of the large cell or histiocytic type, it often can be diagnosed by cytology. In a patient with previously diagnosed lymphoma, aspiration biopsy aids in staging, confirming recurrence, diagnosing new and unrelated malignancy, and assessing evolution of a lymphoma to a more aggressive form. If the spleen is of normal size, we frequently obtain carcinoma cells on fine needle aspiration biopsy. These usually represent metastases, which may come from a known or unknown primary source and, occasionally, from a primary source that is never discovered. Apart from lymphomas and carcinomas, retroperitoneal sarcomas such as leiomyosarcoma and liposarcoma are also candidates for NAB.

Gastrointestinal Tract

Traditionally, tumors of the gastrointestinal tract are diagnosed by barium contrast studies and endoscopic biopsy. We have performed fine needle aspiration biopsies on many occasions for lesions in the stomach, small bowel, and colon. If the lesion is clearly of bowel origin (the sonographic target sign of barium within the lesion on a computed tomography scan), there is usually no point in performing a percutaneous aspiration biopsy. However, sometimes it is important to differentiate other causes of bowel-wall thickening from a malignancy. Sometimes, a lesion arising from the gastrointestinal tract is subject to biopsy because it does not have the typical appearance of a gastrointestinal lesion. In this case, a specific diagnosis can be obtained by cytologic biopsy before barium studies. Occasionally, a percutaneous NAB is done because an endoscopic biopsy cannot be performed or attempts at endoscopic biopsy fail because too superficial a "bite" is obtained. Some patients may be too ill to undergo surgical excision, and the NAB can provide a diagnosis and help determine prognosis. In patients with previous colorectal carcinoma, computed tomography is recommended as a routine follow-up procedure and recurrence can be readily confirmed by a fine needle aspiration biopsy.[13,14]

Kidney

Renal biopsy by fine needle is not as widely practiced in North America as in Europe[15,16] because a nephrectomy will be performed even if there is a possibility that they are benign. This is due, in part, to the inability of a "benign" cytologic diagnosis to exclude with absolute certainty a malignant lesion. However, a preoperative renal biopsy plays an important role in the following situations. If the lesion is too widespread to justify surgical excision, a fine needle aspiration biopsy can supply adequate proof of the nature of the lesion. If the patient has a known condition such as lymphoma or carcinoma and presents with a renal mass detected by ultrasound or computed tomography a fine needle aspiration biopsy can differentiate lymphomatous involvement or metastatic carcinoma from an independently arising renal cell carcinoma. If the mass is shown to be cystic by ultrasound, needle aspiration of the cyst followed by examination of the aspirated fluid may obviate the need for surgical excision.

Patients on long-term intermittent hemodialysis have a higher incidence of renal cysts and neoplasms, creating a problem in diagnosis and management.[17] Nunez and associates[18] reported the successful use of fine needle aspiration biopsy in the differential diagnosis of the various mass lesions of the kidney in this group of patients.

Adrenal

Adrenal lesions can be detected by computed tomography on a regular basis, especially in patients who are referred for evaluation of spread of bronchogenic carcinoma. It becomes important to differentiate secondary malignant involvement of adrenal glands from the more common benign adenoma. If the lesion is large, the needle can often be easily guided by placing an ultrasound transducer in either a subcostal position anterolaterally or aiming a needle from an intercostal approach laterally or even posterolaterally. However, the majority of adrenal lesions are now biopsied using CT. The right adrenal masses are generally approached with the patient placed supine passing through the liver, or prone taking a posterior approach. Lesions in the left adrenal, however, are biopsied either prone or in the left decubitus position. The left decubitus position has the advantage of decreasing the chance of aerated lung occupying the posterior costophrenic angle in the path of the gland biopsied.[19]

REFERENCES

1. Cooperberg PL, Hutchinson D, Li D, et al: Percutaneous fine needle aspiration biopsy under ultrasound and computed tomographic control. *Br Col Med J* 23:537–541, 1981.

2. Ferrucci JT, Wittenberg J, Mueller PR, et al: Diagnosis of abdominal malignancy by radiological fine needle aspiration biopsy. *AJR* 134:323–330, 1980.

3. Ho CS, Tao LC, McLoughlin MJ: Percutaneous fine-needle aspiration biopsy of intraabdominal masses. *Can Med Assoc J* 119:1311–1314, 1978.

4. Holm HH, Pedersen JF, Kristensen JK, et al: Ultrasonically guided percutaneous puncture. *Radiol Clin North Am* 13:493–503, 1975.

5. Pereiras RV, Meiers A, Kunhardt B, et al: Fluoroscopically guided thin needle aspiration biopsy of the abdomen and retroperitoneum. *AJR* 131:197–202, 1978.

6. Sundaram M, Wolverson MK, Heiberg E, et al: Utility of CT-guided abdominal aspiration procedures. *AJR* 139:1111–1115, 1982.

7. Von Schreeb T, Arner O, Skovsted G, et al: Renal adenocarcinoma: Is there a risk of spreading tumor cells in diagnostic puncture? *Scand J Urol Nephrol* 1:270–276, 1967.

8. Zornoza J, Jonsson K, Wallace S, et al: Fine needle aspiration biopsy of retroperitoneal lymph nodes and abdominal masses: An updated report. *Radiology* 125:87–88, 1977.

9. Hopper KD, Abendroth CS, Sturtz KW, et al: Fine needle aspiration biopsy for cytopathologic analysis: Utility of syringe handles, automated guns, and nonsuction methods. *Radiology* 185:8–19, 1992.

10. Dahnert WF, Hoagland MH, Hamper UM, et al: Fine-needle aspiration biopsy of abdominal lesions: Diagnostic yield for different needle tip configurations. *Radiology* 185:263–268, 1992.

11. Swaroop VS, Gupta SK, Dilwari JB: Fine needle aspiration cytology in the diagnosis of abdominal lumps. *Indian J Med Res* 76:265–271, 1982.

12. Poskitt K, Cooperberg P, Sullivan L: Ultrasound and computerized tomography in the staging of nonseminomatous testicular carcinoma. *AJR* 144:939–944, 1985.

13. Zelas P, Haaga JR, Lavery IC, et al: The diagnosis of percutaneous biopsy with computed tomography of a recurrence of carcinoma of the rectum in the pelvis. *Surg Gynecol Obstet* 151:525–527, 1980.

14. Butch RJ, Wittenberg J, Mueller PR, et al: Presacral masses after abdominoperineal resection for colorectal carcinoma: The needle for needle biopsy. *AJR* 144:309–312, 1985.

15. Juul N, Torp-Pedersen S, Gronvall S, et al: Ultrasonically guided fine needle aspiration biopsy of renal masses. *J Urol* 133:579–581, 1985.

16. Von Schreeb T, Franzen S, Ljungqvist A: Renal adenocarcinoma. Evaluation of malignancy on a cytologic basis: A comparative cytologic and histologic study. *Scand J Urol Nephrol* 1:265–269, 1967.

17. Scanlon MH, Karasick SR: Acquired renal cystic disease and neoplasia: Complications of chronic hemodialysis. *Radiology* 147:837–838, 1983.

18. Nunez D Jr, Yrizarry JM, Nadji M, et al: Renal cell carcinoma complicating long-term dialysis: Computed tomography-guided aspiration cytology. *CT* 10:61–66, 1986.

19. Charboneau JW, Reading CC, Welch TJ: CT and sonographically guided needle biopsy: Current techniques and new innovations. *AJR* 154:1–10, 1990.

3

Retroperitoneum I: Overview

KEY FACTS

▶ By tradition, the term "neoplasms of the retroperitoneum" refers to those tumors that do not have an anatomic connection to the major retroperitoneal organs, such as the kidney, adrenal, pancreas, or duodenum.

▶ Because of the rigidity of the posterior, cephalad, and caudad boundaries of the retroperitoneal space, large retroperitoneal tumors tend to expand and invade anteriorly into the abdominal cavity.

▶ Malignant tumors of the retroperitoneum are four to five times more common than benign tumors. The former generally fall into one of the four major categories: lymphoma, sarcoma, germ cell tumor, and metastatic carcinoma of somatic origin.

▶ Schwannoma is the most frequently diagnosed benign retroperitoneal tumor.

▶ In young adults, when an undifferentiated carcinoma of unknown primary site is diagnosed, the pathologist must make an effort to rule out germ cell tumor or lymphoma because these tumors are highly responsive to modern chemotherapy.

▶ The cytopathologist must be aware of the atypical, reactive mesothelial cells that are commonly present in aspirate samples, and may be mistaken for cells of adenocarcinoma.

EMBRYOLOGY AND ANATOMY

To understand the retroperitoneal space and its diseases, an appreciation of the embryology and anatomic boundaries of the region is essential.[1,2] The retroperitoneal space is primarily of mesodermal origin. The embryonic mesoderm is divided into three distinct zones in relation to the notochord in the midline. Immediately adjacent to the notochord is the paraaxial mesoderm, from which skeletal muscle, bone, and dermis of the skin develop. Lateral to the paraaxial mesoderm is the intermediate mesoderm, from which portions of the urinary and genital systems are formed (see Chapter 10). The outermost zone is the lateral plate mesoderm, which splits into a somatic (parietal) layer and a splanchnic (visceral) layer. These layers ultimately become the tissue lining the pleural, pericardial, and peritoneal cavities. The splanchnic mesoderm also gives rise to the smooth muscle and connective tissue of the digestive tract, the mesentery, and the cardiovascular and lymphatic systems.

The retroperitoneum is the space between the peritoneal cavity and the posterior body wall. Various structures protrude into the peritoneal cavity from the posterior body wall, carrying the peritoneum before them. Those that protrude sufficiently to be completely covered by peritoneum, and thus to have a mesentery, are said to be intraperitoneal. Those that bulge for a distance so short that they are covered by the peritoneum only on one surface, and thus have no mesenteries, are said to be retroperitoneal. The boundaries of the retroperitoneal space are defined superiorly by the diaphragm; inferiorly by the pelvic levator muscles; and posteriorly by the spinal column, psoas and quadratus lumborum muscles. The anterior boundary of this space is not limited by the posterior parietal peritoneum, but extends into the spaces between the leaves of the various mesenteries of the large and small intestines. Because of the rigidity of the posterior, cephalad, and caudad boundaries, large retroperitoneal tumors tend to expand and invade anteriorly into the abdominal cavity.

Within these anatomic boundaries exist both an actual and a potential space. The actual space contains large organs, including the pancreas, kidneys, adrenals, part of the duodenum, aorta, and inferior vena cava. The potential space consists of a loose mesh of fibroadipose tissue with nerve bundles, small blood vessels, and lymphatics. Numerous lymph nodes are present along the aorta and in the iliac fossa.

GENERAL CONSIDERATIONS

By tradition, the term "neoplasms of the retroperitoneum" is reserved for those tumors that are independent of and therefore not anatomically arising from the large retroperitoneal organs such as the pancreas, kidneys, and adrenals. Tumors arising from these large visceral organs are classified separately.

A variety of diseases may occur within the retroperitoneal space. Neoplasms may arise primarily from the retroperitoneum, may invade the retroperitoneum directly from the adjacent organs, or may metastasize to the retroperitoneum from elsewhere. Inflammatory diseases may be localized to this space and cause compression of adjacent organs, mimicking a neoplasm. Abdominal trauma may injure vascular structures, resulting in retroperitoneal hematoma.

The most common indication for NAB of the retroperitoneum is the discovery of a mass lesion. The majority of masses at this location are neoplastic, with malignancies occurring at least four times as often as benign lesions.[2-4] These malignancies generally fall into one of the four major tumor types: malignant lymphoma, soft tissue sarcoma, metastatic carcinoma of somatic origin, and germ cell neoplasm (**Table 3.1**). In some reports, soft tissue sarcoma is listed as the most common primary tumor of the retroperitoneum,[5-7] while in other series malignant lymphoma is the most common.[8-11] Schwannoma is the most commonly diagnosed benign neoplasm of the retroperitoneum.[12] These neoplasms will be discussed more fully in subsequent chapters.

When consulting a pathologist, the clinician should provide all pertinent information

TABLE 3.1. Frequency Distribution of Various Retroperitoneal Tumors

```
                      Retroperitoneal Masses

Benign (10–15%)                        Malignant (85–90%)


                Lymphoma       Sarcoma        GCT      MCSO
```

GCT = germ cell tumor; MCSO = metastatic carcinoma of somatic origin.

regarding the case, including the patient's age and sex, the details of the present illness, and the past history. Information about any recent or remote trauma to the abdomen, neoplastic disease, or familial disease should be included. Any abnormal physical findings should be noted. In particular, the presence of peripheral lymphadenopathy or a testicular mass should be ascertained, as this information may provide clues to the nature of the retroperitoneal mass. Any radiologic studies and laboratory data should be available for review, if needed.

The cytopathologist who is called upon to interpret the aspirate material must be familiar with the diseases that present as a mass in the retroperitoneum. Knowledge of surgical pathology of the various lesions found at this site helps to narrow the differential diagnosis; only then can the pathologist interpret the NAB accurately and suggest relevant investigations to confirm the cytologic interpretation if the NAB is not absolutely diagnostic. For example, a so-called undifferentiated carcinoma of unknown primary site discovered in the retroperitoneum of a young male should arouse suspicion that the tumor is of germ cell origin. The clinician should be asked to examine the testicles carefully, and appropriate serum markers, such as alpha-fetoprotein and beta-human chorionic gonadotropin, should be obtained. Similarly, an ABC diagnosis of lymphoma should prompt the clinician to examine the patient for enlarged lymph nodes outside the retroperitoneum, which may be more accessible for surgical biopsy to confirm the ABC diagnosis.

NEEDLE ASPIRATION BIOPSY

Role of Needle Aspiration Biopsy

Indications for fine needle aspiration biopsy of the retroperitoneum are outlined in **Table 3.2.**

The diagnosis of retroperitoneal lesions has traditionally been approached with an air of pessimism because the retroperitoneal space is one of the parts of the body least accessible to conventional investigation. Exploratory laparotomy was often the only means available for excluding or confirming a retroperitoneal malignancy. With the advent of ultrasound, computed tomography, and magnetic resonance imaging, together with the use of fine needle aspiration biopsy, this pessimistic view is rapidly changing. Knowing the diagnosis before surgery permits an individualized treatment plan and allows proper pretreatment staging in cases of malignancy. Standard metastatic workup can be carried out on an outpatient basis before definitive surgery is

TABLE 3.2. Indications for Fine Needle Aspiration Biopsy of Retroperitoneal Masses

In Malignant Tumors
1. Establishing a diagnosis in inoperable patients, or patients of poor surgical risk
2. Documenting tumor recurrence or metastasis
3. Staging of tumors
4. Identification of unknown neoplasms

In Benign Conditions
1. Cyst (evacuate)
2. Abscess (culture)
3. Granulomas, i.e., tuberculosis, fungus (culture)
4. Identification of unknown neoplasms

undertaken. The lung is a frequent site of spread for retroperitoneal sarcomas; therefore, when NAB suggests a sarcoma, preoperative staging should include whole-lung tomography or computed tomography of the chest. A bone marrow biopsy is mandatory in suspected lymphomas. In cases of metastatic carcinoma to the retroperitoneum, probable primary sites, as suggested on ABC, can be investigated.

When the NAB diagnosis is suggestive but not diagnostic, the need for and the type of ancillary studies are anticipated. So when further biopsy material becomes available, priorities for various special studies (such as microbiologic, flow cytometric, cell surface marker, and electron microscopic examinations) can be set with a view to establishing a correct diagnosis. In cases in which testicular tumor, neuroblastoma, or pheochromocytoma is diagnosed or suspected on ABC, various secretory products that may be present in the patients' serum or urine can be measured to confirm the cytologic diagnosis. Examples are measurements of serum alpha-fetoprotein and human chorionic gonadotropin in patients suspected to have a germ cell tumor, and measurements of catecholamines in serum or urine and vanillylmandelic acid in urine in patients suspected to have neuroblastoma or pheochromocytoma.

Furthermore, by using NAB many other patients with advanced or metastatic diseases can be spared the trauma and expense of a laparotomy. In one series of 106 patients with abdominal lesions (including pancreas and hepatic lesions) NAB was instrumental in avoiding 61 planned invasive investigations and 11 surgical explorations.[13] Similarly, in a study reported by Smith and Butler,[14] results of NAB obviated the need for a diagnostic laparotomy in 51 (65%) of the 78 patients with a malignant neoplasm. There were no false-positive results. The specificity was 100% and sensitivity was 90%.

Fine Needle Aspiration Biopsy Versus Cutting (Core) Needle Biopsy

In the past few years there has been a movement toward using larger cutting needles that provide a core of tissue for histologic examination of abdominal and retroperitoneal lesions. Orell and associates[15] believe that this may reflect the pressure on tissue pathologists, including those without sufficient training and experience in diagnostic cytology, to make specific and definitive diagnoses on fine needle aspiration cytology

TABLE 3.3. Advantages of Fine Needle Aspiration Biopsy of
Retroperitoneal Masses

1. Minimal patient discomfort and minimal complications.
2. Immediate microscopic assessment of specimen adequacy is feasible, thereby reducing the number of unsatisfactory reports.
3. Easily repeated and can be used for multiple lesions.
4. Suitable for poor-risk patients.
5. Aspirate material is suitable for microbiologic culture and other special studies.
6. Cost-effective by reducing the number of diagnostic laparotomies.

in all kinds of disease processes in all body sites. In a report based upon a literature review, Roussel and coworkers[16] showed that the use of core needles carried a higher risk of complications than simple fine needles (22 to 23 gauge), without necessarily improving diagnostic accuracy. A major advantage of NAB is the ease of immediate evaluation of the adequacy of the cytologic material following aspiration. The merits of NAB are outlined in **Table 3.3.**

It is our view that core needle biopsy has a place but it should be reserved for specific situations.[17] We agree with Hall-Craggs et al.[18] and Jonasson et al.[19] that diagnosis is best attempted first by fine needle cytology and only when this fails to provide an answer, or more information is required for management decisions, is a properly planned core needle biopsy carried out.

Complications of Needle Aspiration Biopsy

Although complications of fine needle aspiration biopsy are very rare, death, exsanguination, peritonitis, and tumor implantation along the needle tract have been observed following abdominal NAB.[20–24] The complication rate of fine needle aspiration biopsy resulting in major morbidities or mortalities is from 0.05% to 0.18%,[21,24] as compared to 0.5% for core needle biopsy.[25] The safety of needle biopsy appears to be related to the degree of invasiveness of the procedure. The risk is minimal with the use of a fine needle no larger than 22 gauge and with the reduction of the number of passes to a minimum by immediate examination of the aspirate for adequacy of the sample.[26]

ASPIRATION CYTOLOGY OF NORMAL AND REACTIVE CELLS

During the aspiration process, the needle may pass through normal abdominal organs such as the liver, pancreas, stomach, intestine, kidneys, and adrenals with no apparent complications.[27] Familiarity with these normal cell types is essential for proper interpretation of NAB specimens.

The surface mucosal epithelia of the stomach, intestine, and pancreatic duct are represented on the smears by monolayered or multilayered sheets or clusters of uniform columnar cells, which display a palisade arrangement when they are seen on profile and a honeycomb arrangement when viewed *en face* (**Figs. 3.1A** and **B**).

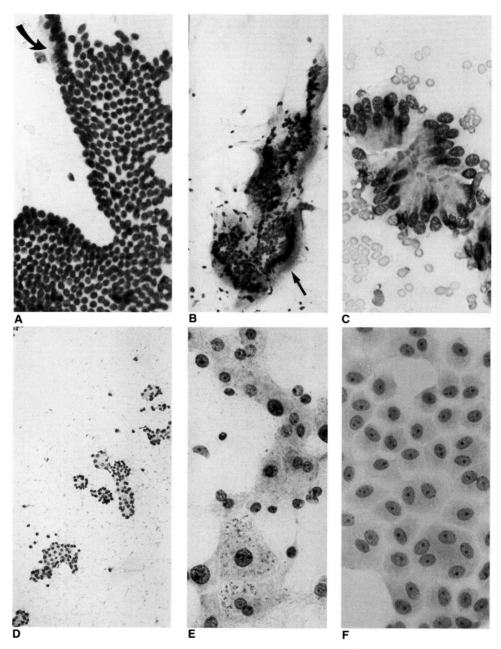

Fig. 3.1. Normal cellular components as seen in abdominal ABC. **A.** Ductal epithelium of pancreas. Note *en face* cells showing a honeycomb arrangement. The peripheral cells in picket-fence arrangement are seen on profile (*arrow*),. (H & E preparation; ×310). **B.** Gastric epithelium. Arrow indicates picket-fence arrangement of the tall columnar cells. (H & E preparation; ×125). **C.** Normal gland of gastrointestinal tract. Note columnar cells arranged around a lumen. The nuclei are basal, located away from the luminal surface. (H & E preparation; ×500). **D.** Pancreatic acinar cells. Note numerous acini, simulating carcinoid or islet cell tumor. (H & E preparation; ×125). **E.** Hepatocytes. Note abundant eosinophilic cytoplasm with pigment granules and central nuclei. (H & E preparation; ×500). **F.** Mesothelial cells. Monolayered sheet of large polygonal cells with prominent intercellular gaps. (H & E preparation; ×500).

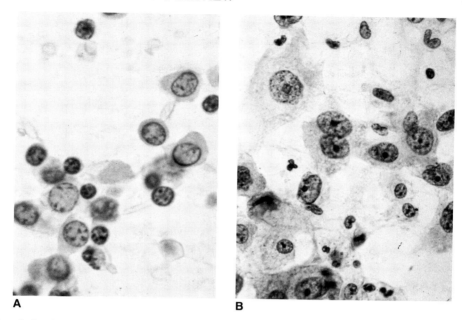

A   **B**

Fig. 3.2. Contrast ABC. **A.** Atypical reactive mesothelial cells. Note bland nuclei with smooth nuclear membranes. Cytoplasm is dense. **B.** Metastatic adenocarcinoma. Note irregular coarse chromatin, uneven nuclear membranes, and prominent nucleoli. Cytoplasm is diffusely vacuolated. (H & E preparation; A: ×500; B: ×500).

Glands of the stomach and intestine are represented by tall columnar cells arranged radially around a space (lumen), with polar nuclei characteristically located away from the luminal surface **(Fig. 3.1C)**. Acinar cells of the pancreas present as small, cuboidal cells arranged in acinar formation **(Fig. 3.1D)**. They may be mistaken for carcinoid tumor by the unwary (see Chapter 7, section on Carcinoid Tumor). Hepatocytes occur in thin cords, flat sheets, or as single cells. They are large polygonal cells with abundant eosinophilic granular cytoplasm and a central round nucleus containing a conspicuous but small nucleolus **(Fig. 3.1E)**. Small brown granules (probably lipofuscin) are often seen in the cytoplasm, and binucleation is not uncommon, particularly in the elderly. The normal ABC of the kidney and adrenal is described in Chapters 9 and 10, respectively.

Mesothelial cells are frequently aspirated in abdominal NABs. They are large, uniform, polygonal cells that often display nucleoli when irritated. They form rather large, monolayered sheets with prominent intercellular spaces or gaps created by the numerous long microvilli that are present on the cell surfaces **(Fig. 3.1F)**. In long-standing ascites or after abdominal surgery, the reactive mesothelial cells can display cellular atypia and may be confused with cells of adenocarcinoma **(Fig. 3.2)**. Mesothelial cells are not stainable with mucicarmine or periodic acid-Schiff (PAS)-diastase reaction and show no immunostaining for carcinoembryonic antigen and B72.3 antigen (see Chapter 8 for more detailed discussion.)

REFERENCES

1. Pack GT, Tabah EJ: Collective review. Primary retroperitoneal tumors: A study of 120 cases. *Surg Gynecol Obstet* 99:209–231, 313–341, 1954.

2. Felix EL, Wood DK, Das Gupta TKD: Tumors of the retroperitoneum. *Curr Probl Cancer* 6:3–47, 1981.

3. Donnelly BA: Primary retroperitoneal tumors. A report of 95 cases and a review of the literature. *Surg Gynecol Obstet* 83:705–717, 1946.

4. Klein EA, Streem SB, Novick AC: Intraoperative consultation for the retroperitoneum and adrenal glands. *Urol Clin North Am* 12:411–421, 1985.

5. Braasch JW, Mon AB: Primary retroperitoneal tumors. *Surg Clin North Am* 47:663–675, 1967.

6. Storm FK, Sondak VK, Economou JS: Sarcomas of the retroperitoneum. In Eilber FR, Morton DL, Sondak VK, et al (ed): *Soft Tissue Sarcomas*. Orlando, FL, Grune & Stratton, 1987, p. 239.

7. Mihatsch MJ: Tumoren des retroperitoneums. *Helv Chir Acta* 56:315–322, 1989.

8. Johnson AH, Searls HH, Grimes OF: Primary retroperitoneal tumors. *Am J Surg* 88:155–161, 1954.

9. Smith RB: Surgical management of retroperitoneal tumors. In Crawford ED, Das S (eds): *Current Genitourinary Cancer Surgery*. Philadelphia, Lea & Febiger, 1990, p 129.

10. Harbrecht B, Gosche JR, Larson GM: Sarcomas of the retroperitoneum. *J Kentucky Med Assoc* 85:29–32, 1987.

11. Adams JT: Abdominal wall, omentum, mesentery, and retroperitoneum. In Schwartz SI (ed): *Principles of Surgery*, ed. 4. New York, McGraw-Hill, 1984, pp 1449–1452.

12. Perhoniemi V, Anttinen I, Kadri F, et al: Benign retroperitoneal schwannoma. *Scand J Urol Nephrol* 26:85–87, 1992.

13. Bret PM, Fond A, Casola G, et al: Abdominal lesions: A prospective study of clinical efficacy of percutaneous fine needle biopsy. *Radiology* 159:345–346, 1986.

14. Smith C, Butler JA: Efficacy of directed percutaneous fine-needle aspiration cytology in the diagnosis of intra-abdominal masses. *Arch Surg* 123:820–824, 1988.

15. Orell SR, Sterrett GF, Walters MNI, et al: *Manual and Atlas of Fine Needle Aspiration Cytology*, ed. 2. Edinburgh, Churchill Livingstone, 1992, p 2.

16. Roussel F, Dalion J, Benozio M: The risk of tumoral seeding in needle biopsies. *Acta Cytol* 33:936–939, 1989.

17. Suen KC: Fine needle biopsy (correspondence). *Histopathol* 17:486, 1990.

18. Hall-Craggs MA, Lees WR: Fine needle biopsy: Cytology, histology, or both? *Gut* 28:233–236, 1987.

19. Jonasson JG, Wang HH, Porter DH, et al: Image-directed percutaneous biopsy. A comparison of cytologic and histologic findings. *Cancer* 70:2187–2191, 1992.

20. Mueller P, Ferruci J Jr: Fine needle aspiration biopsy of abdominal masses. *Semin Roentgenol* 16:52–61, 1981.

21. Livraghi T, Damascelli B, Lombardi C, et al: Risk in fine needle abdominal biopsy. *J Clin Ultrasound* 11:77–81, 1983.

22. Yankaskas B, Staab E, Craven M, et al: Delayed complications from fine-needle biopsies of solid masses of the abdomen. *Invest Radiol* 21:325–328, 1986.

23. Malberger E, Edoute Y, Nagler A: Rare complications after transabdominal fine needle aspiration. *Am J Gastroenterol* 79:458–460, 1984.

24. Fornari F, Civardi G, Cavanna L, et al: Complications of ultrasonically guided fine-needle abdominal biopsy. Results of a multicenter Italian study and review of the literature. *Scand J Gastroenterol* 24:949–955, 1989.

25. Rode J: Fine needle cytology versus histology. *Histopathol* 15:435–439, 1989.

26. Schultenover SJ, Ramzy I, Page CP, et al: Needle aspiration biopsy: Role and limitations in surgical decision making. *Am J Clin Pathol* 82:405–410, 1984.

27. Tao LC, Sanders DE, McLoughlin MJ, et al: Current concepts in fine needle aspiration biopsy cytology. *Hum Pathol* 11:94–96, 1980.

4

Retroperitoneum II: Lymphoproliferative Disorders

KEY FACTS

▶ Diagnosis of lymphoma on ABC is chiefly cellular and not structural. Diagnosis of high-grade lymphomas by NAB is accurate because the cells are cytologically "dysplastic."

▶ Development of knowledge of monoclonal antibodies, flow cytometry, and molecular genetics will continue to expand our abilities in accurately diagnosing lymphoma.

▶ In the diagnosis of lymphoma, the cytopathologist must pay special attention to the patient's age. Small lymphocytic lymphoma and follicular lymphoma occur rarely in patients under 40 years of age, while lymphoblastic lymphoma and Burkitt's lymphoma occur mostly in adolescents and young adults. Hodgkin's disease affects predominantly young adults between the age of 20 and 30 years.

▶ In children and young adults, moderate lymphoid hyperplasia may by regarded as physiological, but the diagnosis of reactive hyperplasia without an apparent cause in a significantly enlarged lymph node of an older person should be made with caution. Malignant lymphomas that may be mistaken for reactive lymphoid hyperplasia on ABC include small lymphocytic lymphoma, follicular lymphoma, mixed small and large cell lymphoma, T-cell lymphoma, and Hodgkin's lymphoma.

▶ Sites of involvement of disease frequently correlates with histologic types of non-Hodgkin's lymphoma. Extranodal presentation (e.g., stomach, intestine, kidney, soft tissue, and bone) is common in large-cell and high-grade lymphomas, whereas follicular and low-grade lymphomas are node-based.

▶ Certain unusual sites (anorectum, brain, heart) of extranodal lymphoma are preferentially involved in patients with AIDS.

▶ A lymphoma in the retroperitoneum may be part of an as yet undiscovered generalized involvement. In such cases, bone marrow biopsy, liver biopsy, or peripheral node biopsy is often helpful and may suffice to confirm the cytologic diagnosis.

▶ A characteristic feature of retroperitoneal lymphomas is the presence of sclerosis in over half to two-thirds of the cases. The sclerosis is a major cause of false-negative cytologic reports.

49

MALIGNANT LYMPHOMAS: GENERAL REMARKS

In the retroperitoneum, the majority of malignant lymphomas are non-Hodgkin's lymphomas (NHL); Hodgkin's disease (HD) arising primarily in the retroperitoneum is uncommon. The incidence of non-Hodgkin's lymphomas has been rising steadily; between 1973 and 1988, the incidence increased by 57%.[1,2] This increase affected not only persons with the acquired immune deficiency syndrome (AIDS), where a 100-fold increase has been observed,[3] but also the general population, suggesting that other environmental and occupational risk factors (e.g., exposure to radiation, pesticides, organic chemicals, and solvents) have been responsible for the overall increase.

Classification of Malignant Lymphoma

Many different histologic classifications of NHL are being used throughout the world (the Rappaport, the Lukes and Collins, the Kiel, and the Working Formulation).[4–8] The proliferation of classification systems attests to the imperfection of our understanding of this diverse group of lymphoid malignancies. The terminologies used in this book are based on the Working Formulation,[8] which is the most widely used classification scheme in North America. In the case of Hodgkin's disease diagnosed by NAB, it is usually not feasible to further subclassify in accordance with the Rye classification.[9]

The Working Formulation[8] **(Table 4.1)** is a purely morphologic classification, which focuses on reproducible light microscopic morphology, and does not differentiate between B- and T-cell phenotypes. The scheme is closest to the Rappaport classifica-

TABLE 4.1. A Working Formulation of Non-Hodgkin's Lymphoma for Clinical Use*

Low-grade
Small lymphocytic
Small cleaved cell (follicular)
Mixed small cleaved and large cell (follicular)
Intermediate-grade
Small cleaved cell (diffuse)
Mixed small and large cell (diffuse)
Large cell
a. Cleaved cell
b. Noncleaved cell
High-grade
Large cell, immunoblastic
Small noncleaved cell
a. Burkitt's
b. Non-Burkitt's
Lymphoblastic

*From ref. 8.

Note: NAB cannot differentiate between follicular and diffuse growth pattern.

tion, familiar to North American pathologists, and easy to use on ABC. The Working Formulation divides non-Hodgkin's lymphomas according to their aggressiveness into low, intermediate, and high grades. In general, the large and median-sized cell types are biologically more aggressive than the small cell types.[10] The scheme also recognizes two histologic growth patterns: diffuse and follicular. The diffuse pattern indicates a more aggressive behavior than the follicular pattern of the same tumor type. Unfortunately, these patterns cannot be determined on ABC.

Clinical Data Relevant to Cytologic Interpretation

In the diagnosis of malignant lymphoma, the cytopathologist must pay special attention to the age of the patient because there are striking differences in the age-dependent incidence of non-Hodgkin's lymphoma by histologic types. Histopathologic types commonly diagnosed in adults are rare in children and vice versa. Follicular lymphoma and small lymphocytic lymphoma seldom affect patients under 40 years of age, while Burkitt's and lymphoblastic lymphomas are found commonly in children and adolescents. In young adults, diffuse large cell lymphomas are the most common type encountered. With increasing age, the incidence of follicular lymphomas and intermediate grade lymphomas continues to rise.[11] While the incidence of NHL rises steadily with age, especially after age 40, the age distribution of Hodgkin's disease is bimodal, with its greatest incidence between 20 and 30 years of age; then its occurrence falls off until the age of 50 when the incidence rises again and continues to increase.

Sites of disease frequently correlate with histologic type of non-Hodgkin's lymphoma. Follicular and low-grade lymphomas are node-based; they infrequently present as primary extranodal disease.[12,13] In contrast, extranodal infiltration or extranodal presentation is common in diffuse large cell and high-grade lymphomas, which may involve the stomach, intestine, soft tisse, lung, CNS, skin, or bone.[14] NHL associated with acquired immunodeficiency syndrome is characteristically high-grade and extranodal, involving unusual sites, such as the rectum, heart, epicardium, and brain. In Hodgkin's lymphoma, primary extranodal disease is exceedingly uncommon. In the majority of cases HD presents as a superficial lymph node disease, involving usually the cervical and supraclavicular lymph nodes.[15] Abdominal lymph nodes generally are not affected in the absence of cervical or mediastinal lymph node involvement.

ROLE OF FINE NEEDLE ASPIRATION BIOPSY

Fine needle aspiration is very useful in the initial investigation of patients with lymphadenopathy. When the lymphadenopathy is predominantly within the abdomen and is not readily accessible for surgical biopsy, percutaneous NAB will at least distinguish metastatic carcinoma to lymph nodes from malignant lymphoma. At times, the clinician may not consider lymphoma in the differential diagnosis, particularly if the clinical presentation is atypical. Not uncommonly it is the cytopathologist interpreting the aspirate who is the first to suggest that the patient may have lymphoma. In the ideal

TABLE 4.2. Applications of Aspiration Cytology to Lymphomas

1. As the sole morphologic diagnostic tool, so as to avoid major surgery in cases of advanced disease, in frail patients, and in patients with AIDS
2. To document recurrence of a previously diagnosed lymphoma
3. To document transformation of a previously diagnosed low-grade lymphoma to a high-grade lymphoma
4. To assess the staging of the disease following histologic diagnosis
5. To exclude an unrelated malignancy or an infectious process

situation the initial diagnosis of lymphoma by NAB would be confirmed by histologic examination of the resected lesion. However, retroperitoneal lymphoma is primarily a disease of older patients,[16] some of whom may be too frail to undergo surgery. The extent and vigor of investigation must therefore be tailored to fit the circumstances of each patient. In a modern cytology laboratory, the cytologic diagnosis of lymphoma by ABC can often be confirmed by the ancillary techniques of immunocytochemistry, flow cytometry, or molecular genetic analysis performed on aspiration specimens, without resorting to laparotomy to obtain tissue. Furthermore, a lymphoma in the retroperitoneal space may be part of an as yet undiscovered generalized involvement. A cytologic diagnosis of a retroperitoneal mass as malignant lymphoma will considerably revitalize the clinician's search for peripheral enlarged lymph nodes which are more accessible for surgical biopsy. Different types of NHL show different propensity for dissemination. About 20 to 25% of the large cell and 70 to 90% of the small cell lymphomas will have disseminated disease (stage III or IV) at the time of diagnosis,[12,13,16,17] and in such cases a relatively minor procedure, such as a bone marrow biopsy, liver biopsy, or peripheral lymph node biopsy will often suffice to confirm the cytologic diagnosis.

Another use of NAB is in the diagnosis of lymphoma in patients with AIDS. AIDS-related lymphomas are almost always diffuse in histology and high-grade. NAB as a primary diagnostic tool is ideally suited to this setting.[18,19] **Table 4.2** enumerates further the clinical utilities of NAB in lymphoma diagnosis.

One of the drawbacks of NAB in the diagnosis of NHL is its inability to identify the histologic growth pattern (follicular versus diffuse), on which basis some of the lymphoma types are graded. More recently, DNA ploidy and S-phase fraction (a measure of tumor proliferation) analyzed by flow cytometry have been proposed as additional parameters in assessing the aggressiveness (and hence the grade) of the lymphoma.

ANCILLARY DIAGNOSTIC PROCEDURES

The accuracy rate of cytodiagnosis of lymphoma can be greatly enhanced by supplementing cytomorphology with the judicious use of specialized diagnostic techniques. A discussion of these special techniques has been presented in Chapter 1; only those aspects of immediate clinical relevance to the diagnosis of lymphoproliferative disorders are included in the following sections.

Immunocytochemistry

There is little doubt that the use of surface markers in lymphoma diagnosis is exceedingly useful, particularly to distinguish between malignant lymphoma and lymphoid hyperplasia, and between malignant lymphoma and some poorly differentiated nonlymphoid malignances. The following antibodies are commonly used in the differential diagnosis of lymphoproliferative disorders.

Antibodies to Leukocyte Common Antigen (LCA)

Leukocyte common antigen is a predominantly surface antigen (about 200,000 daltons), which is present on virtually all nucleated hematopoietic cells. However, LCA is not detectable in plasma cells. Reed-Sternberg cells and the mononuclear variants are also LCA-negative. Several monoclonal antibodies to LCA are commercially available. The major use of these antibodies is in the identification of the lymphoid lineage of the cells in question; hence they are very useful in distinguishing lymphomas from poorly differentiated nonlymphoid malignancies that mimic lymphoma (**Fig. 4.1**), but they cannot distinguish benign from malignant lymphoid cells. The commercially available anti-LCA monoclonal antibodies have persistently showed good sensitivity and excellent specificity. False-positive results for LCA are very uncommon, but a small number of large cell lymphomas and some Ki-1 anaplastic lymphomas are LCA-negative.

Anti-kappa and Anti-lambda Antibodies

Each B-lymphocyte possesses immunoglobulin of a single light chain type: either kappa (κ) or lambda (λ). A neoplastic population of lymphocytes arising from a single progenitor B cell will exhibit restricted light chain expression, i.e., either κ or λ. Thus the demonstration of monotypic light chain expression is presumptive evidence of B-cell neoplasia, as opposed to the polyclonal proliferation found in reactive lymphoid hyperplasia. The normal ratio of κ-bearing lymphocytes to λ-bearing lymphocytes is 2:1. We define B cell monoclonality as a κ:λ ratio greater than 6 or less than 0.25. There are no immunophenotypic markers for T-cell clonality, and immunophenotypic evidence of T-cell malignancy rests on the identification of abnormal or aberrant expression of T cell associated antigens.[20]

Leu-M1 Antibody

Monoclonal Leu-M1 antibody detects an antigen which is primarily a myelomonocytic marker. The antibody also reacts with Reed-Sternberg cells of Hodgkin's disease and hence has been used for the identification of these cells.[21] Interestingly, a high percentage (60–90%) of adenocarcinoma also express Leu-M1 antigen whereas mesotheliomas do not (see Chapter 8).

Nonlymphoid Markers

These antibodies are used to elucidate the histogenetic origin of a LCA-negative tumor. Cytokeratin antibodies are used to confirm the epithelial origin of a poorly

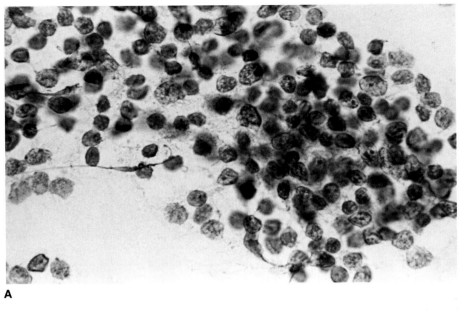

A

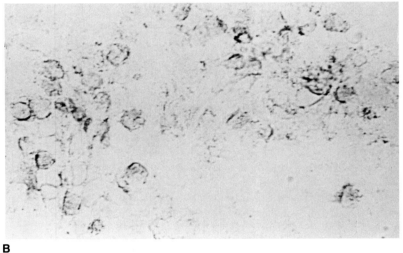

B

Fig. 4.1. Aspirate of a retroperitoneal mass in a 74-year-old man. **A.** Note many large atypical round cells, morphologically consistent with a large cell lymphoma. However, the patient had a melanoma of the right leg, excised 18 months previously. (H & E preparation; ×500). **B.** Cytospin specimen of the same case. The tumor cells show immunoreactivity for leukocyte common antigen. The reaction product appears as cytoplasmic brown granules. Immunostaining with an antimelanoma antibody (HMB45) shows a negative reaction (not depicted). These findings confirm the diagnosis of lymphoma and rule out melanoma. (Immunoperoxidase stain with anti-LCA; ×500).

differentiated carcinoma. Other antibodies can be used to demonstrate lineage-restricted (but not necessarily lineage-specific) antigens; examples are carcinoembryonic antigen expressed by many adenocarcinomas, alpha-fetoprotein expressed by germ cell tumors, S100 antigen by melanoma, and prostate-specific antigen by prostatic carcinoma. The applications of these antibodies are listed in **Table 1.6,** Chapter 1.

When an immunocytochemical method is used to support a diagnosis, it is always advisable to use a carefully selected panel of antibodies rather than a single antibody, because there is virtually no single marker that is absolutely diagnostic for any particular neoplasm. Conversely, it is neither practical nor economical to use a large battery of antibodies routinely since most problems can be resolved by using a limited number of antibodies. Different types of information are provided by judicious selection of different panels of antibodies; attention to the clinical and cytologic data will permit the cytopathologist to tailor the immunocytochemical study in each case. For example, high-grade lymphomas are cytologically atypical and unlikely to be confused with reactive lymphoid processes. However, they may be so poorly differentiated that confusion with other undifferentiated malignancies may occur. In these circumstances, some authors advocate using antibodies to both cytokeratin and S100 protein in addition to anti-LCA.[22] The use of the first two antibodies serves to exclude carcinoma and melanoma respectively. On the other hand, low-grade lymphoma may be difficult to distinguish from reactive lymphoid hyperplasia. In this instance, using anti-κ and anti-κ antibodies to demonstrate either a polyclonal or monoclonal immunoglobulin pattern would provide additional information to assist in the evaluation of such a lesion.[23]

Flow Cytometry

Flow cytometric data should be used as an adjunct to good cytomorphology and not as a substitute. There are two broad areas of analysis by flow cytometry as applied to lymphoma diagnosis: immunologic marker analysis and DNA content and cell cycle kinetics analysis.[24] **Table 4.3** summarizes the clinical applications of flow cytometry to lymph node pathology.

Immunologic Marker Analysis

Lymphocytes are characterized by the presence of surface antigens, which means that the cells can be readily tagged with fluoresceinated antibodies and analyzed by flow cytometry for immunophenotyping. Flow cytometric methodology is able to detect a monoclonal population of lymphocytes when they comprise as little as 10% of the cells present. This small number may not always be detectable by use of immunocytochemical technique on cytocentrifuge smears.

Immunologic marker analysis can be used to confirm or exclude the lymphoid origin of a tumor using antibodies against LCA and cytokeratin, to confirm B-cell monoclonality (see **Fig. 1.5)** using anti-κ and anti-λ antibodies (B cell monoclonality is generally defined as a κ : λ ratio greater than 6 or less than 0.25), and to subclassify the lymphoma using antibodies against various lymphocyte differentiation antigens.

TABLE 4.3 Clinical Applications of Flow Cytometry in Lymph Node Pathology*

Differential Diagnosis	Flow Cytometric Analysis	Comments
Lymphoma vs. metastasis	Surface marker studies	LCA, cytokeratin, EMA, S100
Lymphoma vs. benign reactive hyperplasia	Surface immunoglobulin studies	Abnormal $\kappa:\lambda$ ratio
B-cell vs. T-cell lymphoma	Immunophenotype	Abnormal T-cell antigen expression; B- and T-cell differentiation antigens
Low vs. high-grade lymphoma	DNA analysis Cell kinetics	Abnormal DNA index % Proliferative cells (S-phase fraction)

*Modified from Vielh P: *Flow Cytometry. Guides to Clinical Aspiration Biopsy.* New York, Igaku-Shoin, 1991, p 75.
LCA = leukocyte common antigen; EMA = epithelial membrane antigen.

DNA Content and Cell Cycle Kinetics Analysis

Flow cytometric analysis of DNA content, which is assessed by staining cells in suspension with special DNA-binding fluorescent dyes, is used to aid in the diagnosis and gauge the prognosis of lymphomas. **Table 4.4** lists the criteria used for the interpretation of flow cytometry results. Normal diploid DNA content (DNA index = 1) is generally found in benign lymphoid hyperplasia, low-grade NHL, and Hodgkin's disease **(Fig. 4.2),** while aneuploidy is frequently found in high-grade NHL **(Fig. 4.3).**[25,26] In addition to quantification of DNA content, flow cytometry also measures the various phases of the cell cycle, including the S-phase fraction. The latter is linked to the rate of cell proliferation (see the section on Flow Cytometry in Chapter 1). Many investigators[27,28] have found that the three prognostic categories of NHL designated by the Working Formulation, i.e., low, intermediate, and high grades, can be discriminated by the proliferation rate of the tumors. In one study the mean proportion of S-phase cells was shown to be 4.75% in low-grade, 9.57% in intermediate grade, and 18.12% in high-grade NHLs.[29] Interestingly, Hodgkin's disease had normal DNA

TABLE 4.4. Criteria for Interpreting a Flow Cytometry DNA Histogram as Abnormal*

1. Presence of a distinctive DNA aneuploid population.
2. Increased percentage of cells in G2 and cells beyond that region which could be proliferating cells of the abnormal population.
3. An increased proliferation rate of a diploid population (S + G2/M% = 13% for fine needle aspirates).†

*Adapted from Fuhr JE, Sullivan TA, Nelson HS, Jr. *Am J Pathol* 141:211, 1992, with permission.
†Each laboratory must establish its own baseline for the proliferation rate value. The proliferation rate value varies among laboratories, depending on the types of specimen and computer software program used.

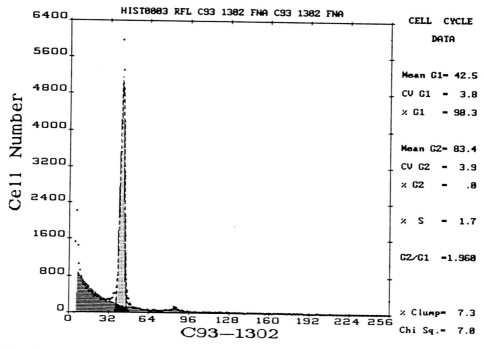

Fig. 4.2. DNA histogram of a low-grade, small cleaved cell non-Hodgkin's lymphoma. No DNA abnormality is detected (DNA index = 1).

content and unremarkable S-phase percentage in all but one of eight cases studied by Diamond et al.[27]

Molecular Genotypic Studies

Aspirates obtained by NAB are suitable for molecular genetic analysis,[30–32] which is far more sensitive and specific for diagnostic purposes than immunophenotyping. However, the techniques of DNA sequence analysis (Southern blotting or polymerase chain reaction using radiolabeled or biotinylated commercially available DNA probes) are complex and expensive and should be restricted to those cases that lack detectable surface or cytoplasmic immunoglobulin or have an otherwise ambiguous immunophenotype. Two areas of investigation by molecular methods are particularly useful for lymphoma diagnosis: (1) detection of rearrangements of immunoglobulin and T-cell receptor genes (to establish clonality), and (2) detection of chromosomal translocations (to identify specific oncogene rearrangements as tumor markers for histologically defined subgroups of NHL).

Rearrangements of immunoglobulin and T-cell receptor genes occur at the earliest stages of lymphoid differentiation. A vast variety of immunoglobulin molecules exist, each corresponding to a unique antigenic epitope. This diversity is produced by genetic recombination within the immunoglobulin gene loci of B lymphocytes. Immunoglobulin genes are encoded by discontinuous segments of DNA. During development, a potential antibody-producing cell must rearrange variable (V), diversity (D),

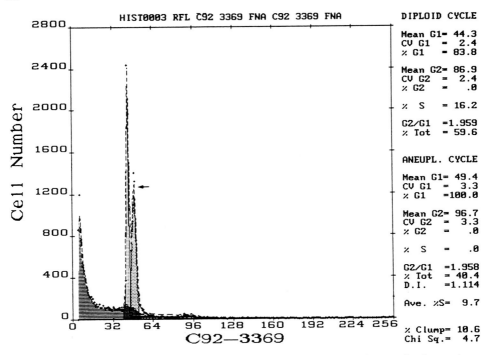

Fig. 4.3. DNA histogram of a small cleaved cell NHL containing an abnormal cell population with DNA index = 1.11 (*arrow*). It is unusual to see an abnormal DNA component in low-grade lymphoma unless the lesion is in the process of transforming into a higher grade lymphoma.

and joining (J) genes, which are then linked to the constant region locus. The numbers of potential recombinants of V,D,J regions are enormous. These rearrangements can be detected by Southern blot hybridization using DNA probes specific for heavy and light chains of immunoglobulin genes. Since cancer is a clonal process, clonal rearrangements of light chain genes are therefore an extremely sensitive tool to identify B-cell lymphomas.[30] A gene rearrangement of the same type (clonal) is seen as a discrete, nongermline band of hybridization on Southern blotting (see **Fig. 1.11**). In contrast, in reactive lymphoid hyperplasia numerous gene rearrangements occur (polyclonal), resulting in a diffuse smear pattern on Southern blot hybridization. In addition, molecular techniques using probes specific for the T-cell receptor (TRC) β chain genes can establish clonality in T-cell lymphomas by demonstrating clonally rearranged TCR-β genes.[31] However one should note that monoclonality does not always imply malignancy, and gene rearrangement must be considered in the context of clinical and morphologic data. Clonal B-cell gene rearrangements have been reported in patients with AIDS, and in certain cases of benign lymphoid hyperplasias of the skin (lymphomatoid papulosis, pityriasis lichenoides et varioliformis acuta), salivary gland (Sjögren's disease), thyroid, and orbit.[33]

Specific chromosomal translocations (another form of tumor markers) can identify histologically defined groups of NHL, such as t(8;14) in Burkitt's lymphoma, (t(14;18) in follicular lymphoma, and t(11;14) in small cell lymphoma/chronic lymphocytic leukemia.[32] Southern blot analysis, by employing a battery of gene probes, can detect chromosomal translocation without conventional chromosomal morphologic analysis.

NON-HODGKIN'S LYMPHOMA

Aspirates of lymphoma often yield a generous sample of cells. Unlike epithelial cells, lymphocytes lack intercellular cohesion and present themselves on the smears as singly dispersed cells. In the majority of cases, the neoplastic lymphocytes are of a single series, hence a monomorphic population of lymphocytes is observed. It must be recognized, however, that "monomorphism" is a relative term and that a small number of histiocytes and other morphologic types of lymphocytes are often present, in addition to the predominant one. In Lennert's opinion, the microscopic diagnosis of lymphoma is chiefly cellular and not structural.[6] The size and shape of the nuclei, the number, position and prominence of the nucleoli, and the chromatin texture are all important morphologic criteria that must be carefully evaluated in the diagnosis of non-Hodgkin's lymphoma. The type of NHL in which the tumor belongs is indicated by the type of lymphoid cells present (Fig. 4.4). The descriptions of NHL in the following sections adopt the terminologies of the Working Formulation (Table 4.1), with no reference to immunophenotypes.

Although any type of NHL can be found in the retroperitoneum, the most frequent types are large cell, cleaved or noncleaved, and large cell, immunoblastic.[34,35] The neoplastic cells from these lymphoma types are morphologically atypical and can be recognized with a high degree of accuracy on ABC.

Malignant Lymphoma, Small Lymphocytic

This lymphoma is the tissue manifestation of chronic lymphocytic leukemia. It is a low-grade, indolent lymphoma afflicting predominantly patients over 45 years of age. The ABC shows small, uniform, round cells resembling normal small lymphocytes (Fig. 4.5). Nuclear chromatin is compact, clumped, and darkly stained. Nucleoli are not usually present, but in some instances, during a phase of accelerated growth, the chromatin becomes more dispersed and a distinct nucleolus may be seen. The cytoplasm is scanty. Since the neoplastic lymphocytes are indistinguishable cytologically from normal small lymphocytes, the diagnosis is suspected primarily on the basis of a monotonous population of small cells. The ABC diagnosis must be substantiated by examination of peripheral blood, bone marrow, and serum proteins. The bone marrow is involved in from 75% to almost 100% of cases.[36,37] A positive bone marrow biopsy will therefore readily confirm the ABC diagnosis.

A small proportion of small cell lymphocytic lymphomas can convert to diffuse large cell lymphoma (Richter's syndrome). These patients often present with abdominal masses and experience short survival.[38,39]

When increased numbers of plasma cells and/or plasmacytoid lymphocytes are present in the background of a small lymphocytic lymphoma, the designation "small lymphocytic-plasmacytoid NHL" is used (Fig. 4.6). When the lymphoma is accompanied by IgM monoclonal dysproteinemia, the condition is known specifically as "Waldenström's macroglobulinemia."

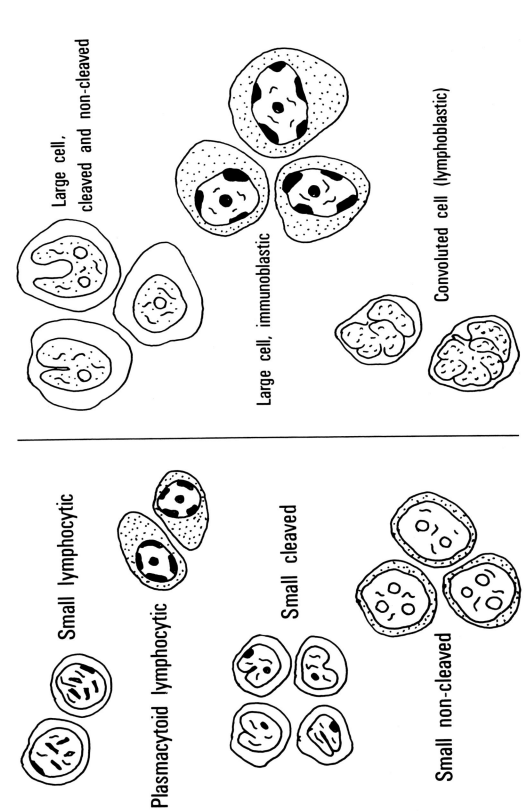

Large cell, cleaved and non-cleaved

Large cell, immunoblastic

Convoluted cell (lymphoblastic)

Small lymphocytic

Plasmacytoid lymphocytic

Small cleaved

Small non-cleaved

Fig. 4.4. Non-Hodgkin's lymphoma cell types.

60

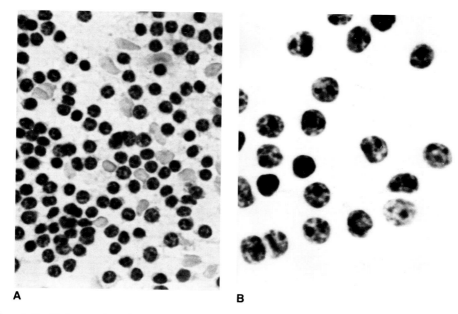

Fig. 4.5. Malignant lymphoma, small lymphocytic, ABC. **A.** Note dispersed small lymphocytes. **B.** Note characteristic clumped chromatin pattern, similar to that of normal small lymphocytes. (H & E preparation; A ×500; B ×1,250).

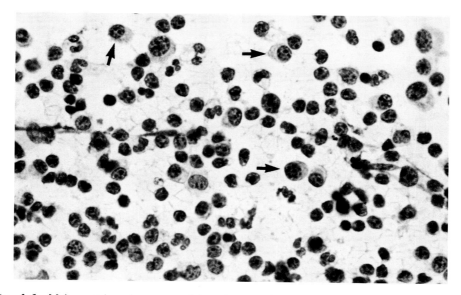

Fig. 4.6. Malignant lymphoma, small lymphocytic-plasmacytoid, ABC. Note admixture of small lymphocytes and plasmacytoid lymphocytes (*arrows*) characterized by eccentric nuclei and abundant basophilic cytoplasm. (H & E preparation; ×500).

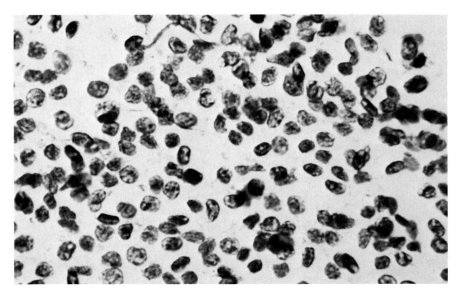

Fig. 4.7. Malignant lymphoma, small cleaved cell, ABC. Note irregular nuclei with linear cleavage planes and coarse chromatin. (H & E preparation; ×500).

Malignant Lymphoma, Small Cleaved Cell

Most cases of small cleaved cell lymphoma represent neoplastic proliferation of follicular center B cells derived from lymph nodes. The cells (8 to 12 μm in size) with clumped chromatin resemble small or medium-sized lymphocytes but they show nuclear indentations and clefts, resulting in pronounced variations in nuclear shape **(Fig. 4.7).** Nucleoli are not prominent. The cytoplasm is scanty, with a variable degree of basophilia. Small cleaved cells, by definition, have nuclei which are smaller than those of a histiocyte. There may be a few larger cells containing oval nuclei with fine chromatin and nucleoli related to the nuclear membrane, corresponding to the noncleaved follicular center cells (centroblasts). Peripheral blood and bone marrow involvements are common at the time of diagnosis in small cleaved cell lymphoma.[40]

When the histologic pattern of the small cleaved cell lymphoma is follicular, it is categorized as low-grade in the Working Formulation; when diffuse it is classified as intermediate grade. However, this distinction cannot be made in aspirate material. Determination of proliferative rate of the lymphoma cells by flow cytometric method has been reported to be useful. Low-grade lymphomas have a low S-phase fraction, while intermediate-grade lymphomas show a statistically significantly higher S-phase fraction.[41]

Molecular genotypic studies have revealed t(14;18) chromosomal translocations in as many as 90% of low-grade, follicular lymphomas.[42,43] The translocation brings the *bcl-2* gene from chromosome 18 into association with the joining region (J_H) of the immunoglobulin heavy-chain gene on chromosome 14. In its new position, the *bcl-2* gene causes prolonged survival of resting cells;[44] the associated lymphoma is low-grade and is relatively nonproliferative.

Malignant Lymphoma, Mixed Small and Large Cell

This category of non-Hodgkin's lymphoma includes cases in which there is no clear-cut preponderance of one cell type (large or small), and it embraces a diverse group of lymphomas. The proportions of large and small cells present in the tumor are not stated in the Working Formulation but probably there should be about equal numbers **(Fig. 4.8)**. The lymphoma can be low-grade or intermediate grade, depending on whether it has a follicular or diffuse growth pattern. When the tumor is of the follicular center cell origin, the small lymphoid cells have features of small cleaved cells. In others, the small cells have noncleaved but irregular nuclei and may bear T-cell markers. The large cells have nuclei which are larger than those of a histiocyte. They may be cleaved and/or noncleaved. Nucleoli are usually not prominent in the large cleaved cells, while the large noncleaved cells always exhibit readily identifiable nucleoli and dispersed chromatin.

Malignant Lymphoma, Large Cell, Cleaved and Noncleaved

This is an intermediate grade lymphoma in the Working Formulation, regardless of whether the pattern is follicular or diffuse. ABC shows both large cleaved and large noncleaved cells **(Fig. 4.9)**, but at times one type may predominate. The large cleaved cell nuclei are irregular and often very elongated, imparting a "dysplastic" appearance. The chromatin tends to be more dispersed than in the small cleaved cells, but prominent nucleoli are absent. The large noncleaved cells have large vesicular nuclei. Nucleoli are always present, are often multiple, and lie next to the nuclear membranes.

Malignant Lymphoma, Large Cell, Immunoblastic

This type of lymphoma is a high-grade tumor, with a diffuse growth pattern. Those tumors with a B-immunophenotype are characterized by large immunoblasts showing plasmacytoid features **(Fig. 4.10)**. The nuclei are large, measuring about 20 μm or more in diameter, and are frequently eccentrically placed. The nuclear membranes are thick. Nucleoli are prominent, eosinophilic and centrally placed. They are often single but may be multiple. Sometimes, the nucleoli are placed peripherally. The cytoplasm is moderate to abundant, deeply staining, and basophilic or pyroninophilic. There may be some admixed large noncleaved cells present. Normal and abnormal plasma cells may also be evident. The clear cell variant has immunoblasts with abundant pale or clear cytoplasm and shows T-cell phenotype.

Malignant Lymphoma, Small Noncleaved Cell (Burkitt's and Non-Burkitt's)

The small noncleaved cell lymphoma is a high-grade tumor. The term "small cell" used for this category of lymphoma is a misnomer because the cells are of intermediate size, larger than the small cleaved cells but smaller than those of the large cell lymphoma. There are two subsets: Burkitt's and non-Burkitt's.

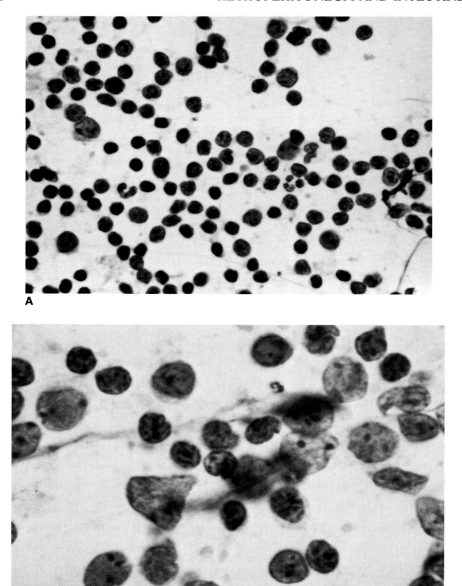

Fig. 4.8. Malignant lymphoma, mixed small and large cell, ABC. **A,B.** Note two populations of lymphocytes, small and large. (H & E preparation; A ×500; B ×1,250).

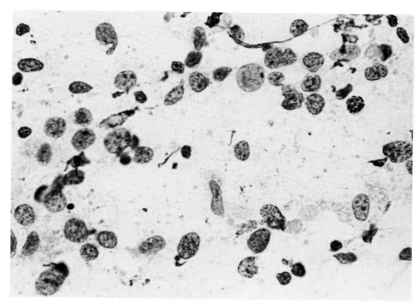

Fig. 4.9. Malignant lymphoma, large cell, ABC. The tumor is composed mostly of large cells with noncleaved vesicular nuclei and multiple nucleoli. (H & E preparation; ×500).

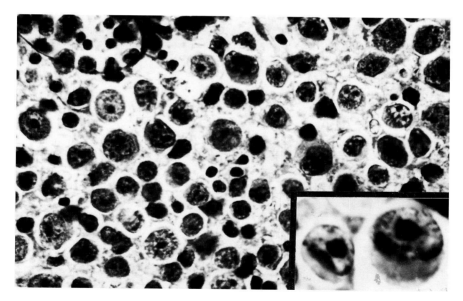

Fig. 4.10. Malignant lymphoma, large cell, immunoblastic, ABC. Note many large round cells with prominent central nucleoli. *Inset* shows higher magnification view of two large cells with plasmacytoid features, characterized by eccentric nuclei and abundant basophilic cytoplasm. (H & E preparation; ×500, inset × 1,250).

Burkitt's lymphoma occurring in North America commonly presents as an abdominal mass, frequently involving the small bowel, in children and adolescents. The aspirates **(Fig. 4.11)** contain intermediate-sized lymphocytes that are characteristically monomorphic with respect to nuclear size, shape, and prominence of nucleoli. The nuclei are round and uniform, with coarsely reticulated chromatin, and contain two to four distinct, central nucleoli. The nuclear membrane is prominent. The thin rim of cytoplasm is amphophilic or basophilic and intensely pyroninophilic due to high content of ribonucleic acid. There is rapid cell turnover, reflected by a high mitotic rate and many scattered macrophages with ingested nuclear debris.

Burkitt's lymphoma is one of the first human malignancies in which chromosomal translocation and oncogene activation have been related. The human oncogene (*c-myc*), located on the region of chromosome 8, is translocated to either chromosome 2, 14, or 22. In the most common translocation, t(8;14), the segment of chromosome 8 carrying the *c-myc* gene is brought into close proximity with the locus on chromosome 14 that encodes immunoglobulin heavy chains. The overexpression of the *c-myc* gene confers a proliferative advantage on the cells, resulting in a rapidly proliferating tumor.[45,46]

In small noncleaved cell lymphoma of the non-Burkitt's type, the neoplastic cells exhibit greater variability in nuclear size and shape, finer and less clumped chromatin, and fewer and sometimes solitary nucleoli. The tumor is more closely related to the other aggressive large cell lymphomas, and some pathologists undoubtedly diagnose small noncleaved cell lymphoma of the non-Burkitt's type where others would diagnose a large noncleaved cell lymphoma.

Lymphoblastic Lymphoma

Lymphoblastic lymphoma, a high-grade malignancy, is a disease seen usually in children and young adults. Involvement of the anterior mediastinum is common but involvement of the retroperitoneum is unusual. Virtually all lymphoblastic lymphomas that occur in the mediastinum in children are of T-cell (thymic) lineage. On the aspirate smears **(Fig. 4.12)**, the cells are medium-sized blasts with a high mitotic rate. Characteristically, many nuclei are convoluted or gyrated (knoblike projections and bulging protrusions). Nucleoli are small or inconspicuous. Chromatin is finely dispersed and has a dusty appearance. The fine chromatin pattern distinguishes the convoluted lymphoblasts from the cleaved lymphocytes, whose chromatin is characteristically more coarse.

Non-Hodgkin's Lymphoma Types Not Specified in the Working Formulation

T-cell Lymphoma

T-cell neoplasms account for about 15 to 20% of all non-Hodgkin's lymphomas. There is no provision for T-cell lymphomas in the Working Formulation and they are placed under several categories: diffuse small cleaved cell, diffuse mixed, diffuse large cell, diffuse large cell immunoblastic, and lymphoblastic. Nearly all lymphoblastic lymphomas occurring in the mediastinum of children and adolescents are T-cell neoplasms, presumably of thymic origin. Peripheral (postthymic) T-cell lymphoma, a

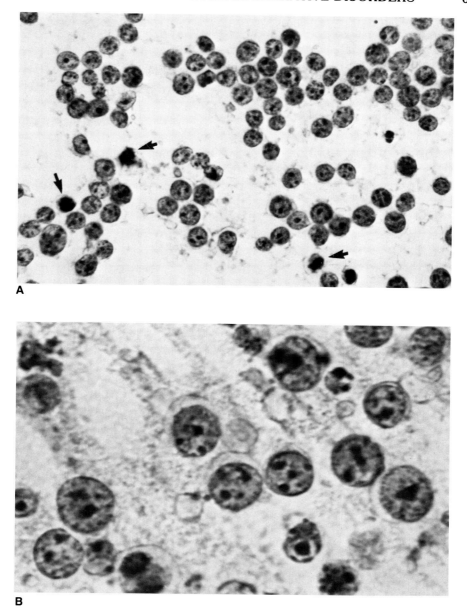

Fig. 4.11. Malignant lymphoma, small noncleaved cell, Burkitt's type, ABC. **A.** Note cellular monotony and mitotic figures (*arrows*). (H & E preparation; ×500). **B.** Note noncleaved nuclei with two to four distinct nucleoli and thick nuclear membranes. (H & E preparation; ×1,250).

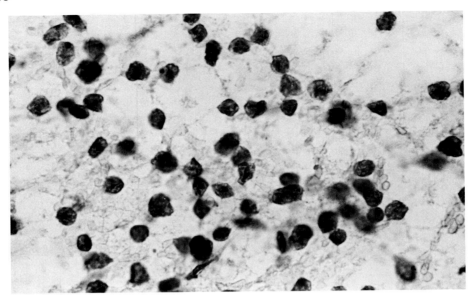

Fig. 4.12. Malignant lymphoma, lymphoblastic, ABC. Note lymphocytes with nuclear convolutions. The convoluted lymphocytes can be distinguished from small cleaved cell lymphoma by their fine chromatin pattern and from large cell lymphoma by the absence of prominent nucleoli. (H & E preparation; ×500).

term used to distinguish it from lymphoblastic lymphoma, is derived from peripheral T cells in lymph nodes and other sites. Unlike lymphoblastic lymphoma, peripheral T-cell lymphoma occurs mainly in adults (median age 57 years) and exhibits a broad spectrum of cell types. A number of morphologic features **(Fig. 4.13)** characterize T-cell lineage but none is considered specific.[47–49] They include: (1) small or medium-sized atypical lymphocytes with irregular or folded nuclei; (2) large pale to "water-clear" cells with round nuclei and central nucleoli, and without plasmacytoid differentiation (T-immunoblasts); (3) large cells with polylobated nuclei; (4) an admixture of benign reactive cells (plasma cells, eosinophils, and macrophages) and epithelioid histiocytes.

Morphologic classification of peripheral T-cell lymphoma is difficult and arbitrary. The above-mentioned morphologic criteria identify no more than two-thirds of T-cell lymphomas and do not exclude B-cell tumors.[50] Undoubtedly, immunophenotyping contributes considerably to the diagnosis of T-cell tumors. Peripheral T-cell lymphomas express T cell antigens and are negative for B cell markers. Many show aberrant phenotypes, such as loss of one or several pan-T cell antigens, loss of both the helper (CD4) and the suppressor (CD8) antigens, or coexpression of the CD4 and CD8 antigens. Molecular analysis demonstrated clonal rearrangements of the β chain of the T-cell receptor gene in 12 of 14 cases studied by Ramsay et al.[48]

Despite the usefulness of immunologic data in diagnosing T-cell lymphoma, attempts to incorporate them into classification schemes have been met with some hesitation because their clinical relevance to treatment and prognosis is still being debated. Many investigators have shown that immunophenotype has little independent prognostic value when compared with that of the grade of tumor evaluated by

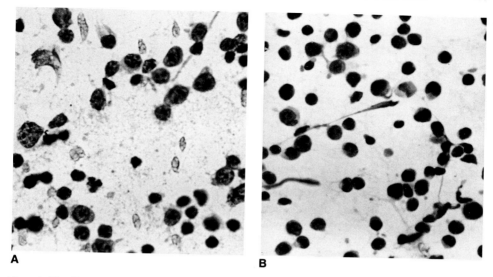

A   B

Fig. 4.13. Two cases of peripheral T-cell lymphoma, ABC. **A.** Note a mixture of small, intermediate, and large cells with no particular cell type predominating. This cytologic pattern can be easily confused with reactive lymphoid hyperplasia. However, there is nuclear dysplasia, particularly in the larger cells. This feature is not seen in reactive benign conditions. (H & E preparation; ×500). **B.** Note admixture of dysplastic small and large cells. If no immunopheno-typing data were available, this case would have been classified as mixed small and large cell lymphoma in the Working Formulation. (H & E preparation; ×500).

conventional morphology.[51] Some authors believe that the poor survival in patients with peripheral T-cell lymphoma can be accounted for by an excess of high-grade histology (many cases are large cell immunoblastic or diffuse mixed in the Working Formulation).[52] Others have indicated that the stage of a T-cell lymphoma at the time of diagnosis is a better prognostic indicator than the immunophenotypic data.[50,53]

Anaplastic Large Cell (Ki-1) Lymphoma

Anaplastic large cell (Ki-1) lymphoma is a newly recognized entity,[54] estimated to comprise 1–8% of non-Hodgkins's lymphomas.[55] The clinical features of this lymphoma are quite unusual, and include a young median age at onset and frequent extranodal disease affecting the skin, gastrointestinal tract, and bone. The cytologic spectrum ranges from large cells with pleomorphic nuclei, clumped chromatin, one or more nucleoli, and abundant, often vacuolated cytoplasm to cells with more regular rounded vesicular nuclei (usually containing a single prominent nucleolus) and baso-philic cytoplasm. Multinucleated wreathlike and Reed-Sternberg-like giant cells are frequently present **(Fig. 4.14).** A retrospective study of cases originally diagnosed as lymphocyte depletion Hodgkin's disease has revealed a high proportion that today would instead be classified as anaplastic large cell lymphoma, although the distinction between the two is indeed arbitrary in some cases.[56] Another diagnostic problem is caused by the tumor cells frequently growing in a sheetlike, cohesive manner, mimick-ing metastatic anaplastic carcinoma, sarcoma, or malignant melanoma.

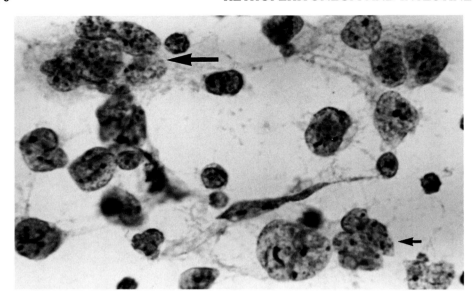

Fig. 4.14. Anaplastic large cell (Ki-1) lymphoma, ABC. Note large round cells with irregular nuclear contour, coarse chromatin, and multiple nucleoli. Bizarre multinucleated cells (*arrows*) are seen. (H & E preparation; ×500).

Immunophenotyping may be necessary to confirm the diagnosis. Large cell anaplastic lymphomas express Ki-1 (CD30) and epithelial membrane antigen, but are negative for cytokeratin and other epithelial markers. Some, but not all, are positive for leukocyte common antigen, which distinguishes them from carcinomas, which are not marked by leukocyte common antigen.

Lymphomas Associated with AIDS

Patients with AIDS have an increased risk of developing aggressive, high-grade NHLs, usually of the Burkitt's and Burkitt's-like (small noncleaved cells) and immunoblastic types.[57,58] A disproportionate fraction of these patients present with extranodal disease. The gastrointestinal tract, central nervous system, and liver are the common sites of involvement, and unusual sites of disease reported include the rectum, heart and pericardium, and common bile duct. Patients presenting with these types of extranodal lymphoma should be screened for antibody to human immunodeficiency virus (HIV). This information is of paramount importance in planning treatment (patients with AIDS are poor candidates for surgery), estimating prognosis, and monitoring for infectious complications. Malignant lymphomas occurring in AIDS patients can be readily and accurately diagnosed by NAB because (1) the cytologic types are almost invariably high-grade and therefore easily recognized as malignant, and (2) the histologic growth pattern of the NHL is always diffuse.[19,59–61] Similarly, the diagnosis of Hodgkin's disease in AIDS patients can be readily made on NAB because the disease usually features abundant Reed-Sternberg cells.

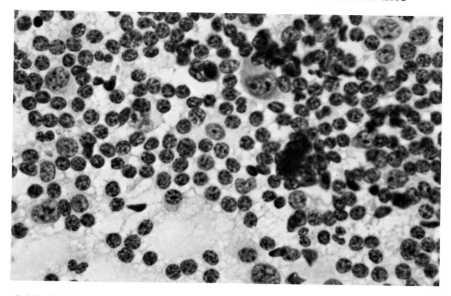

Fig. 4.15. Hodgkin's disease, ABC. Note many normal small lymphocytes, a few bilobed eosinophils, and a diagnostic Reed-Sternberg cell with "mirror-image" nuclei, and prominent nucleoli. (H & E preparation; ×500).

HODGKIN'S DISEASE

Hodgkin's disease (HD) is the most common type of malignant lymphoma in young adults between the ages of 20 and 30 years. HD is essentially a superficial lymph node disease, involving most frequently the cervical lymph nodes. Intrathoracic involvement is also more common than in non-Hodgkin's lymphoma. Abdominal lymph nodes are seldom affected in the absence of cervical or mediastinal lymph node involvement. The diagnosis of HD on aspirates is quite easy and reliable.[62,63] Morphologically, it is composed of Reed-Sternberg (R-S) cells admixed with benign small lymphocytes and other cells of the immune system, such as plasma cells, eosinophils, and histiocytes **(Fig. 4.15).** The R-S cell is a large cell, measuring 25 μm or more. It is much more readily discernible on aspirate smears than on tissue sections, because a whole cell is seen on a smear but due to its large size, usually only a portion of it is seen on section. In the classical form **(Fig. 4.16A),** two large, "mirror-image" nuclei are opposed to each other in the same cell. The nucleus has an overall clear vesicular appearance. In the center of each nucleus there is a single huge eosinophilic nucleolus. The nuclear chromatin is condensed to the periphery with the result that the nuclear membrane appears thickened and a clear halo is commonly evident about the nucleolus. If the R-S cell has only one nucleus, the latter must be bilobed and must contain two typical nucleoli, with the same peripheral condensation of chromatin. A bilobed nucleus with one typical nucleolus is not diagnostic.

In any case of Hodgkin's disease there are variable numbers of large atypical mononuclear cells, which share some of the nuclear characteristics of the R-S cell.

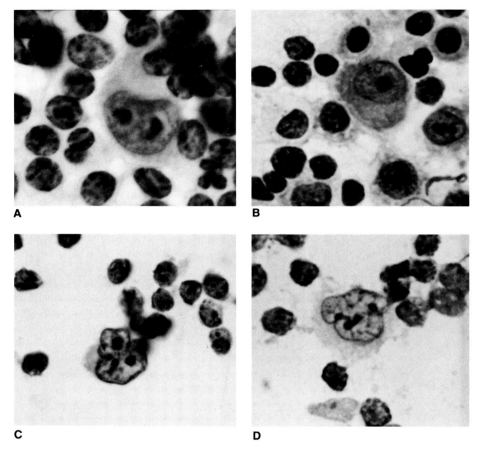

Fig. 4.16. ABC of Hodgkin's disease showing Reed-Sternberg cell and its variants. **A.** Note typical Reed-Sternberg cell with bilobed nucleus, macronucleolus in each lobe, and perinuclear halos. **B.** Note "Hodgkin cell" structurally similar to R-S cell but with only a single, round nucleus. **C,D.** Note hyperlobated mononucleated cells, corresponding to the lacunar cells in histologic sections. (H & E preparation; all magnifications ×1,250).

These mononuclear cells have a distinct nuclear membrane, a vesicular nucleus, and a large central eosinophilic nucleolus. This type of cell has been referred to as the "Hodgkin cell" **(Fig. 4.16B).** They may outnumber R-S cells but are not considered diagnostically reliable since they may be closely simulated by reactive immunoblasts in the lymphoid reactions of viral infections.

The lacunar cells and L & H (lymphocytic and histiocytic) cells resemble each other on ABC. They are large, mononucleated cells having folded, overlapping nuclear lobes (polylobated) and delicate lacy chromatin. The nucleoli are more prominent in the lacunar cells than in the L & H cells **(Figs. 4.16C&D).** The presence of these R-S cell variants should alert the pathologist to the possibility of Hodgkin's disease, and a search should be made for more typical RS cells.

REACTIVE LYMPHOID HYPERPLASIA

Significant enlargement of lymph nodes with abdominal pain, and weight loss are the common presentations of malignant retroperitoneal lymphomas.[34] In contrast, retroperitoneal lymph nodes with reactive lymphoid hyperplasia generally are much smaller, and therefore are not usually targets for needle aspiration biopsy, unless the involved nodes are substantially enlarged, producing a mass effect or other symptoms. Tuberculous lymphadenitis and giant lymph node hyperplasia (Castleman's disease) are examples of lymphoid hyperplasia that may present as a mesenteric or retroperitoneal mass.

Acute Lymphadenitis

Acute lymphadenitis is a reactive condition generally secondary to inflammation of a viscus, such as the kidney (pyelonephritis), large bowel (diverticulitis), and appendix (appendicitis). The signs and symptoms refer to the primary diseased organ and the lymphadenitis is not a target for aspiration biopsy. At times, a large abscess may result and in these cases, the aspirates show large numbers of polymorphonuclear leukocytes with necrotic debris. Culture of the aspirate usually shows coliform bacteria.

Chronic Lymphadenitis and Lymphoid Hyperplasia

Reactive lymphoid hyperplasia is not a disease entity, but rather a description of a lymphoid reaction. In many instances, the cause of the hyperplasia is not known. On histologic sections, reactive lymphoid hyperplasia exhibits follicular and/or paracortical hyperplasia. Follicular hyperplasia (formation of secondary germinal centers) is characterized by a predominance of large, basophilic, transformed type lymphocytes (large noncleaved cells) and many tingible body macrophages with nuclear debris. Cleaved cells are more prominent in follicles showing lesser degree of reactivity, and in regressing or resting reactive centers. Follicular hyperplasia is typically seen in HIV infection, syphilis, toxoplasmosis, and autoimmune disorders such as rheumatoid arthritis. Paracortical hyperplasia is characterized by a population of cells with an abundance of cytoplasm. These cells have a plasmacytoid appearance, and range from mature plasmacytoid lymphocytes to large immunoblasts. The hyperplastic paracortical pattern is most prominently seen in some viral conditions such as infectious mononucleosis or following vaccination, drug-induced lymphadenopathy (Dilantin), and some autoimmune disorders such as systemic lupus erythematosis. More often, reactive lymph nodes expand as a result of combined follicular and paracortical hyperplasia.

The aspirates obtained from lymph nodes with reactive lymphoid hyperplasia (**Fig. 4.17**) show a polymorphous population of cells consisting of small and large, cleaved and noncleaved, lymphocytes; plasma cells; immunoblasts; and tingible body macrophages. There is no real cellular atypia. The important cytologic features that distinguish non-Hodgkin's lymphoma, Hodgkin's disease, and lymphoid hyperplasia are listed in **Table 4.5.**

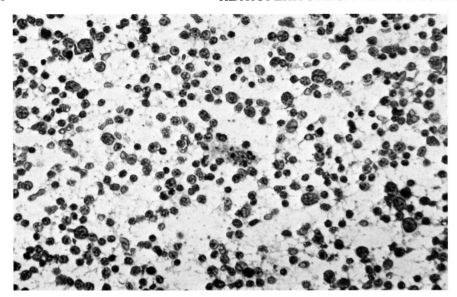

Fig. 4.17. Reactive lymphoid hyperplasia, ABC. Note lymphocytes in various stages of maturation. A phagocytic histiocyte is seen at the center. (H & E preparation; ×310).

Giant Follicular Hyperplasia (Castleman's Disease)

This is a very rare disease in the retroperitoneum. The hyaline-vascular type usually presents as a single mass in the anterior mediastinum in asymptomatic patients. The plasma-cell type may appear in the retroperitoneum, with associated hematologic abnormalities such as anemia and hyperglobulinemia. The aspirate consists of many plasma cells, immunoblasts and lymphocytes. The differential diagnosis includes a plasma cell neoplasm or a malignant lymphoma with plasma cell differentiation. Monoclonality of plasma cells has been reported in some cases of Castleman's disease and its presence, therefore, does not rule out this disease.[64] The multicentric form of the disease may run a progressive course complicated by infection and lymphoma.[65]

TABLE 4.5 Cytologic Differences between Non-Hodgkin's Lymphoma, Hodgkin's Disease, and Lymphoid Hyperplasia

Non-Hodgkin's Lymphoma	Hodgkin's Disease	Lymphoid Hyperplasia
Monomorphic cell population (exception: mixed type NHL)	Mixed cell population (with small lymphocytes predominating)	Mixed cell population (lymphocytes in various stages of transformation)
Cytologic atypia present (exception: small lymphocytic NHL)	Atypical monocytes and Reed-Sternberg cells	Cytologic maturity

NHL = non-Hodgkin's lymphoma.

Tuberculous Lymphadenitis

The cytologic features of tuberculosis are discussed in Chapter 5 in the section on Benign Tumors and Tumor-like Lesions. In the past two years, we have encountered more patients with tuberculosis who presented initially with massive abdominal and/ or retroperitoneal lymphadenopathy, clinically mimicking lymphoma. The outbreak has been partly caused by an increase in immigrants from countries where tuberculosis is prevalent. Another important factor is the continuing increase in the number of HIV-infected persons. In general, people who have a depressed cellular immune system are at highest risk to develop active disease and more rapidly progressive disease.

INTERPRETATIVE PITFALLS

Problems Related to Histologic Types

Which aspects of lymphoma diagnosis by NAB are sufficiently reproducible and provide useful information to the clinician? The literature has shown that modern cytopathologists can regularly diagnose various subtypes of large cell lymphomas, small noncleaved cell lymphoma, and lymphoblastic lymphoma.[26,66] Moreover, they are able to differentiate true lymphoma from undifferentiated carcinoma and other nonlymphoid tumors that mimic lymphoma. On the other hand, malignant lymphomas that can be potentially confused with benign lymphoid hyperplasia include small lymphocytic NHL, mixed small and large cell NHL, follicular NHL, peripheral T-cell lymphoma, and Hodgkin's disease (if R-S cells are not identified).

In malignant lymphoma of the small lymphocytic type, the neoplastic lymphocytes are morphologically indistinguishable from normal small lymphocytes. The ABC diagnosis is suggested by the monotonous pattern of small lymphocytes and must be substantiated by other diagnostic means, such as differential peripheral blood count, bone marrow biopsy, immunophenotyping, and/or surgical biopsy.

In mixed small and large cell lymphoma, two predominant types of cells (small and large) are seen, whereas in lymphoid hyperplasia a broad spectrum of cell types at varying stages of development is characteristic. Demonstration of a monoclonal population of cells by immunophenotypic or genotypic analysis helps confirm the diagnosis of malignant lymphoma.

Follicular lymphoma as seen on ABC may show either a monomorphous or a polymorphous cell population. The latter situation will occur if benign reactive lymphoid cells present in between the neoplastic follicles are included in the aspirates. A recent report[67] from our laboratory showed that follicular lymphoma could be diagnosed or suspected when the smears showed a monomorphous cell population (eight cases, or 66%), whereas a polymorphous cell population contributed to false-negative results (four cases, or 33%). This study showed that the ABC diagnosis of follicular lymphoma was less accurate than that of NHL in general, but the accuracy rate was similar to that of all low-grade NHL. Although most of the malignant lymphomas in the retroperitoneum are diffuse varieties, follicular lymphomas do occasionally occur. The currently accepted approach is that negative results in the face of a clinical suspicion of lymphoma should be followed by an open surgical biopsy. Alternatively, routine use of immunophenotyping and/or flow cytometry on the aspirate material would allow a more accurate diagnosis of many of the otherwise equivocal cases.[26] If facilities for molecular genetic analysis are available, demonstration of antigen receptor gene rearrangement or chromosomal translocation may be carried out on the aspirates.[31] About 80–90% of the follicular lymphomas will demonstrate specific chromosomal translocation, t(14;18).

Another area of difficulty is the distinction between the polymorphous cell pattern of peripheral T-cell lymphoma and reactive hyperplasia. In T-cell lymphoma **(Fig. 4.13)**, even though the cellular pattern is polymorphous, the cells for the most part are morphologically atypical, with irregularity of nuclei in small, intermediate, and large lymphoid cells. There are clinical differences as well. Features that favor T-cell neoplasm include the older age of patients, the frequent extranodal involvement, and the advanced stage of the disease at presentation. It should be noted that a moderate degree of reactive hyperplasia in children and young adults can be accepted as physiological. In older patients, especially those over 60 years of age, the immune response is subdued, and physiological lymphoid hyperplasia resulting in significant lymph node enlargement is quite unusual. Any lymph node hyperplasia without an apparent cause in an older person should be viewed with suspicion. In a study of 58 patients who were aged 60 or over and whose lymph node biopsies had shown lymphoid follicular hyperplasia, 18 (31%) either had concurrent lymphoma or developed NHL over an interval of 1 month to 9 years.[68] Hence, when reactive lymphoid hyperplasia is diagnosed in a significantly enlarged lymph node of an elderly person, the clinician must follow the patient closely.

Problems Related to Sclerosis

Extensive sclerosis is a common finding in retroperitoneal NHLs[34,69,70] and was observed in 74% of the cases in the series reported by Waldron et al.[69] The sclerosis is essentially an extranodal phenomenon, with a relatively abrupt zone between the nonsclerotic lymph node tissue and the sclerosing infiltrate, beginning in the region of, and usually incorporating, the nodal capsule.[69] Zellers et al[70] reviewed seven cases of retroperitoneal lymphomas whose NABs were interpreted as nondiagnostic, and found sclerosis evident on the histologic sections. It must be remembered that if a bulky lymph node yields a hypocellular sample consisting of only a few lymphocytes, one must not diagnose reactive lymphoid hyperplasia without considering the possibility of a sclerosing lymphoma. Hypocellularity may be due to aspiration of the sclerotic area of the lymphoma, hence multiple sampling is essential to ensure representative cellular material. In contrast, aspirates of reactive hyperplasia of a significantly enlarged lymph node are cell-rich and show different morphologic forms of transformed lymphocytes (cleaved and noncleaved cells), immunoblasts, and tingible body histiocytes.

Another disorder in the retroperitoneum that may yield aspirates of small lymphocytes of low cellularity is idiopathic retroperitoneal fibrosis.[71] The pathogenesis of the disorder is unknown, but may be related to autoimmunity or hypersensitivity to drugs such as methysergide maleate. Medial deviation of the ureters is a characteristic finding on intravenous urography, as opposed to lateral displacement in other retroperitoneal mass lesions. The aspirate sample **(Fig. 5.20** in Chapter 5) shows fibrous tissue fragments admixed with small mature lymphocytes, a few plasma cells and eosinophils. At times the plasma cells may be numerous. The cytologic features are entirely nonspecific, but the important finding is that no malignant cells are present after adequate sampling.

Problems in Hodgkin's Disease

A false-negative report may result from aspirating the nodular sclerosis variant of Hodgkin's disease due to dense fibrosis. At other times, the classic R-S cells may not be present, and if the pathologist is not familiar with the appearance of R-S cell variants (the hyperlobated mononucleated cells), the diagnosis of Hodgkin's disease may not be suspected.

A false-positive report may occur if atypical cells present in other diseases are interpreted as R-S cells by the unwary. It must be remembered that the diagnosis of HD is made only when R-S cells are identified in an appropriate cellular milieu and in an appropriate clinical setting. Large, Reed-Sternberg-like cells (reactive immunoblasts) may be seen in viral lymphadenopathy, postvaccination reaction, and phenytoin (Dilantin) therapy. As well, malignant cells resembling R-S cells may be found in high-grade lymphoma, malignant melanoma, and some anaplastic carcinomas.[63,72] To prevent mistakes, the pathologist must adhere to strict morphologic criteria for diagnosing R-S cells as described earlier.

The reactive lymphadenopathy that most likely contains cells simulating R-S cells is infectious mononucleosis, in which the number of large immunoblasts is often greater and the degree of cellular atypia more pronounced than in most other forms of viral lymphadenitis.[73] If the atypical immunoblasts are binucleated, then there is a risk in overinterpreting them as R-S cells. Immunoblasts do not stain with Leu M-1 antibodies, while true R-S cells do. Moreover, smears from infectious mononucleosis show a continuum of cytologic forms ranging from small mature plasmacytoid cells to highly atypical immunoblasts, as opposed to HD in which there is a hiatus between the surrounding reactive cells and the large neoplastic cells (compare **Fig. 4.18** and **Fig. 4.19**). The atypical cells seen in reactive conditions disappear after resolution of the disease or discontinuation of the drug.

Lymphoma versus Nonlymphoid Neoplasms

Many carcinomas, melanomas, and even some sarcomas metastasize to lymph nodes. In most cases, the distinction from lymphoma is obvious because slides of the primary tumor are available for comparison or the metastatic tumors are well enough differentiated to form glands, contain mucin, or produce keratin. In general, cells of metastatic carcinomas are arranged in clusters or cohesive sheets on the smears, whereas lymphoma cells are characteristically dispersed. Although both malignant lymphomas and metastatic carcinomas may display necrosis, extensive necrosis is more commonly seen in metastatic carcinoma than in lymphoma (with the exception of Hodgkin's disease). The types of metastatic tumor that closely mimic primary lymphoid malignancy are all undifferentiated tumors composed of round or polygonal cells. The small round cell tumors that morphologically simulate lymphoma include small cell anaplastic carcinoma, neuroblastoma, Ewing's sarcoma, and embryonal rhabdomyosarcoma. These tumors are discussed in detail in Chapter 5. Mimics of large cell lymphoma are often melanoma and poorly differentiated carcinoma. The timely use

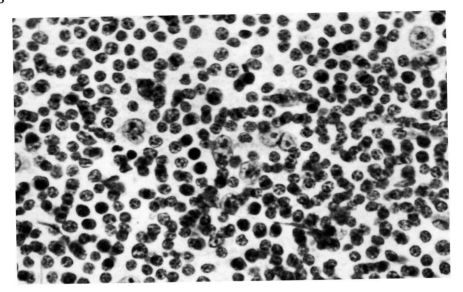

Fig. 4.18. Hodgkin's disease, ABC. Note admixture of small mature lymphocytes and large R-S cells and their variants. There is a morphologic hiatus between the small and the large cells. (H & E preparation; ×500).

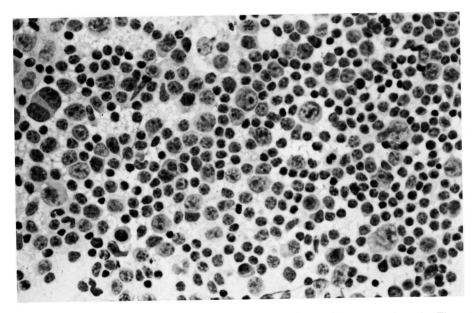

Fig. 4.19. Infectious mononucleosis. This aspirate was obtained from a neck node. There is admixture of small mature lymphocytes and variably-sized larger stimulated lymphocytes. The latter show a spectrum of morphologic forms, ranging from small plasmacytoid lymphocytes to large immunoblasts with macronucleoli and binucleation.

of monoclonal antibodies (anti-LCA, anti-keratin, and anti-S100 protein/HMB43) and electron microscopy may resolve many of these diagnostically difficult cases.

RESULTS OF ASPIRATION BIOPSY CYTOLOGY

The accuracy rate of NAB diagnosis of lymphoma at all body sites varies according to the type and location of the lymphoma. For high-grade lymphomas, the accuracy rate ranges from 80 to 94%, but drops to around 65% for low-grade lymphomas.[67,74–76] This can be explained by the fact that high-grade lymphomas consist of neoplastic cells that are cytologically recognizable as atypical, while cells of low-grade lymphomas may resemble normal lymphocytes.

The accuracy rate for diagnosing retroperitoneal lymphomas varies markedly, ranging from 50% to almost 100%.[70,77–82] This extremely marked variation reflects the wide variation in the experience of the aspirators who performed the aspirations and of the cytopathologists who interpreted the smears, as well as the ancillary special techniques employed and case selections. It is to be expected that the diagnostic accuracy rate will be lower in retroperitoneal than in superficially located lymphomas, given the deep location and the sclerosing nature of many retroperitoneal lymphomas. However, these disadvantages are compensated for by the fact that the majority of retroperitoneal lymphomas are cytologically atypical (large cell and immunoblastic types).[34,35,69]

One of the largest series of fine needle aspiration biopsy of intraabdominal and retroperitoneal lymphomas, consisting of 238 cases, was reported by Cafferty et al. at the M.D. Anderson Cancer Center, Texas.[81] The sensitivity of diagnosis of lymphomas by NAB for all patients in the study was 66% (63% for patients with prior chemotherapy versus 74% for patients without prior therapy). The predictive value of a positive result was 99% (100% in cases where immunocytochemistry had been performed). There was 86% agreement between the cytologic and surgical biopsy in classification of the lymphomas, 8% discrepancy rate when the two examinations were separated by chemotherapy (usually several courses given over a period of several months), and 6% concurrent discrepancy. False-negative results due to sampling error were not uncommon, giving a predictive value of a negative result as 42%. The authors attributed this partly to the referral nature of their cases, which included a high percentage of previously treated lymphomas.

Analysis of 54 retroperitoneal, intraabdominal, and pelvic lymphomas examined by NAB at the Vancouver General Hospital from 1984 to 1989 inclusive showed that 11 (20%) did not yield sufficient material for interpretation. Of the remaining 43 cases, 30 were diagnosed as lymphoma and 13 were suggestive of lymphoma. If the "suggestive" group was included as positive, the sensitivity rate was 80% (43 of 54 cases). Confirmation of the lymphomas was obtained by surgical biopsies, autopsies, or follow-up clinical data. Among the 42 positive cases, histologic slides were available for review in 31 cases; agreement between cytologic and histologic diagnosis (using the Working Formulation scheme but excluding diffuse versus follicular) was found to exist in 28 cases (90%), discrepancy in lymphoma classification occurred in two cases (7%), and one case proved on follow-up to be a metastatic small cell anaplastic carcinoma of the lung (this case was seen in the early part of our study, without the benefit of immunocytochemical studies). Nine of the patients who had had unsatisfactory aspirates underwent surgical biopsies of the retroperitoneal lymphomas. Sclerosis was evident on the histologic sections from six cases.

The NAB diagnosis of malignant lymphoma is very reliable, especially when immunocytochemistry or other special diagnostic techniques are employed, but diagnosis of the absence of lymphoma in deep sites is often unreliable and should be accepted with caution.

REFERENCES

1. Weisenburger DD: An epidemic of non-Hodgkin's lymphoma: Comments on time trends, possible etiologies, and the role of pathology. *Mod Pathol* 5:481–482, 1992.

2. Reis LAG, Hankey BF, Miller BA, et al: *Cancer Statistics Review 1973–88*. Bethesda, MD, National Cancer Institute, NIH Pub. No. 91-2789, 1991.

3. Biggar RJ, Rabkin CS: The epidemiology of acquired immunodeficiency syndrome-related lymphomas. *Curr Opin Oncol* 4:883–893, 1992.

4. Rappaport H: *Tumors of the Hematopoietic System. Atlas of Tumor Pathology, Fascicle 8*. Washington, DC, Armed Forces Institute of Pathology, 1966.

5. Lukes RJ, Collins RD: Immunologic characterization of human malignant lymphomas. *Cancer* 34:1488–1503, 1974.

6. Lennert K: *Histopathology of Non-Hodgkin's Lymphomas: Based on the Kiel Classification*. New York, Springer-Verlag, 1981.

7. Gerard-Marchant R, Hamlin I, Lennert K, et al: Classification of non-Hodgkin's lymphomas. *Lancet* 2:406–408, 1974.

8. The Non-Hodgkin's Lymphoma Pathologic Classification Project: NCI sponsored study of classifications of Non-Hodgkin's lymphoma: Summary and description of working formulation for clinical usage. *Cancer* 49:2112–2135, 1982.

9. Lukes RJ, Craver LF, Hall TC, et al: Report of the nomenclature committee. *Cancer Res* 26:1311, 1966.

10. Rosenberg SA: Non-Hodgkin's lymphoma—selection of treatment on the basis of histologic type. *N Engl J Med* 301:924–928, 1979.

11. Menck HR, Garfinkel L, Dodd GD: Preliminary report of the National Cancer Data Base. *CA* 41:7–18, 1991.

12. Moormeier JA, Williams SF: The staging of non-Hodgkin's lymphomas. *Semin Oncol* 17:43–50, 1990.

13. Chabner BA, Fisher RI, Young RC, et al: Staging of non-Hodgkin's lymphoma. *Semin Oncol* 7:285–291, 1980.

14. Paryani S, Hoppe RT, Burke JS, et al: Extralymphatic involvement in diffuse non-Hodgkin's lymphoma. *J Clin Oncol* 1:682–688, 1983.

15. Ultmann JE, Moran EM: Clinical course and complications in Hodgkin's disease. *Arch Intern Med* 131:332–353, 1973.

16. Lee YTN, Spratt JS Jr: *Malignant Lymphoma: Nodal and Extranodal Diseases*. New York, Grune & Stratton, 1974, p 5.

17. Chabner BA, Johnson RE, Young RC, et al: Sequential nonsurgical and surgical staging of non-Hodgkin's lymphoma. *Ann Intern Med* 85:149–154, 1976.

18. Ferguson D, Borrow P, Gallo L, et al: Fine needle aspiration as a primary diagnostic approach in HIV-associated lymphomas. *Mod Pathol* 6:29A, 1993.

19. Martin-Bates E, Tanner A, Suvarna SK, et al: Use of fine needle aspiration cytology for investigating lymphadenopathy in HIV positive patients. *J Clin Pathol* 46:546–566, 1993.

20. Picker LJ, Weiss LM, Medeiros LJ, et al: Immunophenotypic criteria for the diagnosis of non-Hodgkin's lymphoma. *Am J Pathol* 128:181–201, 1987.

21. Pinkus GS, Thomas P, Said JW: Leu-M1—A marker for Reed-Sternberg cells in Hodgkin's disease. *Am J Pathol* 119:244–252, 1985.

22. Michie SA, Spagnolo DV, Dunn KA, et al: A panel approach to the evaluation of the sensitivity and specificity of antibodies for the diagnosis of routinely processed histologically undifferentiated human neoplasms. *Am J Clin Pathol* 88:457–462, 1987.

23. Levitt S, Cheng L, DuPuis MH, et al: Fine needle aspiration diagnosis of malignant lymphoma with confirmation by immunoperoxidase staining. *Acta Cytol* 29:895–902, 1985.

24. Vielh P: Flow Cytometry. Guides to Clinical Aspiration Biopsy. New York, Igaku-Shoin, 1992.

25. Barlogie B, Raber MN, Schumann J, et al: Flow cytometry in clinical cancer research. *Cancer Res* 43:3982–3997, 1983.

26. Katz RL: Cytologic diagnosis of leukemia and lymphoma. *Clinics Lab Med* 11:469–499, 1991.

27. Diamond LW, Braylan RC: Flow analysis of DNA content and cell size in non-Hodgkin's lymphoma. *Cancer Res* 40:703–712, 1980.

28. Joensuu H, Klemi PJ, Eerola E: Diagnostic value of DNA flow cytometry combined with fine needle aspiration biopsy in lymphomas. *J Pathol* 154:237–245, 1988.

29. Christensson B, Tribukait B, Linder IL, et al: Cell proliferation and DNA content in non-Hodgkin's lymphoma. Flow cytometry in relation to lymphoma classification. *Cancer* 58:1295–1304, 1986.

30. Hu E, Horning S, Fynn S, et al: Diagnosis of B-cell lymphoma by analysis of immunoglobulin gene rearrangement in biopsy specimens obtained by fine needle aspiration. *J Clin Oncol* 4:278–283, 1986.

31. Katz RL, Hirsch-Ginsberg C, Childs C, et al: The role of gene rearrangements for antigen receptors in the diagnosis of lymphoma obtained by fine-needle aspiration. *Am J Clin Pathol* 96:479–490, 1991.

32. Williams ME, Frierson HF, Tabrarah S, et al: Fine needle aspiration of non-Hodgkin's lymphoma: Southern blot analysis for antigen receptor, bcl-2, and c-myc rearrangements. *Am J Clin Pathiol* 92:754–759, 1990.

33. Sklar J: What can DNA rearrangements tell us about solid hematolymphoid neoplasms. *Am J Clin Pathol* 14 (Suppl 1):16–25, 1990.

34. Waldron JA, Magnifico M, Duray PH, et al: Retroperitoneal mass presentations of B-immunoblastic sarcoma. *Cancer* 56:1733–1741, 1985.

35. Ampil FL: Malignant lymphoma presenting in the retroperitoneum. *Oncol* 46:198–200, 1989.

36. Dick F, Bloomfield C, Brunning R: Incidence, cytology and histopathology of non-Hodgkin's lymphoma in the bone marrow. *Cancer* 33:1382–1398, 1974.

37. Foucar K, McKenna R, Frizzera G, et al: Incidence and patterns of bone marrow and blood involvement of lymphoma in relationship to the Lukes-Collins classification. *Blood* 54:1417–1422, 1979.

38. Ben-Ezra J, Burke JS, Swartz WG, et al: Small lymphocytic lymphoma: A clinicopathologic analysis of 268 cases. *Blood* 73:579–587, 1989.

39. Horning SJ, Rosenberg SA: The natural history of initially untreated low grade non-Hodgkin's lymphoma. *N Engl J Med* 311:1471–1475, 1984.

40. Coller BS, Chabner BA, Gralnick HR: Frequencies and patterns of bone marrow involvement in non-Hodgkin's lymphomas. *Am J Hematol* 3:105–119, 1977.

41. Griffin NR, Howard MR, Quirke P, et al: Prognostic indicators in centroblastic-centrocytic lymphoma. *J Clin Pathol* 41:866–870, 1988.

42. Weiss LM, Warnke R, Sklar J, et al: Molecular analysis of the t(14;18) chromosomal translocation in malignant lymphomas. *N Engl J Med* 317:1185–1189, 1987.

43. Cossman J, Uppenkamp M, Sundeen J, et al: Molecular genetics and the diagnosis of lymphoma. *Arch Pathol Lab Med* 112:117–127, 1988.

44. Hockenberry D, Nunez G, Milliman C, et al: Bcl-2 is an inner mitochondrial membrane protein that blocks programmed cell death. *Nature* 348:334–336, 1990.

45. Inghirami G, Grignani G, Sternas L, et al: Down-regulation of LFA-1 adhesion receptors by *c-myc* oncogene in human B lymphoblastoid cells. *Science* 250:682, 1990.

46. Lombardi L, Newcomb EW, Dalla-Favera R: Pathogenesis of Burkitt's lymphoma. Expression of an activated *c-myc* oncogene causes the tumorigenic conversion of EBV-infected human B lymphoblasts. *Cell* 49:161–170, 1987.

47. Katz RL, Gritsman A, Cabanillas F, et al: Fine needle aspiration cytology of peripheral T-cell lymphoma. *Am J Clin Pathol* 91:120–131, 1989.

48. Ramsay AD, Smith WJ, Earl HM, et al: T-cell lymphomas in adults. A clinicopathological study of eighteen cases. *J Pathol* 152:63–76, 1987.

49. Hastrup N, Hamilton-Dutoit S, Ralfkiaer E, et al: Peripheral T-cell lymphomas. *Histopathol* 18:99–105, 1991.

50. Aisenberg AC: Surface markers in non-Hodgkin's lymphoma. In *Malignant Lymphoma.* Philadelphia, Lea & Febiger, 1991, pp 319–331.

51. Kawk LW, Wilson M, Weiss LM, et al: Similar outcome of treatment of B-cell and T-cell diffuse large cell lymphomas: The Stanford experience. *J Clin Oncol* 9:1426–1431, 1991.

52. Cheng AL, Chen YC, Wang CH, et al: Direct comparison of peripheral T-cell lymphoma with diffuse B-cell lymphoma of comparable histological grades—Should peripheral T-cell lymphoma be considered separately? *J Clin Oncol* 7:725–731, 1989.

53. Noorduyn LA, van der Valk P, van Heerde P, et al: Stage is a better prognostic indicator than morphologic subtype in primary noncutaneous T-cell lymphoma. *Am J Clin Pathol* 3:49–57, 1990.

54. Kadin ME, Said JW: Pathology of malignant lymphomas. *Curr Opin Oncol* 2:822–831, 1990.

55. Stein H, Mason DY, Gerdes J, et al: The expression of Hodgkin's disease associated antigen Ki-1 in reactive and neoplastic lymphoid tissue: Evidence that Reed-Sternberg cells and histiocytic malignancies are derived from activated lymphoid cells. *Blood* 66:848–858, 1985.

56. Leoncini L, Del Vecchio MT, Kraft R, et al: Hodgkin's disease and CD30-positive anaplastic large cell lymphoma—a continuous spectrum of malignant disorders. *Am J Pathol* 137:1047–1057, 1990.

57. Knowles DM, Chamulak G, Subar M, et al: Clinicopathologic, immunophenotypic, and molecular genetic analysis of AIDS-associated lymphoid neoplasia. *Pathol Annu* 23:33–67, 1988.

58. Lowenthal DA, Straus DJ, Campbell SW, et al: AIDS-related lymphoid neoplasia. The Memorial Hospital experience. *Cancer* 61:2325–2337, 1988.

59. Shabb N, Katz RL: Exfoliative and fine-needle aspiration cytology of human immunodeficiency virus infection: A systems review. *Cytopathol Annu* 119–153, 1992.

60. Shabb N, Katz R, Ordonez N, et al: Fine-needle aspiration evaluation of lymphoproliferative lesions in human immunodeficiency virus-positive patients. *Cancer* 67:1008–1018, 1991.

61. Bottles K, McPhaul LW, Volberding P: Fine needle aspiration biopsy of patients with the acquired immunodeficiency syndrome: Experience in an outpatient clinic. *Ann Intern Med* 108:42–45, 1988.

62. Friedman M, Kim U, Shimaoka K, et al: Appraisal of aspiration cytology in management of Hodgkin's disease. *Cancer* 45:1653–1663, 1980.

63. Kardos TF, Vinson JH, Behm FG, et al: Hodgkin's disease: Diagnosis by fine needle aspiration. *Am J Clin Pathol* 86:286–291, 1986.

64. Radaszkiewicz T, Hansmann ML, Lennert K: Monoclonality and polyclonality of plasma cells in Castleman's disease of the plasma cell variant. *Histopathol* 14:11–24, 1989.

65. Kessler E: Multicentric giant lymph node hyperplasia. *Cancer* 56:2446–2451, 1985.

66. Kern WH: Exfoliative and aspiration cytology of malignant lymphomas. *Semin Diag Pathol* 3:211–218, 1986.

67. McNeely TB: Diagnosis of follicular lymphoma by fine needle aspiration biopsy. *Acta Cytol* 36:866–868, 1992.

68. Osborne BM, Butler JJ: Clinical implications of nodal reactive follicular hyperplasia in the elderly patient with enlarged lymph nodes. *Mod Pathol* 4:24–30, 1991.

69. Waldron JA, Newcomer LN, Katz ME, et al: Sclerosing variants of follicular center cell lymphomas presenting in the retroperitoneum. *Cancer* 52:712–720, 1983.

70. Zellers RA, McClure SP: Fine needle aspiration of intraabdominal sites in 160 patients with emphasis on utility in diagnosis of malignant lymphoma. *Am J Clin Pathol* 89:436–437, 1988.

71. Jones J, Ross E, Matz L, et al: Reptroperitoneal fibrosis. *Am J Med* 48:203–208, 1970.

72. Dorfman RF, Warnke R: Lymphadenopathy simulating the malignant lymphomas. *Hum Pathol* 5:519–550, 1974.

73. Kardos TF, Kornstein MJ, Frable WJ: Cytology and immunocytology of infectious mononucleosis in fine needle aspirates of lymph nodes. *Acta Cytol* 32:722–726, 1988.

74. Kline TS, Kannan V, Kline IK: Lymphadenopathy and aspiration biopsy cytology. *Cancer* 54:1076–1081, 1984.

75. Suhrland MJ, Wieczorek R: Fine needle aspiration biopsy in the diagnosis of lymphoma. *Cancer Invest* 9:61–68, 1991.

76. Carter TR, Feldman PS, Innes DJ, et al: The role of fine needle aspiration cytology in the diagnosis of lymphoma. *Acta Cytol* 32:848–853, 1988.

77. Droese M, Altmannsberger M, Kehl A, et al: Ultrasound-guided percutaneous fine needle aspiration biopsy of abdominal and retroperitoneal masses. *Acta Cytol* 28:368–384, 1984.

78. Zornoza J, Cabanillas TF, Altoff TM, Ordonez N, Cohen MA: Percutaneous needle biopsy in abdominal lymphoma. *Am J Roentgenol* 136:97–103, 1981.

79. Zornoza J, Johnsson K, Wallace S, Lukeman JM: Fine needle aspiration biopsy of retroperitoneal lymph nodes and abdominal masses: An updated report. *Radiology* 125:87–88, 1977.

80. Buscarini L, Cavanna L, Fornari F, et al: Ultrasonically guided fine needle biopsy: A new useful technique in pathological staging of malignant lymphoma. *Acta Haematol* 73:150–152, 1985.

81. Cafferty LL, Katz RL, Ordonez NG, et al: Fine needle aspiration diagnosis of intraabdominal and retroperitoneal lymphomas by a morphologic and immunocytochemical approach. *Cancer* 65:72–77, 1990.

82. Liliemark J, Tani E, Christiansson B, et al: Fine-needle aspiration cytology and immunocytochemistry of abdominal Non-Hodgkin's lymphomas. *Leukemia Lymphoma* 1:65–69, 1989.

5

Retroperitoneum III:
Soft Tissue Tumors

Key Facts

▶ Next to the extremities, the retroperitoneal space is the second most common site for soft tissue sarcomas to occur. Benign soft tissue neoplasms of the retroperitoneum are uncommon. The ratio of sarcomas to benign neoplasms is about 5:1.

▶ Histologic classification of sarcomas is based on histogenesis. Liposarcoma, leiomyosarcoma, and malignant fibrous histiocytoma are the histogenetic types most often found in the retroperitoneum.

▶ In cytologic specimens, classification of sarcomas is based on cell morphology. Four general categories are recognized: spindle cell, pleomorphic cell, round cell, and polygonal cell.

▶ In each cytologic category, histogenetic typing is feasible if specific morphologic features of differentiation can be identified. Additionally, immunocytochemistry and electron microscopy are helpful in classification of sarcomas.

▶ The retroperitoneum is a common primary site of cellular schwannomas, which may be mistaken for sarcoma clinically and cytologically.

RETROPERITONEAL SARCOMAS: GENERAL CONSIDERATIONS

Few pathologists have extensive experience of soft tissue sarcomas. Compared with other solid tumors, such as breast or prostate carcinoma, soft tissue sarcomas are rare, comprising 1% of all cancers in men and 0.6% in women.[1] However, in children younger than 15 years, 6.5% of all malignant tumors are soft tissue tumors.[2] Next to the extremities, the retroperitoneal space is the second most common site for soft tissue sarcomas to occur—about 15–20% of all soft tissue sarcomas of the body arise in the retroperitoneum.[3,4] A large abdominal mass is the most frequent presentation. In a series of 30 tumors reported by Bose,[5] the mean diameter was 14.6 cm and none measured less than 8 cm. The natural history of retroperitoneal sarcomas is characterized by aggressive local invasion and a high tendency for local recurrence. When they metastasize, the liver and lung are most commonly involved. Although the histogenesis of the various types of sarcomas is individually distinct, their biologic behavior as a group is quite similar and therefore they are treated similarly. The prognosis of sarcomas is related more to the tumor grade and the completeness of excision than to the histologic type.[6] Cody et al[7] found that survival for 5 years was 40% after complete surgical excision of the tumors versus 3% after incomplete excision. Five-year survival for low-grade tumors is 70% and for high-grade tumors is 10%.

CLASSIFICATION AND PATHOLOGY

The most widely used histologic classification scheme for soft tissue sarcomas is based on histogenesis, i.e., the type of tissue a tumor differentiates into, rather than on the type of tissue from which it arose. For example, a malignant tumor that produces bone, even though it arises from a skeletal muscle, is classified as a soft tissue osteosarcoma, not a rhabdomyosarcoma.[8,9] **Table 5.1** lists the distribution of various histologic types of retroperitoneal sarcomas. In Hajdu's series, published in 1979, liposarcoma, leiomyosarcoma, rhabdomyosarcoma, and fibrosarcoma were the most frequent histologic types in this location.[10] However, in Lane's 1989 report the most common tumor was malignant fibrous histiocytoma due to a change in morphologic criteria and reclassification.[11] Pleomorphic rhabdomyosarcoma and fibrosarcoma have become almost nonexistent.[11-13] On the other hand, there has been an increasing recognition of germ cell tumors as a primary extragonadal retroperitoneal tumor[14] (see Chapter 6).

Although in general each histologic type of sarcomas reflects the morphologic appearance of the cells into which the tumor has differentiated, some tumors are so poorly differentiated that no specific features can be identified. Indeed, it is not unusual for pathologists to disagree on the histogenesis of an individual sarcoma. In a peer review of the histopathology of 207 cases of sarcomas, there was full agreement between the primary pathologist and the review panel in only 66% of the cases.

TABLE 5.1. Frequency Distribution of Primary Retroperitoneal Sarcomas

Histopathologic Type	Hajdu* 1979	Lane† 1989
Liposarcoma	28%	19%
Leiomyosarcoma	18%	16%
Malignant schwannoma (neurofibrosarcoma)	10%	8%
Fibrosarcoma	16%	0.2%
Rhabdomyosarcoma	18%	0.2%
Malignant fibrous histiocytoma	—	29%
Others	9%	27.6%

*Data from ref. 10.

†Data from ref. 11.

Twenty-seven percent were considered to be a different type of sarcoma and 6% not to be sarcomas at all.[15]

The American Joint Committee on Cancer has devised a uniform staging system for sarcomas, which bypasses the problem of histogenesis.[6,16,17] The parameters used in the classification are tumor grade, size of the primary tumor ($\leq$ or $>$ 5 cm), and other clinical characteristics such as status of lymph nodes and presence or absence of distant metastases. Tumor location, however, is not incorporated into the scheme. Sarcomas of the retroperitoneum incur a poor prognosis by virtue of their large size at presentation. The specific histology of the tumor appears not to be a critical variable for either prognosis or treatment. High-grade tumors are characterized by a high mitotic count, high cellularity, scant stroma, tumor necrosis, and cellular pleomorphism, while low-grade sarcomas show minimal cellular anaplasia, a rich stroma, and no necrosis.[17] Low-grade sarcomas are capable of aggressive, locally invasive growth but are not prone to early metastasis. In contrast, high-grade tumors are more likely to metastasize early.

Immunocytochemistry and Electron Microscopy

Although the use of immunocytochemical techniques in the study of soft tissue sarcomas has become widely accepted since the 1980s, the number of tissue markers available for soft tissue sarcomas is still relatively limited. Several antibodies (**Table 5.2**) can be effectively used as an aid to their diagnosis and differential diagnosis, provided the results are carefully correlated with the morphologic features of the tumor.[18,19] Vimentin is a broad-spectrum mesenchymal tissue marker. It is a highly sensitive but not a specific marker for mesenchymal tumors; other tumors such as mesothelioma, melanoma, renal cell carcinoma, some anaplastic giant cell carcinomas, and some lymphomas also express vimentin.[20,21] Desmin is an excellent marker of myogenic differentiation and has been found to be extremely useful for the diagnosis of rhabdomyosarcoma (**Plate 5.1**), especially when, as is usually the case, smooth muscle tumors can be excluded from the differential diagnosis.[22] Myoglobin is specific for striated muscle, but it is no longer widely used because the immunoreactivity tends to be focal and limited to a few tumor cells.[23] S100 protein and neurofilaments are useful in identifying peripheral nerve sheath tumors.[24]

TABLE 5.2. Immunocytochemistry of Soft Tissue Tumors

Antibody	Soft Tissue Tumor
Vimentin	All mesenchymal tumors
Desmin, MSA	Smooth and striated muscle tumors
Myoglobin, SMA	Striated muscle tumors
S100 protein	Neural tumors, chordoma, chondrosarcoma
Alpha-1-antitrypsin and alpha-1-antichymotrypsin	Malignant fibrous histiocytoma
Factor VIII	Endothelial cell tumors
Cytokeratin	Synovial sarcoma and epithelioid sarcoma

MSA = muscle specific actin; SMA = skeletal muscle actin.

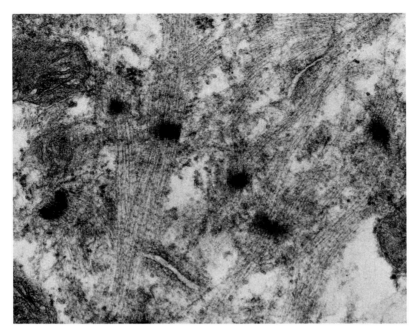

Fig. 5.1. Electron micrograph of an embryonal rhabdomyosarcoma. This portion of rhabdo-myoblast shows remnants of sarcomeres. Note characteristic Z disks. (Uranyl acetate and lead citrate preparation; ×41,900).

Cases that fail to be resolved by immunocytochemical and histochemical techniques may be studied by electron microscopy, which can be used effectively (1) to differentiate sarcomas from neoplasms that may be confused with sarcomas, e.g., pseudosarcomatous carcinoma, melanoma, and lymphoma, and (2) to classify and establish the histogenesis of sarcomas by revealing specific ultrastructural features of the tumors.[25,26] Examples include the identification of Z-band substance in rhabdo-myosarcomas **(Fig. 5.1)** and of thin actin filaments with dense bodies in leiomyosarcomas **(Fig. 5.2)**. However, electron microscopy cannot establish whether a given soft tissue neoplasm is benign or malignant. This distinction is made on the basis of light microscopic morphology.

NEEDLE ASPIRATION CYTOLOGY

Cytologic criteria for diagnosing sarcomas have continued to develop in the last few years. Many soft tissue tumors can now be diagnosed on ABC using the recently developed criteria published in the literature.[27-34] The classification of sarcomas on ABC is based on a scheme which was published in the first edition of this monograph and was further refined in 1992 by Gonzalez-Campora et al.[28] Unlike the histologic classification, which classifies sarcomas on a histogenetic basis, the ABC classification is based on the morphologic appearance of the tumors. **Table 5.3** shows the four main categories of sarcoma classified on ABC: spindle cell, pleomorphic cell, round

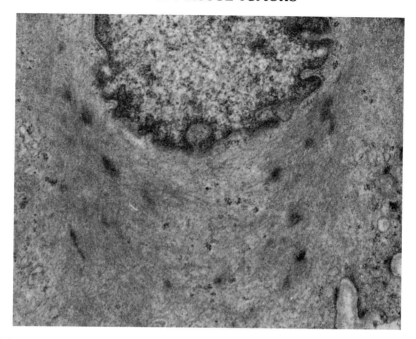

Fig. 5.2. Electron micrograph of a leiomyosarcoma. This portion of the tumor cell shows bundles of actin microfilaments with characteristic fusiform dense bodies. (Uranyl acetate and lead citrate preparation; ×22,800).

TABLE 5.3. Aspiration Cytology Classification of Soft Tissue Sarcomas

1. **Spindle cell sarcomas** Leiomyosarcoma Liposarcoma, well-differentiated and myxoid types Malignant schwannoma Fibrosarcoma Angiosarcoma* 2. **Pleomorphic sarcomas** Malignant fibrous histiocytoma Pleomorphic liposarcoma* Pleomorphic rhabdomyosarcoma* 3. **Round cell sarcomas** Embryonal rhabdomyosarcoma Ewing's sarcoma (peripheral neuroectodermal tumor) Round cell liposarcoma* 4. **Polygonal cell sarcomas** Eipthelioid leiomyosarcoma Epithelioid sarcoma* Paraganglioma Chordoma

*Unlikely to be encountered in the retroperitoneum.

cell, and polygonal cell. In each category, histogenetic typing of the tumor is feasible if specific morphologic features of differentiation are identified.

Fine needle aspiration biopsy is particularly useful in the initial investigation of retroperitoneal lesions, when open biopsy would require a major operation.[35] By obtaining several aspirates one can employ a variety of diagnostic stains to aid in interpretation. Even when a specific histologic subtype cannot be made on NAB a diagnosis of general class of tumor such as lymphoma, sarcoma, or metastatic carcinoma can frequently be established. Quite often a suggestive cytologic diagnosis is sufficient to guide the clinician's decision on what further action should be taken.

SPINDLE CELL SARCOMAS

Leiomyosarcoma

The frequent sites for leiomyosarcomas to occur are the uterus and gastrointestinal tract. Leiomyosarcomas of soft tissue are relatively uncommon and the majority arise in the retroperitoneum. Grossly, the tumors are firm, solid, bulky masses; occasionally they may be partly cystic. Histologically, the tumors show spindle cells with a degree of cytologic atypia ranging from low to moderate in the majority of cases. Absolute minimal criteria for the diagnosis of soft tissue leiomyosarcoma have not been established, but most authors would agree that the size of the primary tumor (>7.5 cm) is probably a good indicator of malignancy and that a tumor with as few as 1 mitosis/ 10 high-power fields is capable of metastasis.[36,37]

Aspirates obtained from leiomyosarcomas **(Fig. 5.3)** are moderately to markedly

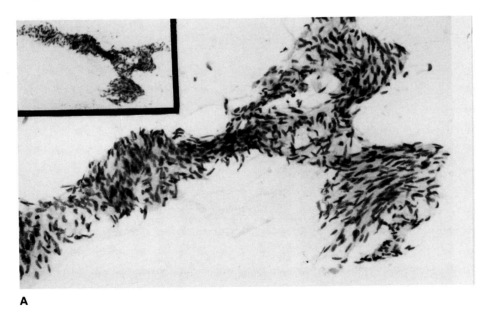

A

Fig. 5.3. Leiomyosarcoma. **A.** ABC. Note cohesive tissue fragments composed of fascicles of spindle cells. (H & E preparation; ×160, inset ×60).

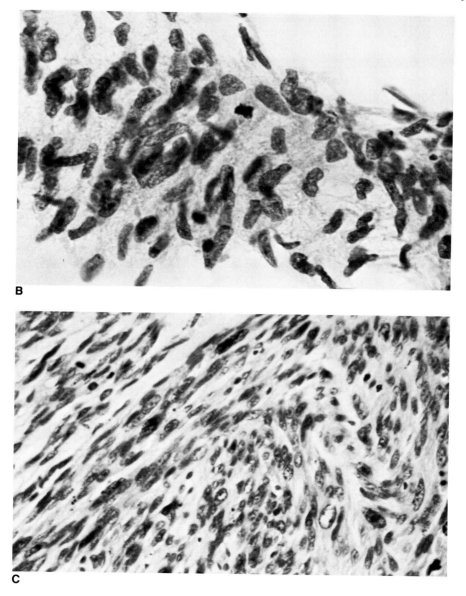

Fig. 5.3. B. ABC. Note elongated nuclei with blunted ends, irregular chromatin distribution, and mitoses. (H & E preparation; ×500). **C.** Histologic section of leiomyosarcoma. Note hypercellularity consisting of atypical spindle cells with nuclear palisading. (H & E preparation; ×500).

cellular. The tumor cells are spindle-shaped and have scanty and ill-defined cytoplasm. The nuclei are characteristically cigar-shaped or blunt ended. The chromatin may be finely or coarsely granular. The degree of nuclear atypia is dependent on the histologic grade of the tumor. In high-grade leiomyosarcomas there is considerable cellular pleomorphism with frequent mitoses, large bizarre cells, and cells showing prominent nucleoli. The cells are dyshesive and therefore scattered single cells are often seen. In well-differentiated leiomyosarcomas scattered single cells are less frequent, the tumor cells tend to form cohesive tissue fragments, due to a relatively strong intercellular cohesion among the spindle cells. The tissue fragments are of variable size, composed of tightly packed, cohesive, overlapping spindle cells arranged in parallel rows **(Fig. 5.4A)**. The spindle cells are relatively uniform, with only a modest degree of nuclear atypia. Hypercellularity and irregularity in chromatin distribution may be the only clues to the malignant nature of the cells in some cases.

Differentiation of low-grade leiomyosarcoma from leiomyoma is at times difficult on ABC. In the series of Dahl et al[38] three of 11 cases of soft tissue leiomyosarcoma were misinterpreted as benign because the conventional criteria of malignancy were minimal in the three cases. More recently, Tao and Davidson[30] compared the cytologic features of low-grade leiomyosarcoma and leiomyoma. They concluded that the presence of highly cellular tissue fragments composed of closely packed spindle cells in side-by-side, parallel arrangements (i.e., a fascicular pattern) would strongly support the diagnosis of leiomyosarcoma **(Fig. 5.4A)**. By contrast, aspirates of leiomyomas **(Fig. 5.4B)** reveal cell groups with loosely and irregularly arranged nuclei, resulting in a syncytial appearance.

Moreover, one should be careful not to misinterpret normal smooth muscle frag-

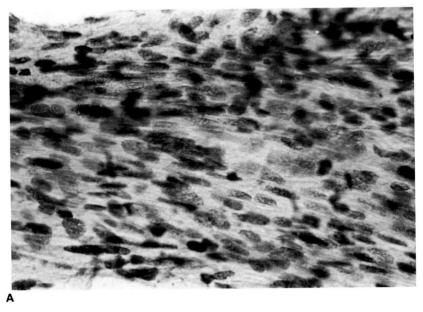

A

Fig. 5.4. Contrast ABC. **A.** Leiomyosarcoma. Hypercellular tissue fragment composed of densely packed spindle cells, arranged in parallel rows. (H & E preparation; ×500).

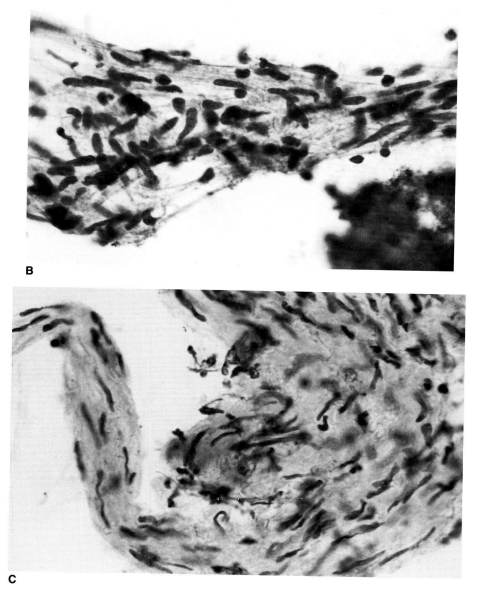

B

C

Fig. 5.4. B. Leiomyoma. Tissue fragment composed of loosely and irregularly arranged spindle cells. (H & E preparation; ×500). **C.** Tissue fragment of normal smooth muscle cells derived from bowel wall. Note serpentine thin nuclei with pointed ends. The nuclei are equidistant from one another without undue crowding. (H & E preparation; ×500).

ments derived from the bowel wall as well-differentiated leiomyosarcoma. Normal smooth muscle fragments **(Fig. 5.4C)** consist of spindle cells having delicate, serpentine nuclei with pointed ends. The nuclei are bland, are uniformly spaced from one another without undue crowding, and are all oriented uniformly in one direction. Although the tissue fragments can be quite large in size, they are few in number. Normal muscle cells are not present as single cells. In contrast, aspirates of smooth muscle tumors give rise to both scattered single cells and tissue fragments in much greater quantity.

Low-grade Liposarcoma

The low-grade liposarcomas grow slowly, have a low incidence of metastases, and may attain a large size before they are recognized. There are two histologic subtypes: myxoid and well-differentiated. The gross appearance of the tumor tends to reflect the histologic appearance. The myxoid type appears as slimy grayish-white tumors, while the well-differentiated liposarcomas resemble lipomas.

Myxoid Liposarcomas

Myxoid liposarcoma is one of the commonest sarcomas encountered in the retroperitoneum. Aspirates obtained from these tumors **(Plate 5.2** and **Fig. 5.5)** consist of gelatinous, myxoid material derived from the tumor matrix, which is rich in acid mucopolysaccharides. There may be many networks of small capillaries surrounded by tumor cells embedded within the myxoid stroma. The number of tumor cells present is quite variable, depending on the area of the lesion aspirated. The tumor cells may be spindle, stellate, or oval in shape. The nuclei are only minimally atypical. The spindle and stellate cells have nonvacuolated cytoplasm and are referred to as prelipoblasts. The lipoblasts are characterized by the presence of a variable amount of fat in the form of well-defined intracytoplasmic vacuoles, which may be of univacuolated or multivacuolated type.[39] The diagnostic lipoblasts are distinguished from lipid-laden histiocytes by the presence of distorted or scalloped nuclei caused by the pressure of the expanding lipid vacuoles. In most cases, the spindle prelipoblasts are the predominant cells. Lipoblasts are few, but can usually be found if diligently searched for. The diagnosis of myxoid liposarcoma is based on the combination of morphologic features of myxoid stroma, network of capillaries, spindle and stellate cells, and lipoblasts with atypical or hyperchromatic nuclei.

Both lipoblasts and myxoid matrix can be encountered separately in other conditions. Benign lipoblasts may be seen in fat necrosis and atypical lipomas, but the nuclei of the malignant lipoblasts are much more hyperchromatic and show greater degrees of atypia. Similarly, myxoid stroma is not found exclusively in myxoid liposarcoma; it may be found in schwannoma, myxoma, and the myxoid variant of malignant fibrous histiocytoma.

Well-differentiated Liposarcomas

The aspirates of well-differentiated liposarcomas reflect the histology of the tumor. The diagnosis is made by finding mature adult fat admixed with a variable amount

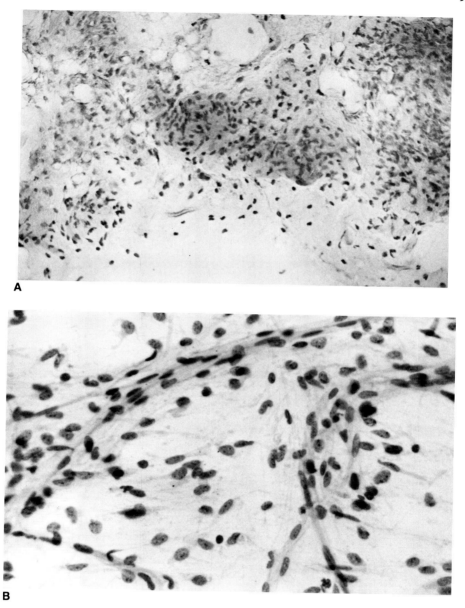

Fig. 5.5. Myxoid liposarcoma. **A.** ABC. Note hypercellularity consisting of spindle and stellate cells in a myxoid background. (H & E preparation; ×125). **B.** ABC. Note network of arborizing capillaries and spindle cells (prelipoblasts) with minimal atypia. (H & E preparation; ×310).

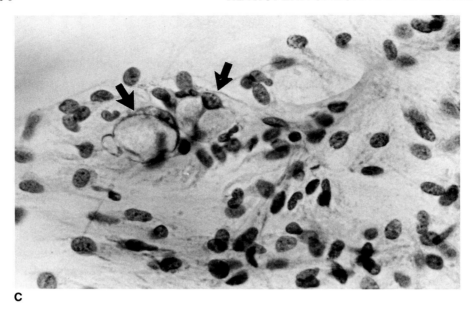

C

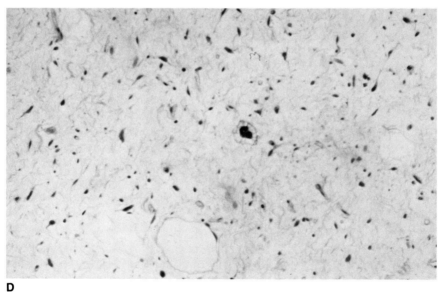

D

Fig. 5.5. C. ABC. Note many oval shaped prelipoblasts and two lipoblasts (*arrows*) with large cytoplasmic vacuoles distorting the nuclei. (H & E preparation; ×500). **D.** Histologic section of myxoid liposarcoma. Note abundant loose myxoid stroma, spindle cells, and a multivacuolated malignant lipoblast at the center. (H & E preparation; ×125).

of fibrous and myxoid tissues containing atypical spindle cells with hyperchromatic enlarged nuclei **(Fig. 5.6)**. If the aspirate contains only adult fat without the atypical cells, the diagnosis of well-differentiated liposarcoma is not possible. On the other hand, the cytopathologist must be careful not to misinterpret smooth muscle cells and fat cells derived from a renal angiomyolipoma as cells from liposarcoma (see Chapter 10, section on Angiomyolipoma).

Malignant Peripheral Nerve Sheath Tumor (Malignant Schwannoma)

Malignant peripheral nerve sheath tumor (malignant schwannoma) is not a common tumor, but between 3% and 10% occur in the retroperitoneum. They have few distinctive morphologic features to separate them from other spindle cell sarcomas, such as leiomyosarcoma and fibrosarcoma. A case of NAB of malignant schwannoma reported by Hood et al. showed obviously malignant spindle cells but further classification was not feasible.[40] Our experience has been similar. The neoplastic cells **(Fig. 5.7)** are spindle-shaped, with coarse chromatin, irregular nuclear membranes, and variable prominence of nucleoli. Mitotic figures may be seen. The cytoplasm is indistinct. Immunoperoxidase staining for S100 protein, a marker for Schwann cells, is useful for the identification of the tumor. The presence of von Recklinghausen's neurofibromatosis in a patient who has a spindle cell sarcoma is also a strong indicator of the neurogenic origin of the tumor.

Fibrosarcoma

Fibrosarcoma is a malignant spindle cell tumor composed of fibroblastic cells. The incidence of this tumor has markedly decreased in recent years and it is now seldom diagnosed in the retroperitoneum. Reviews of cases previously diagnosed as fibrosarcoma have resulted in revised diagnoses in as many as 60% of cases.[41] With the widespread use of immunocytochemistry and electron microscopy many of the cases designated as fibrosarcoma in the past have been shown to be malignant fibrous histiocytoma, leiomyosarcoma, malignant schwannoma, or a monomorphic variant of synovial sarcoma.

PLEOMORPHIC SARCOMAS

Malignant Fibrous Histiocytoma

This is the most common soft tissue sarcoma of late adult life.[42] Of the 18 NAB cases of pleomorphic cell sarcoma reported by Gonalez-Campora et al,[28] 17 were malignant fibrous histiocytomas. The histogenesis of this tumor is still controversial. Many investigators believe that the tumor is of histiocytic nature, but recent studies support the view that malignant fibrous histiocytoma is part of the spectrum of neoplasms of the fibroblasts.[43] Malignant fibrous histiocytomas can occur in a wide variety of anatomic locations, and the most common sites are the extremities, particularly the lower extremity, and the retroperitoneum.

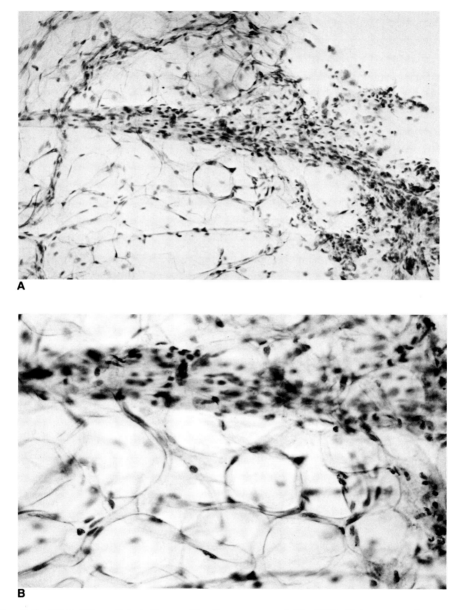

Fig. 5.6. Well-differentiated, lipoma-like liposarcoma. **A,B.** ABC. Note mature fatty tissue intersected by bundles of atypical spindle cells. (H & E preparation; A ×125, B ×300).

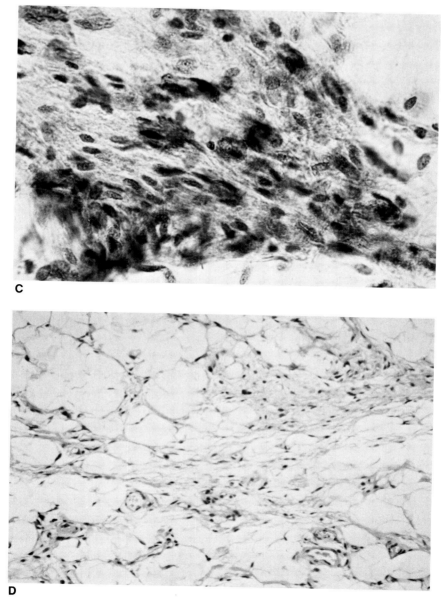

Fig. 5.6. C. ABC. Higher magnification view of the atypical spindle cells. Note malignant nuclei. (H & E preparation; ×500). **D.** Histologic section of lipoma-like liposarcoma. (H & E preparation; ×125).

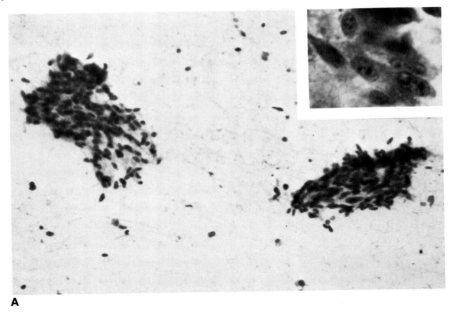

A

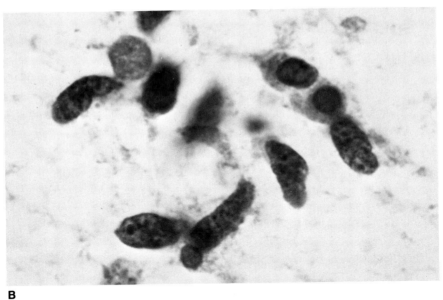

B

Fig. 5.7. Malignant schwannoma. **A.** ABC. Malignant spindle cells arranged in tissue frag-ments. *Inset:* Note multiple, irregular nucleoli. (H & E preparation; ×125, inset ×500). **B.** ABC. Higher magnification view of the spindle cells. Note irregular nuclear membranes and irregular chromatin distribution. (H & E preparation; ×1,250).

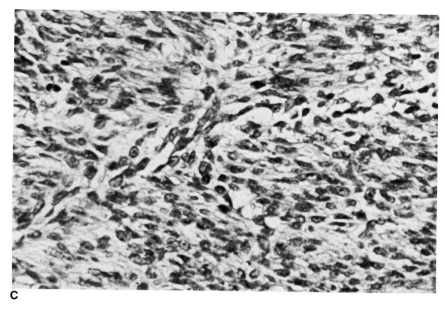

Fig. 5.7. C. Histologic section of malignant schwannoma. (H & E preparation; ×310).

Grossly, malignant fibrous histiocytoma is a white or tan, firm tumor, circumscribed but nonencapsulated. Cytologically, the tumor is well known for its pleomorphic appearance.[44–46] The aspirates are typically hypercellular, consisting of dispersed single cells as well as poorly cohesive cell groups **(Fig. 5.8)**. The classic form of malignant fibrous histiocytoma is characterized by many bizarre, multinucleated giant cells, measuring up to several hundred micrometers in diameter and containing irregular macronucleoli **(Plate 5.3)**. In addition, there are many malignant spindle-shaped cells.

In the myxoid variant of malignant fibrous histiocytoma, the aspirate specimen consists of fibromyxoid stromal tissue fragments with atypical, hyperchromatic stellate cells **(Fig. 5.9)**. The cytologic picture mimics myxoid liposarcoma, except that genuine lipoblasts are lacking.

Pleomorphic Liposarcoma

Unlike the myxoid and well-differentiated variants, pleomorphic liposarcomas are uncommon in the retroperitoneum; they occur more often in the extremities. The aspirates are hypercellular, characterized by a pleomorphic cell population of vacuolated and nonvacuolated cells. The cells show marked variation in size and shape, and may range from small signet ring lipoblasts to large, multinucleated forms with voluminous cytoplasm filled with lipid vacuoles indenting the nuclei, causing a "scalloped" effect **(Fig. 5.10)**. For a detailed description of the lipoblast, the reader is referred to the earlier section on myxoid liposarcoma. Other cell types are also present, including a variety of nonvacuolated spindled and pleomorphic cells with a homogeneous eosinophilic cytoplasm. The morphologic distinction of pleomorphic liposar-

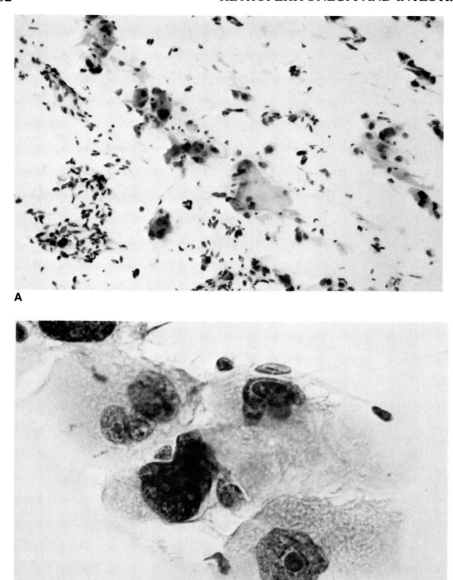

Fig. 5.8. Malignant fibrous histiocytoma. **A.** ABC. Note cell-rich aspirate with admixture of spindle cells and giant cells. (H & E preparation; ×125). **B.** ABC. Note multinucleate giant cells with irregular nuclear contour, macronucleoli, and foamy cytoplasm. (H & E preparation; ×500).

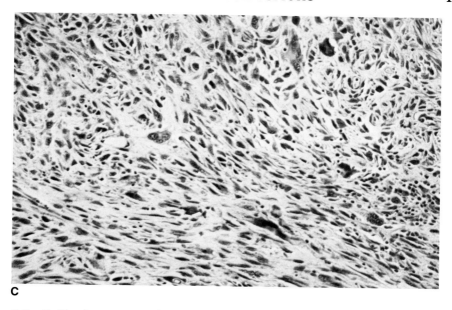

C

Fig. 5.8. C. Histologic section of malignant fibrous histiocytoma. Note storiform arrangement of spindle and giant cells. (H & E preparation; ×125).

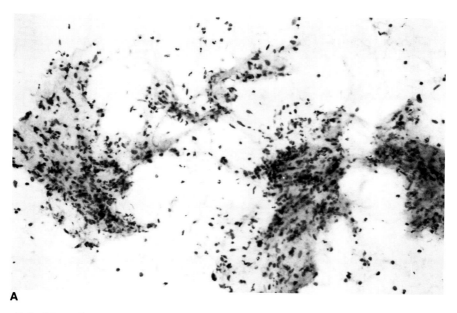

A

Fig. 5.9. Myxoid variant of malignant fibrous histiocytoma. **A.** ABC. Note many myxoid tissue fragments composed of atypical spindle cells. (H & E preparation; ×125).

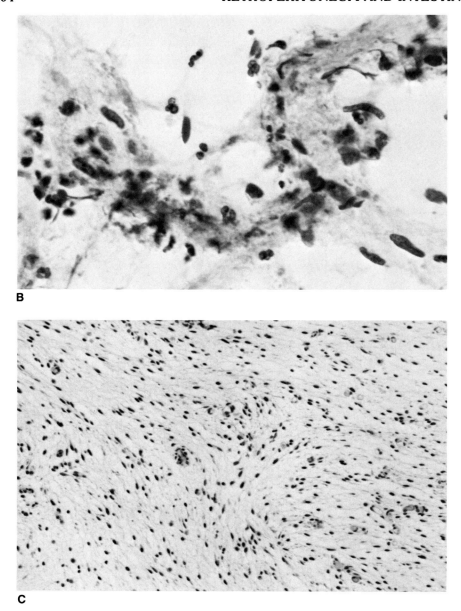

Fig. 5.9. B. ABC. Atypical spindle cells in a fibrillary myxoid background. Note conspicuous absence of capillary network and lipoblasts. (H & E preparation; ×310). **C.** Histologic section of myxoid variant of malignant fibrous histiocytoma. Note loose myxoid stroma. (H & E preparation; ×125).

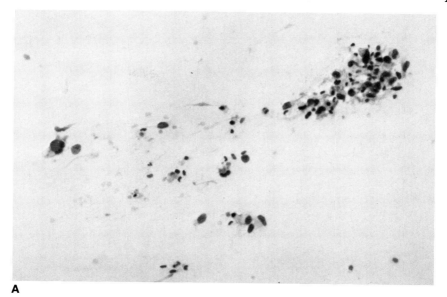

A

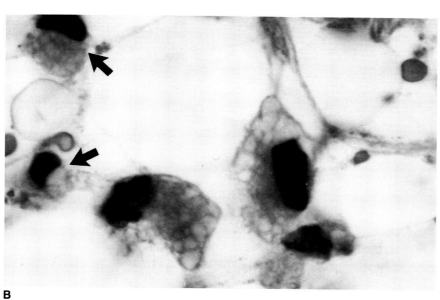

B

Fig. 5.10. Pleomorphic liposarcoma. **A.** ABC. Note many dyshesive pleomorphic oval or spindle cells with vacuolated cytoplasm. (H & E preparation; ×125). **B.** ABC. Note pleomorphic malignant lipoblasts, characterized by well-defined cytoplasmic lipid vacuoles, indenting the nuclei (*arrows*). (H & E preparation; ×500).

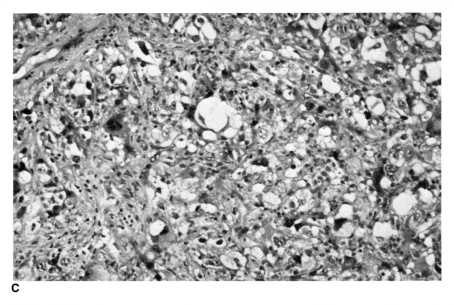

C

Fig. 5.10. C. Histologic section of pleomorphic liposarcoma. Note many pleomorphic lipoblasts with indented nuclei. (H & E preparation; ×310).

coma from malignant fibrous histiocytoma may be difficult, and is contingent upon the identification of malignant lipoblasts. The histiocytic-like tumor cells of malignant fibrous histiocytoma may contain ingested lipid vacuoles in the cytoplasm, but the lipid is more finely dispersed and the vacuoles do not indent the nuclei as they do in lipoblasts.

Pleomorphic Rhabdomyosarcoma

This variant of rhabdomyosarcoma is considered to be extremely rare; some investigators consider that it does not exist.[47] Many previously diagnosed cases are now believed to be examples of malignant fibrous histiocytoma. The tumor occurs in adults and is practically never seen in children. It typically arises in the large muscles of the extremities and is hardly ever encountered in the retroperitoneum. In our NAB file, none of the pleomorphic sarcomas arising in the retroperitoneum proved to be pleomorphic rhabdomyosarcoma. The morphologic picture shown here is from a tumor arising in the lower extremity of an adult male. Histologically, pleomorphic rhabdomyosarcoma displays a striking degree of cellular pleomorphism. On ABC, several cell types can be identified. There are many undifferentiated large round cells **(Fig. 5.11)** containing a single or multiple nuclei, with irregular prominent nucleoli. Chromatin is coarse and irregularly distributed. Bizarre spindle-shaped cells, racquet cells, and strap cells are seen in variable numbers. The cytoplasm is eosinophilic and granular. Cytoplasmic cross-striations are rarely identified. A rather characteristic feature of this tumor is the tandem arrangement of multiple nuclei in some of these cells **(Fig. 5.11B inset)**.

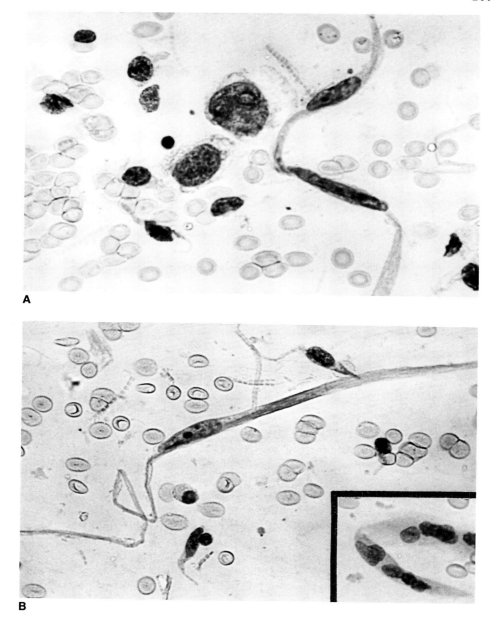

Fig. 5.11. Pleomorphic (adult) rhabdomyosarcoma. **A.** ABC. Note large undifferentiated round cells and bizarre spindle-shaped cells. The nuclei show coarse and irregularly distributed chromatin, prominent nucleoli, and irregular nuclear membranes. (H & E preparation; ×500). **B.** ABC. Note a bizarre strap cell with cytoplasmic cross-striations. *Inset* shows two strap cells featuring tandem arrangement of the nuclei. (H & E preparation; ×500).

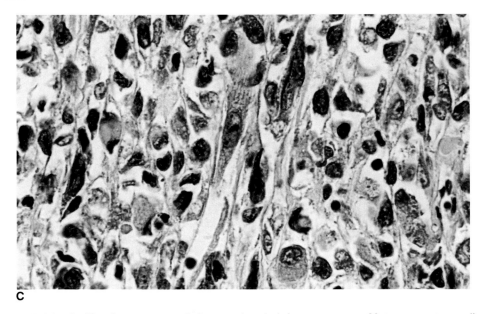

C

Fig. 5.11. C. Histologic section of pleomorphic rhabdomyosarcoma. Note many strap cells with cross-striations. (H & E preparation; ×500).

ROUND CELL SARCOMAS

Embryonal Rhabdomyosarcoma

Embryonal rhabdomyosarcoma is by far the most common variant of rhabdomyosarcoma, accounting for 70% of the cases. It occurs mainly in infants and children, and has an anatomic predilection for the regions of head and neck, the genitourinary tract, and the retroperitoneum. The extremities are less frequently involved.

Grossly, embryonal rhabdomyosarcoma is a fleshy, soft tumor with an irregular, poorly defined border, encroaching on the surrounding tissues. The cut surface is usually gray-white and may show gelatinous myxoid areas and varying degrees of focal necrosis and hemorrhage. The ABC **(Plate 5.1A** and **Fig. 5.12)** is moderately cellular, consisting of small cells diffusely scattered over the smear singly or in small loose clusters and with no distinctive pattern of arrangement. The cells range from undifferentiated small round cells with scant amount of cytoplasm, resembling lymphocytes, to slightly larger elongated or oval cells with deeply eosinophilic cytoplasm. The nuclei are hyperchromatic with irregular membranes. Prominent nucleoli may be present in some cells, but frequently they are obscured by the nuclear hyperchromatism. The larger cells with eosinophilic cytoplasm are reminiscent of the differentiating rhabdomyoblasts of embryonic development. Desmin or (less commonly) myoglobin may be demonstrated in the tumor cells after immunostaining **(Plate 5.1B).**

Ewing's Sarcoma

Although Ewing's sarcoma is primarily a tumor of bone, it can also occur as a primary soft tissue neoplasm. Extraosseous soft tissue Ewing's sarcoma occurs predominantly

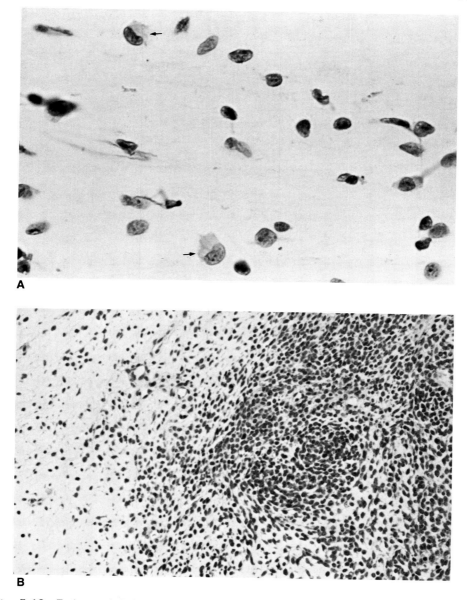

Fig. 5.12. Embryonal rhabdomyosarcoma. **A.** ABC. Note small cells with scant cytoplasm mimicking small lymphocytes and some larger cells with eosinophilic cytoplasm (arrows). (H & E preparation; ×500). **B.** Histologic section of embryonal rhabdomyosarcoma. Note small hyperchromatic cells embedded in a loose myxoid stroma. (H & E preparation; ×125).

in adolescents and young adults. The anatomic sites of predilection are the soft tissues of the paravertebral region, retroperitoneum, chest wall, and lower extremities. Recent ultrastructural observations of some Ewing's sarcomas have revealed neurosecretory granules and microtubules in the tumor cells, suggesting neural differentiation.[48,49] Ewing's sarcoma is now viewed by some workers as a member of a group of neoplasms known as "peripheral neuroectodermal tumors."[50] Ewing's sarcoma has been consistently shown to have the reciprocal chromosome translocation t(11;22), like other members of peripheral neuroectodermal tumors.

The aspirates consist of a rather monotonous population of small round cells that are undifferentiated and are remarkably uniform in size and shape **(Plate 5.4A and Fig. 5.13)**. The cells are arranged singly, or loosely grouped in clusters, or in rosette-like arrangements. Nuclei are oval to round, with dispersed chromatin and well-defined nuclear membranes. Nucleoli are absent or barely discernible. The cytoplasm is pale blue or clear and scanty. Characteristically, the cells of Ewing's sarcoma contain a large amount of cytoplasmic glycogen, which can be demonstrated by a periodic acid-Schiff stain **(Plate 5.4B)**. Although the absence of glycogen distracts from the diagnosis of Ewing's sarcoma, it by no means excludes it.[51,52]

Round Cell Liposarcoma

Round cell liposarcoma is a rare and highly malignant tumor. The aspirates consist of moderate-sized rounded cells with relatively indistinct cytoplasmic borders **(Fig. 5.14)**. Nuclear chromatin is coarse and irregularly distributed. Nuclear membranes are irregular in thickness and contour. The cells are arranged in patternless clusters or dispersed singly. Stroma is scanty and sometimes myxoid. The vascular network is not prominent as it is in other types of liposarcoma. The diagnosis is made by finding microscopic fields that show malignant lipoblasts.

POLYGONAL CELL SARCOMAS

Paraganglioma

Extraadrenal soft tissue paragangliomas are uncommon tumors. They behave more aggressively than their counterparts in the adrenal glands (pheochromocytoma). In a study reported by Sclafani et al[53] half of the extraadrenal retroperitoneal paragangliomas were classified as malignant on the basis of metastasis. However, survival may be prolonged even after metastasis has occurred. Complete tumor resection has been shown to be a good predictor of survival, but tumor size, functional status (catecholamine secretion), and gross and microscopic features are not.[53,54]

The aspirates are cell-rich **(Fig. 5.15)** and consist of uniform polygonal cells, arranged singly or in loose alveolar clusters. The cells have abundant, granular, eosinophilic cytoplasm. Nuclei are round to oval, with prominent nucleoli in some cells. Chromatin is coarsely granular, but evenly distributed. These cells are the prototype of neuroendocrine cells and resemble carcinoid tumor cells. However, in paragangliomas anisonucleosis is often marked. Bare nuclei are sometimes present due to cytoplasmic fragility. Spindle cells and irregular giant cells may be seen. In some cases, cellular pleomorphism can be quite striking, but this does not indicate malignancy.

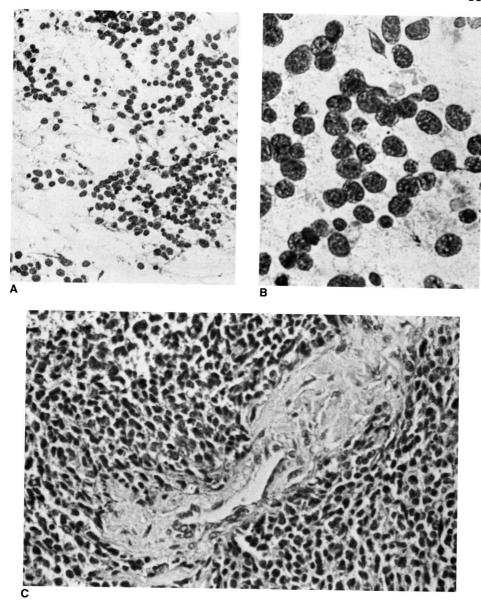

Fig. 5.13. Ewing's sarcoma. **A,B.** ABC. Note cell-rich aspirate showing monotonous appearance of small round cells with inconspicuous nucleoli. (H & E; A ×125, B ×500). **C.** Histologic section of Ewing's sarcoma. (H & E preparation; ×310).

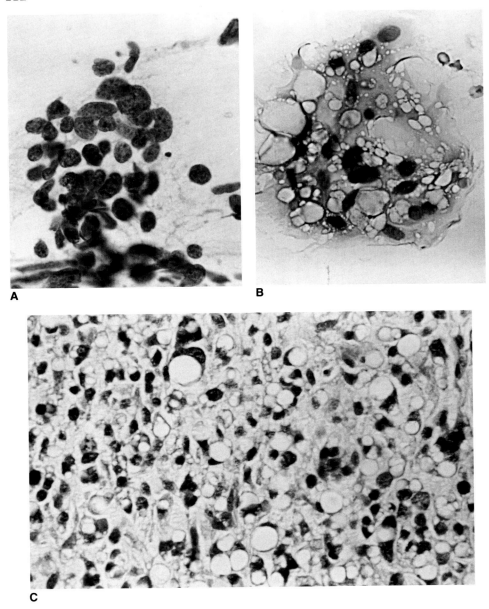

Fig. 5.14. Round cell liposarcoma. **A.** ABC. Note medium sized, round cells, totally undifferentiated. **B.** ABC. In this field, a group of round tumor cells exhibit evidence of lipoblastic differentiation. (H & E preparation; A ×500, B ×500). **C.** Histologic section of round cell liposarcoma. Note numerous malignant lipoblasts. (H & E preparation; ×310).

Chordoma

Chordoma is a rare, slow-growing, locally aggressive neoplasm, with low metastatic potential. The tumors are believed to originate from remnants of the notochord, and are characteristically midline in location. The most frequent location is the sacrococcygeal region, followed by the base of the skull..

The aspirates are hypercellular, with a mucoid background. The diagnostic cells are the physaliphorous (meaning basket in Greek) cells, which are large polygonal cells containing voluminous cytoplasm, ranging from bubbly to clear in appearance with slender septae, imparting a feathery or basket-like appearance (Fig. 5.16). The nuclei are fairly large, round or oval, and multilobulated to multinucleated. The physaliphorous cells resemble lipoblasts to some extent. Bizarre giant nuclei are seen in some cases but these malignant-looking cells are not necessarily associated with a more lethal course. The degree of vacuolation of cells varies from case to case. In addition to the bubbly cells, there is a population of smaller nonvacuolated cells. The diagnosis of chordoma should not be a difficult one if this tumor is always kept in mind when dealing with a midline lesion that arises in sacrococcygeal bone.[55,56]

Chordoma must be differentiated from mucin-producing adenocarcinoma, renal cell carcinoma, liposarcoma, and chondrosarcoma. The immunophenotypic profile of chordoma has been found to be useful in distinguishing it from other tumors. Cells of chordoma stain positively for cytokeratin, epithelial membrane antigen, vimentin, and S100 protein, and negatively for carcinoembryonic antigen.[57]

Epithelioid Leiomyosarcoma

Epithelioid leiomyosarcoma and epithelioid leiomyoma mainly affect the stomach and intestine. They are discussed in Chapter 7.

DIAGNOSTIC PROBLEMS IN SARCOMAS

Spindle Cell Sarcomas

Our ability to diagnose spindle cell sarcomas is dependent on the observation of an adequate, cell-rich aspirate sample containing spindle cells that exhibit cytologic atypia. Depending on the tumor grade, the cytologic atypia present in the tumor may range from modest to severe. A false-negative report may occur if the aspiration is obtained from a spindle cell sarcoma with minimal cellular atypia. Examples include well-differentiated liposarcoma with lipoma-like areas, malignant schwannoma with neurofibroma-like areas, and well-differentiated leiomyosarcoma simulating leiomyoma. Another source of false-negative reports is aspiration from a hypocellular area of a tumor, e.g., myxoid areas of myxoid liposarcoma or embryonal rhabdomyosarcoma.

Conversely, benign spindle cell neoplasms may be mistaken for sarcoma. Examples include some schwanommas, leiomyomas, and renal angiomyolipomas containing areas of hypercellularity and large atypical spindle cells, which can be confused with sarcoma by the unwary (see section on Schwannoma in this chapter, and section on Angiomyolipoma in Chapter 10).

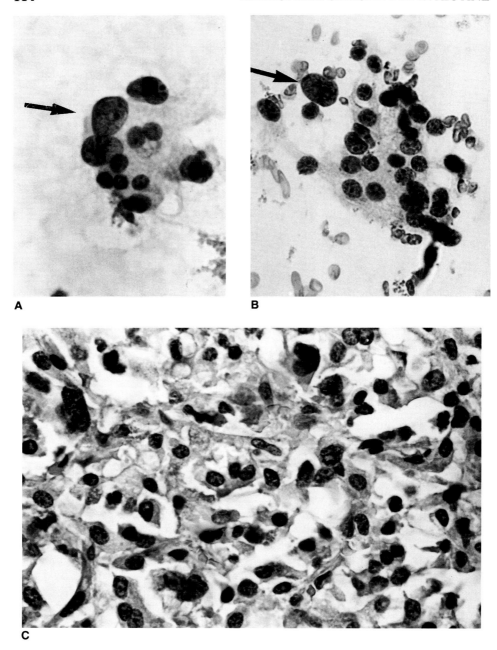

Fig. 5.15. Retroperitoneal paraganglioma. **A,B.** ABC. Note small, uniform, polygonal cells with moderately abundant granular cytoplasm (characteristic of neuroendocrine cells), admixed with much larger atypical cells (*arrows*). Also note alveolar arrangement of cells. (H & E preparation; A ×500, B ×500). **C.** Histologic section of paraganglioma. The prototypic cells are the small to medium sized, uniform, polygonal cells with abundant eosinophilic cytoplasm. Among the uniform cells there are also large cells with hyperlobated, irregular nuclei and spindle-shaped cells. (H & E preparation; ×500).

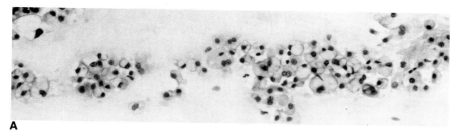

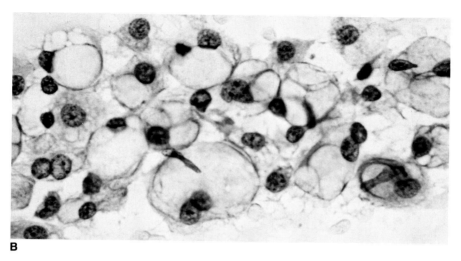

Fig. 5.16. Sacral chordoma. **A,B.** Note physaliphorous cells with abundant, bubbly, septated cytoplasm. (H & E preparation; A ×125, B ×500).

Finally, spindle cell sarcomas must be differentiated from carcinomas and other epithelial tumors that exhibit spindle cell differentiation. Examples are spindle cell squamous carcinomas metastatic to the retroperitoneum, spindle cell melanoma, and renal cell carcinoma. To minimize the chance of misinterpretation, adequate sampling by multiple punctures is essential. In addition, a thorough knowledge of the surgical pathology of various retroperitoneal sarcomas and the judicious use of immunocyto-chemistry and electron microscopy aid the cytopathologist in arriving at a correct diagnosis.

Pleomorphic Sarcomas

In the case of pleomorphic sarcoma, the cytologic diagnosis of malignancy is generally not a problem, due to the presence of marked nuclear atypia and bizarre giant cells. However, pleomorphic sarcomas may be confused with pleomorphic carcinomas, most of which are poorly differentiated adenocarcinomas. The enormous size of some of the tumor cells in pleomorphic sarcomas (e.g., malignant fibrous histiocytoma and pleomorphic liposarcoma) is rarely attained in carcinomas. The prominent nucleoli are more pleomorphic and angulated than those of carcinomas. Even in those pleo-morphic adenocarcinomas in which the smears consist predominantly of scattered solitary cells, some cell clusters exhibiting an epithelial arrangement can usually be found. Immunostaining for cytokeratin is helpful; carcinoma cells stain positively and sarcoma cells do not. However, one must be aware of the recent studies that demonstrated cytokeratin immunoreactivity in some malignant fibrous histiocytomas, leiomyosarcomas, and nerve sheath tumors.[58,59] In general, only scattered or rare sarcoma cells are cytokeratin positive; nevertheless, it is important that an appropriately selected panel of antibodies rather than a single antibody is used to assess the cell of origin of a tumor.

Not all soft tissue neoplasms with pleomorphic tumor cells are malignant. A paraganglioma may contain large bizarre cells that exhibit cytologic features of malignancy and yet the tumor may behave in a benign fashion. A pleomorphic lipoma may show many multinucleated atypical giant cells that can be mistaken for a malignancy by the unwary. Fortunately, pleomorphic lipomas have a clinical presentation distinct from liposarcomas. They tend to occur in superficial soft tissue, such as the subcutis. The common locations for these tumors are the head and upper back, and not the retroperitoneum. This is another example of the importance of possessing a sound knowledge of surgical pathology in order to interpret the cytologic samples properly.

Small Round Cell Sarcomas

From the morphologic point of view, small round cell sarcomas belong in the group of tumors traditionally designated as "small round cell malignancies."[60] These tumors include neuroblastoma, Ewing's sarcoma, embryonal rhabdomyosarcoma, Wilms' tumor, and malignant lymphoma. Other tumors that must also be considered in older patients are undifferentiated small cell carcinoma and similar tumors of neuroendocrine origin, e.g., neuroendocrine carcinoma and carcinoid tumor.

As shown in **Table 5.4,** the patient's age and the site of origin of the tumor with its clinical presentation are useful discriminatory characteristics. **Figure 5.17** is a flow chart for use in the differential diagnosis of small round cell tumors of childhood. Evaluation for unique cytologic features, special stains, electron microscopy, and correlation of clinical data permit a specific diagnosis to be made in most cases.[61]

Neuroblastoma generally occurs in infants and young children whereas Ewing's sarcoma occurs in adolescents and young adults. The cells of Ewing's sarcoma are uniform in size and shape and contain cytoplasmic glycogen, while neuroblastoma cells are less uniform, lack cytoplasmic glycogen, and tend to form rosettes. An eosinophilic fibrillary stroma may be observed in some neuroblastomas. Neuroblastoma cells consistently show positive immunoreactivity for neuron-specific enolase. Moreover, in neuroblastoma there is increased catecholamine secretion in serum or urine.

Embryonal rhabdomyosarcomas affect patients of an age group similar to neuroblastoma, but cytologically they have a more sarcomatous appearance, with some cells showing spindle shape on the smears. The tumor cells exhibit a variable degree of cellular pleomorphism and nuclear hyperchromatism, with coarser nuclear chromatin and prominent nucleoli. There are often larger cells with brightly eosinophilic cytoplasm, representing rhabdomyoblastic differentiation. Recognition of these cells is the key to diagnosis. Intracytoplasmic glycogen, stainable by a diastase-labile periodic acid-Schiff reaction, may be present, but the amount is generally less than that found in Ewing's sarcoma. The use of immunohistochemical stains for desmin, myoglobin,

TABLE 5.4. Differential Diagnosis of Small Round Cell Neoplasms

Neoplasms	Age	Primary Sites	Cytologic Features	Immunostains	Electron Microscopy
Embryonal rhabdomyo-sarcoma	Infants and children	Head and neck, genito-urinary tract, retroperi-toneum	Irregular small cells with eosinophilic cytoplasm	Vim (+) Des (+) Myo (+)	Thick and thin myo-filaments, Z-bands, ±glycogen (mono-particulate form)
Ewing's sarcoma	Adolescents and young adults	Bone, soft tissue, para-vertebral area	Monotonous round cells, PAS-positive cyto-plasmic glycogen	Vim (+) NSE (±)	Primitive cell attach-ments, copious cyto-plasmic glycogen form-ing "lakes"*
Neuroblastoma	Infants and children	Adrenal medulla and paravertebral sympa-thetic ganglia	Rosettes, neurofibrillary matrix	Nf (+) NSE (+) Syn (+)	Microtubules, neurosecre-tory granules, interdig-itating cytoplasmic processes
Wilms' tumor	Children	Kidney	Triphasic pattern: blas-temic cells, tubules, stromal cells	Vim (+) Ker (+) NSE (±)	Tubular differentiation
Lymphocytic lymphoma	Any age	Lymphoid tissue	Round or convoluted nuclei	LCA (+)	Sparse organelles, lack of cell junctions
Undifferentiated small cell car-cinoma	Older adults	Lungs, occasionally other sites	Pleomorphic small cells, nuclear molding, indi-vidual cell necrosis	Ker (+) NSE (±) Syn (±)	Desmosomes, a few neu-rosecretory granules

*Glycogen may be inconspicuous in 10% of cases.

Vim = vimentin; Des = desmin; Myo = myosin; Nf = neurofilament; NSE = neuron-specific enolase; Syn = synaptophysin; LCA = leukocyte common antigen; Ker = keratin; PAS = periodic acid-Schiff.

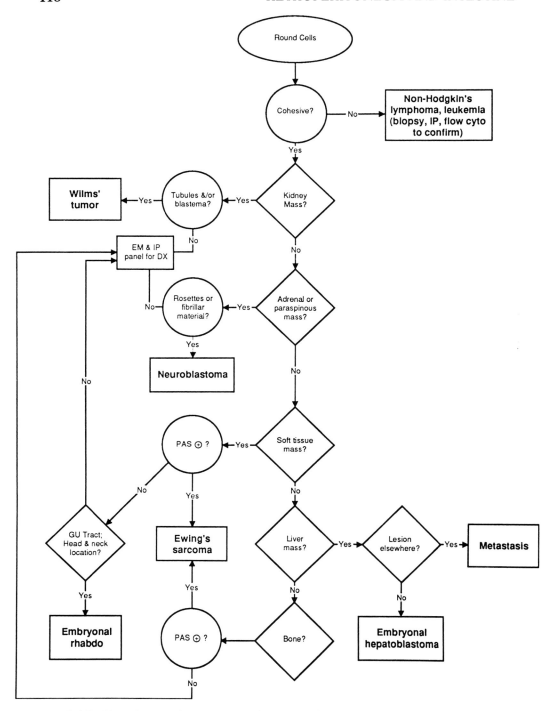

Fig. 5.17. Flow diagram for use in the differential diagnosis of small round cell tumors of childhood. (Reprinted from Howell et al,[61] with permission.)

and skeletal muscle actin may aid in elucidating the myogenic origin of rhabdo-myoblastoma.

Wilms' tumor may occasionally enter into the differential diagnosis of a small round cell tumor of childhood when the predominant cells are the blastemic type (see Chapter 10). Blastemic cells are of moderate size and contain round-to-oval, hyperchromatic nuclei and an indistinct cytoplasm. An important diagnostic clue is evidence of early tubular differentiation and the arrangement of cells in solid columns with well-defined borders. The primitive tubules may take the form of pseudorosettes, which may be mistaken for those of neuroblastoma. However, the fibrillary matrix of neuroblastoma, coupled with the fact that nuclei of neuroblastic rosettes do not form a single layer parallel to one another, will facilitate the diagnosis. In difficult cases, immunostains, ultrastructure, or other special diagnostic tests may be required to establish the correct diagnosis.

Malignant lymphomas occurring in children are usually of immature, blastic cell types (see Chapter 4). The nuclei of lymphoblastic lymphoma are characteristically markedly convoluted and have fine, dusty chromatin; those of Burkitt's lymphoma contain clumped chromatin and two or more prominent nucleoli. Additionally, lymphocytes show a positive immunoreaction for leukocyte common antigen, while other small round cell malignancies do not.

Undifferentiated small cell carcinoma occurs in older patients and the most common primary site is the lung. The ABC is characterized by a more cohesive clustering of tumor cells with nuclear molding. The nuclei are more irregular in size and shape. Tumor necrosis and a high mitotic rate are often present. The demonstration of epithelial or neuroendocrine markers by immunocytochemical stains or electron microscopy (see Fig. 1.10) helps to distinguish this tumor from other small round cell tumors.

Polygonal Cell Sarcomas

Polygonal cell sarcomas must be distinguished from metastatic carcinoma.[28] The dissociated polygonal cells of epithelioid leiomyosarcoma (see Chapter 7) may be easily confused with a metastatic carcinoma. The physaliphorous cells of a chordoma may be mistaken for cells from a metastatic mucin-producing adenocarcinoma, renal cell carcinoma, or liposarcoma.

BENIGN TUMORS AND TUMOR-LIKE LESIONS

Benign tumors and tumor-like lesions arising in the retroperitoneal space are far less common than malignant lesions and constitute only about 15–17% of all the retroperitoneal tumors. They tend to be much smaller in size and are less likely to cause symptoms.

Schwannoma

Schwannoma is a slow-growing encapsulated benign neoplasm of the Schwann cells. Although schwannoma constitutes a small percentage of all retroperitoneal tumors, it is the most common benign soft tissue tumor of the retroperitoneum.[62] The cut surface is tan or gray, often with some irregular myxoid areas and cysts in the larger tumors. In needle aspirates **(Fig. 5.18)** the characteristic cells are spindle shaped. The nuclei are elongated and wavy, with pointed ends. In some cases, both Antoni A and Antoni B tissues can be seen. The former is represented by cellular tissue fragments formed of bands of spindle cells whose nuclei are arranged like a palisade, and there is usually very little intervening stromal tissue. Verocay bodies **(Fig. 5.18C)**, composed of rows of palisading nuclei separated by a fibrillary stroma, may sometimes be discernible. In contrast, the Antoni B tissue is made up of predominantly loose stromal tissue with few spindle cells.

One should be aware that the retroperitoneum and posterior mediastinum are common sites of cellular schwannoma.[63] These tumors differ from the conventional schwannomas in having very cellular Antoni A type tissues with nuclear atypia, lacking verocay bodies, and associated with a histologic appearance resembling a smooth muscle tumor. Aspirates from cellular schwannomas may contain large atypical spindle cells **(Fig. 5.19)**. These cases can be mistaken for leiomyosarcoma by the unwary, and caution is needed in the interpretation of these aspirates. Immunostaining of the tumor cells for S100 protein demonstrates positive reactivity, confirming the Schwann cell origin of these tumors.

Lipoma

Aspirates from lipomas show mature fatty tissue. In the retroperitoneum, lipoma is much less common than what the literature formerly suggested. In general, deep-seated lipomatous neoplasms are more likely to be malignant than superficial ones.

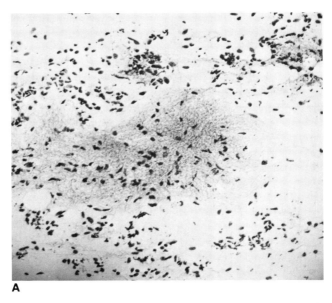

A

Fig. 5.18. Retroperitoneal schwannoma. **A.** ABC. Low magnification view showing abundant spindle cells representing Antoni A tissues, surrounding a hypocellular Antoni B area with fibrillar myxoid stroma (*center of photograph*). (H & E preparation; ×125).

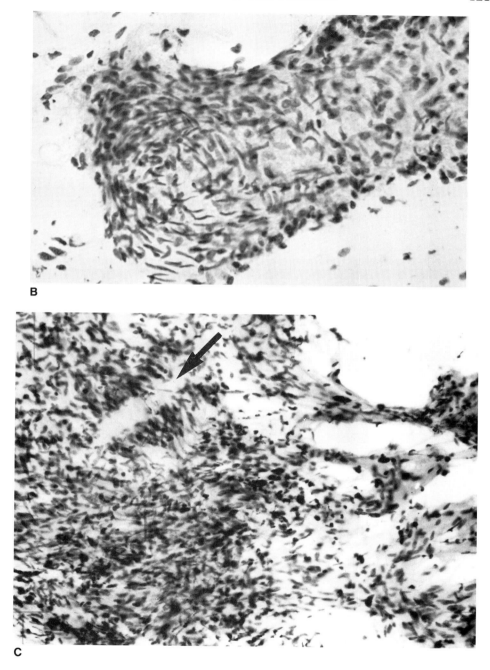

Fig. 5.18. B. ABC. Note Antoni A tissue showing hypercellularity consisting of wavy spindle cells with pointed nuclei. (H & E preparation; ×310). **C.** ABC. Antoni A tissue fragment containing a verocay body (*arrow*). (H & E preparation; ×310).

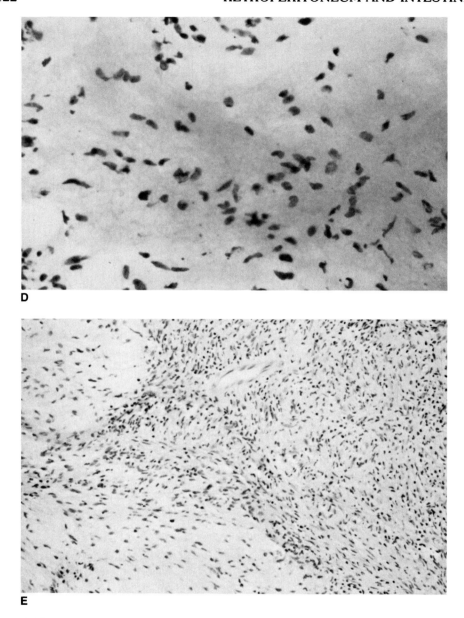

Fig. 5.18. D. ABC. Note Antoni B tissue showing hypocellularity with the spindle cells separated by abundant myxoid stroma. (H & E preparation; ×310). **E.** Histologic section of schwannoma with cellular Antoni A tissue (*right*) and hypocellular myxoid Antoni B tissue (*left*). (H & E preparation; ×160).

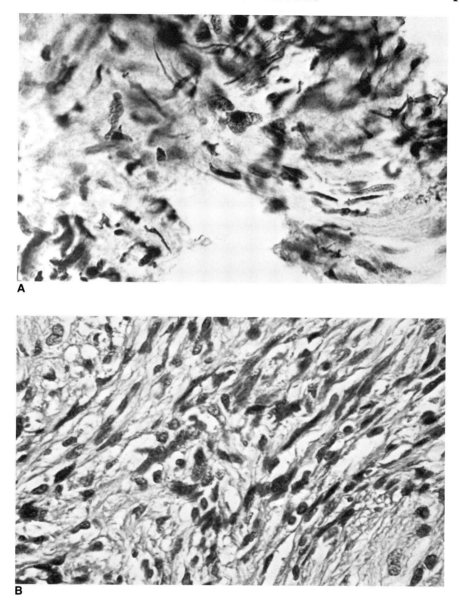

Fig. 5.19. Cellular schwannoma misdiagnosed as leiomyosarcoma. **A.** ABC. Note spindle cells with enlarged, hyperchromatic, atypical nuclei. These nuclei have pointed ends and do not exhibit prominent palisade arrangement as in leiomyosarcoma. (H & E preparation; ×500). **B.** Histologic section of the resected schwannoma showing similar atypical nuclei. No mitoses are present. (H & E preparation; ×500).

Many cases in the retroperitoneum thought to be lipomas subsequently proved to be well-differentiated liposarcomas.[64]

Leiomyoma

Leiomyoma is uncommon as a primary retroperitoneal tumor, although occasionally a uterine or gastric tumor may extend into the retroperitoneal space. On ABC, the cells are benign-appearing, spindle cells with cigar-shaped nuclei. There are no mitoses. The cells form tissue fragments within which the nuclei are not as closely packed as those in leiomyosarcoma (see **Fig. 5.4B**). Unlike its malignant counterpart, nuclear palisading is not a striking feature. Also see Chapter 7, section on Smooth Muscle Tumors.

Idiopathic Retroperitoneal Fibrosis

Idiopathic retroperitoneal fibrosis is a rare tumor-like lesion, which may present as a hard mass in the retroperitoneum. It may be associated with fibrosis in other locations such as the extrahepatic biliary ducts, mediastinum, or orbit. Characteristically, retroperitoneal fibrosis increasingly narrows the lumen of the ureters, with a risk of renal failure. The ureters are displaced medially, as opposed to lateral displacement in most other retroperitoneal tumors. The exact etiology of the disease is still not known; it is most likely related to an autoimmune disorder or to drugs such as methysergide.[65]

The ABC is generally hypocellular and consists of collagen fibers and fibroblasts, admixed with eosinophils, plasma cells, and lymphocytes **(Fig. 5.20)**. The cytologic features are nonspecific, and therefore must be interpreted in the light of the clinical and radiologic findings. In addition, several needle passes must be performed to ensure that one is not missing a sclerosing malignant tumor, especially a malignant lymphoma (see Chapter 4).

Cysts

Cysts can be encountered in the retroperitoneum, mesentery, and omentum. An ultrasound examination discloses a cystic structure, and fluid can be aspirated. The aspirates are not as cellular as those obtained from solid tumors, due to dilution of the cells by the cystic fluid. The content of the aspirates reflects the nature of the cyst. Beahrs and associates[66,67] classify the cystic lesions into four categories: (1) Developmental cysts—these include enteric cysts containing yellowish-brown, mucinous fluid, lymphatic cysts containing lymph and mature lymphocytes, and dermoid cysts containing skin derivatives and even teeth. (2) Traumatic cysts—these result from organization of a hematoma. (3) Infective cysts—these may be bacterial, parasitic, or mycotic in nature. (4) Neoplastic cysts—these may be benign or malignant tumors that have undergone cystic degeneration.

Hematoma

Hematomas give rise to bloody aspirates with many erythrocytes, fibrin, and few scattered leukocytes. If the lesion is old and organized, fibrocytes and hemosiderin-

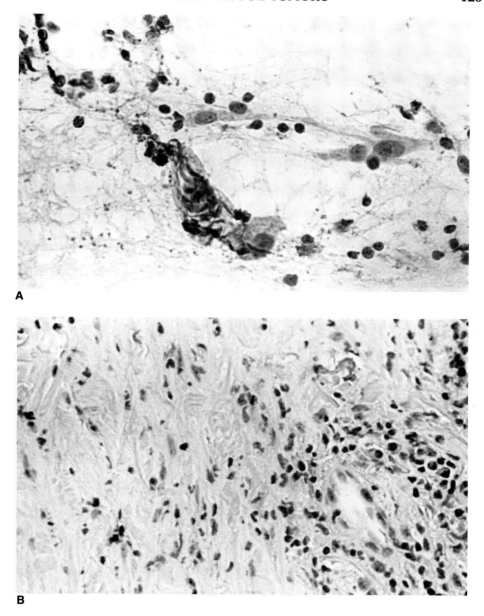

Fig. 5.20. Idiopathic retroperitoneal fibrosis. **A.** ABC. Note a few reactive, plump fibroblasts, some chronic inflammatory cells, and a small fragment of fibrous tissue. (H & E preparation; ×500). **B.** Histologic section of retroperitoneal fibrosis. Note scattered small lymphocytes, plasma cells, and dense fibrosis. (H & E preparation; ×310).

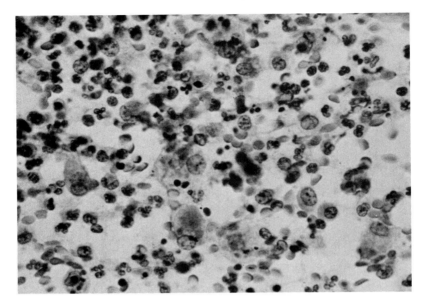

Fig. 5.21. Psoas abscess, aspirate. Note the numerous necrotic polymorphonuclear leukocytes with many phagocytic histiocytes. (H & E preparation; ×500).

laden macrophages are commonly present. The aspirates per se are nondiagnostic.
A history of trauma or surgery is usually obtained. If hematoma is suspected on ABC,
we usually request that the radiologist undertake two or three needle punctures from
different areas of the lesion to ensure that a malignancy is not missed.

Abscess

An aspirate of an abscess yields yellowish, pussy material, cytologic examination of
which shows a large number of degenerated polymorphonuclear leukocytes, phagocytic histiocytes, fibrin, and debris **(Fig. 5.21)**. The patient may have other stigmata
of infection, such as fever, abdominal tenderness, and a high leukocyte count. Gram
stain and culture of the aspirate may permit specific identification of the causative
organism. In selected cases, percutaneous drainage with a larger needle can be accomplished.[68]

Tuberculoma

Tuberculoma is uncommon in developed countries; however, the incidence is increasing due to the increased incidence of acquired immune deficiency syndrome (AIDS)
and the increased number of immigrants from regions where tuberculosis is still prevalent. Tuberculous lymphadenitis can present as multiple retroperitoneal masses, demonstrable by radiologic imaging. The aspirates are characterized by the presence of
many epithelioid histiocytes, in addition to the other cellular elements of chronic

inflammation. The epithelioid histiocytes **(Fig. 5.22)** are plump, elongated or oval cells with abundant pale eosinophilic cytoplasm. The nuclei are oval or elongated, with finely stippled chromatin and small nucleoli. They tend to form small cohesive aggregates, reminiscent of granulomas seen in tissue sections. Necrotic debris is conspicuously present in most cases. Multinucleate histiocytes (Langhans' cells) with peripherally placed nuclei are generally few in numbers and may be overlooked. In patients with AIDS, *Mycobacterium avium intracellulare* infection **(Fig. 5.23)** is common, and numerous acid-fast bacilli, demonstrable by a Ziehl-Neelsen stain, can readily be seen in the cytoplasm of the histiocytes as well as extracellularly.

DIAGNOSTIC ACCURACY

The reports in the literature that evaluated the accuracy rate of cytodiagnosis of soft tissue tumors were based on experience with these tumors in all body sites. Accuracy in cytologic diagnosis of retroperitoneal sarcomas has not specifically been addressed. The largest series was reported by Åkerman et al.[69] In their series of 349 cases of soft tissue tumors of all body sites, the aspirated material was insufficient for diagnosis in 5.7%, and an incorrect cytologic diagnosis was made in 5.8% of adequate smears; 51 of 59 primary sarcomas (86.4%) were correctly diagnosed as such.

In a study of 136 NAB cases of primary soft tissue tumors, Layfield et al[70] reported a sensitivity of 95% and a specificity of 95% for the determination of malignancy. False-positive and false-negative rates were both 2%.

Of the 60 cases of sarcomas studied by Miralles et al,[29] needle aspiration biopsy was able to correctly make the initial diagnosis of malignancy in 22 patients and confirm either a recurrence or metastasis in the remaining 38 patients. Among the 57 benign or nonneoplastic soft tissue lesions, there were two false-positive diagnoses of low-grade sarcomas.

Bennert et al[71] compared the results of NAB with needle core biopsy in diagnosing soft tissue lesions. The 117 NABs were divided into three groups: diagnostic, 53 (37 sarcomas and 16 benign); unsatisfactory, 44; and benign cells present, 20. Of these, 59 had concomitant needle core biopsy. There was 100% correlation between NAB and core biopsy when sarcoma was diagnosed. In seven of these cases, needle core biopsy further specified the type of sarcoma. However, it was found that core biopsy did not contribute more to patient management than NAB. In lesions where anatomic factors (location and needle trajectory) preclude easy accessibility, these authors advocate NAB as the modality of choice.

Barth et al[72] reported that NAB correctly classified 12 of 14 sarcomas and four of 11 benign lesions. Needle core biopsy correctly identified 16 of 16 sarcomas and 10 of 11 benign masses. These workers recommended the use of needle core biopsy for the diagnosis of soft tissue masses and limited use of NAB in selected cases (e.g., retroperitoneal or intraabdominal masses and recurrences). In cases in which a diagnosis of malignancy by NAB obligates either a significant alteration in therapy or a resection that would entail major functional or cosmetic morbidity, these authors recommend the cytologic diagnosis be substantiated by a histologic biopsy.

We reviewed the results of 22 cases of proven sarcomas in the retroperitoneum

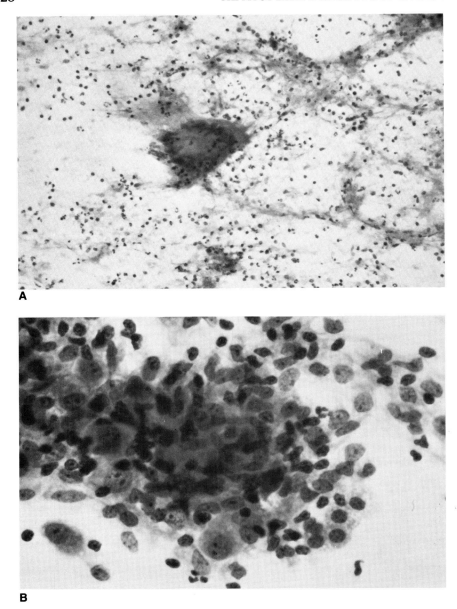

Fig. 5.22. Tuberculous lymphadenitis presenting as retroperitoneal mass. **A.** ABC. Note a Langhans' giant cell in a necrotic inflammatory background. (H & E preparation; ×310). **B.** ABC. Note clusters of elongated, plump epithelioid cells with eosinophilic cytoplasm. (H & E preparation; ×500).

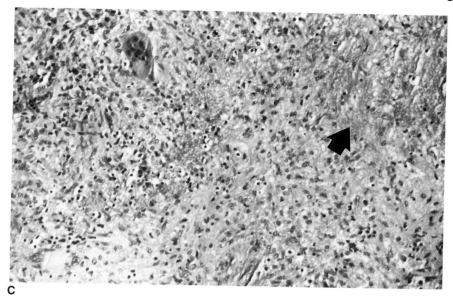

C

Fig. 5.22. C. Tissue section of tuberculosis showing an area of caseous necrosis (*arrow*), many lymphocytes, epithelioid histiocytes, and a Langhans' giant cell. (H & E preparation; ×310).

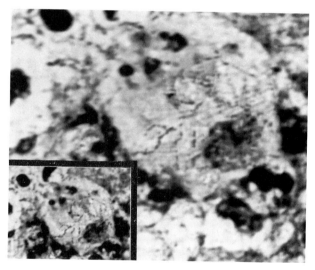

Fig. 5.23. *Mycobacterium avium intracellulare* infection in a patient with acquired immune deficiency syndrome. ABC. Note numerous beaded bacilli within the cytoplasm of a histiocyte as well as lying extracellularly. (Ziehl-Neelsen stain; ×1,250, inset ×500).

that had adequate aspirate smears for interpretation. Nineteen cases (87%) were correctly suspected or diagnosed by NAB; one case of liposarcoma was incorrectly typed as poorly differentiated adenocarcinoma; one embryonal rhabdomyosarcoma was mistyped as malignant lymphoma; and one case was called benign cells present (false-negative). The case misdiagnosed as "poorly differentiated adenocarcinoma" occurred in the early part of the study when immunostains were not routinely used; the diagnosis on the case of "malignant lymphoma" was immediately corrected upon review of the case as requested by the clinician. (Review of the slides showed ovoid and spindly small cells present.) There was one false-positive diagnosis in which a cellular schwannoma was interpreted as leiomyosarcoma.

In addition to these 22 cases having adequate aspirate material for diagnosis, four cases (15% of the total) of retroperitoneal sarcoma contained inadequate material for proper interpretation.

REFERENCES

1. Pories WJ, Murinson DS, Rubin P: Soft tissue sarcoma. In Rubin P: *Clinical Oncology,* ed 6. American Cancer Society, 1983, pp 308–324.

2. Noltenius H: *Human Oncology. Pathology and Clinical Characteristics.* Vol 1. Baltimore-Munich, Urban & Schwarzenberg, 1988, pp 83–203.

3. Chang AE, Rosenberg SA, Glatstein EJ, et al: Sarcomas of the soft tissue. In DeVita VT, Hellman S, Rosenberg SA (eds): *Cancer: Principles and Practice of Oncology.* Philadelphia, JB Lippincott, 1989, pp 1345–1398.

4. Rosenberg SA, Glatstein E: The management of local and regional soft tissue sarcomas. In Carter SK, Glatstein E, Livingston EB (eds): *Principles of Cancer Treatment.* New York, McGraw-Hill, 1982.

5. Bose B: Primary malignant retroperitoneal tumors: Analysis of 30 cases. *Can J Surg* 22:215–220, 1979.

6. Russell WO, Cohen J, Enzinger FM, et al: A clinical and pathological staging system for soft tissue sarcomas. *Cancer* 40:1562–1570, 1977.

7. Cody HS, III, Turnbull AD, Fortner JG, et al: The continuing challenge of retroperitoneal sarcomas. *Cancer* 47:2147–2152, 1981.

8. Mirra JM: Pathology of soft tissue sarcomas. In Eilber FR, Morton DL, Sondak VK, et al (eds): *The Soft Tissue Sarcomas.* Orlando, FL, Grune & Stratton, 1987, pp 11–50.

9. Enzinger FM, Weiss SW: *Soft Tissue Tumors.* St. Louis, CV Mosby, 1988.

10. Hajdu SI: *Pathology of Soft Tissue Tumors.* Philadelphia, Lea & Febiger, 1979, p 284.

11. Lane RH, Stephens DH, Reiman HM: Primary retroperitoneal neoplasms: CT findings in 90 cases with clinical and pathologic correlation. *AJR* 152:83–89, 1989.

12. Harrison LB, Gutierrez E, Fischer JJ: Retroperitoneal sarcomas. The Yale experience and a review of the literature. *J Surg Oncol* 32:159–164, 1986.

13. Storm FK, Sondak VK, Economou JS: Sarcomas of the retroperitoneum. In Eilber FR, Morton DL, Sondak VK, et al (eds): *The Soft Tissue Sarcomas.* Orlando, FL, Grune & Stratton, 1987, pp 239–248.

14. Parkinson MC, Chabrel CM: Clinicopathological features of retroperitoneal tumors. *Br J Urol* 56:17–23, 1984.

15. Presant CA, Russell WO, Alexander RW, et al: Soft tissue and bone sarcoma histopathology peer review. The Southeastern Cancer Study Group Experience. *J Clin Oncol* 4: 1658–1661, 1986.

16. Beahrs OH, Meyers MH: *Manual for Staging of Cancer, American Joint Committee on Cancer*. Philadelphia, JB Lippincott, 1983.

17. Costa J, Wesley RA, Gladstein E, et al: The grading of soft tissue sarcomas. Results of a clinicohistopathologic correlation in a series of 163 cases. *Cancer* 53:530–541, 1984.

18. Roholl PJ, DeJong AS, Ramaekers FC: Application of markers on the diagnosis of soft tissue tumors. *Histopathol* 9:1019–1035, 1985.

19. Gurley AM, Silverman JF, Lassaletta ML, et al: The utility of ancillary studies in pediatric FNA cytology. *Diagn Cytopathol* 8:137–146, 1992.

20. Altmannsberger M, Dirk T, Osborn M, et al: Immunohistochemistry of cytoskeletal proteins in the diagnosis of soft tissue tumors. *Semin Diagn Pathol* 3:306–316, 1986.

21. McNutt MA, Bolen JW, Gown AM, et al: Co-expression of intermediate filaments in human epithelial neoplasms. *Ultrastruct Pathol* 9:31–43, 1985.

22. Molenaar WM, Oosterhuis JW, Oosterhuis AM: Mesenchymal and muscle-specific intermediate filaments (vimentin and desmin) in relation to differentiation in childhood rhabdomyosarcomas. *Hum Pathol* 16:838–843, 1985.

23. Kindblom LG, Seidal T, Karlsson K: Immunohistochemical localization of myoglobin on human muscle tissue and embryonal and alveolar rhabdomyosarcoma. *Acta Pathol Microbiol Immunol Scand [A]* 90:167–174, 1982.

24. Wick MR, Swanson PE, Scheithauer BW, et al: Malignant peripheral nerve sheath tumor: An immunohistochemical study of 62 cases. *Am J Clin Pathol* 87:425–433, 1987.

25. Kindblom LG, Walaas L, Widehn S: Ultrastructural studies in the preoperative cytologic diagnosis of soft tissue tumors. *Semin Diagn Pathol* 3:317–344, 1986.

26. Akhtar M, Bedrossian CWM, Ali MA, et al: Fine-needle aspiration biopsy of pediatric neoplasms: Correlation between electron microscopy and immunocytochemistry in diagnosis and classification. *Diagn Cytopathol* 8:258–265, 1992.

27. Crosby JH, Hoeg K, Hager B: Transthoracic fine needle aspiration of primary and metastatic sarcomas. *Diagn Cytopathol* 1:221–227, 1985.

28. Gonalez-Campora R, Munoz-Arias G, Otal-Salaverri C, et al: Fine needle aspiration cytology of primary soft tissue tumors. Morphologic analysis of the most frequent types. *Acta Cytol* 36:905–917, 1992.

29. Miralles TG, Gosalbez F, Menendez P, et al: Fine needle aspiration cytology of soft-tissue lesions. *Acta Cytol* 30:671–678, 1986.

30. Tao LC, Davidson DD: Aspiration biopsy cytology of smooth muscle tumors. A cytologic approach to the differentiation between leiomyosarcoma and leiomyoma. *Acta Cytol* 37: 300–308, 1993.

31. Akerman M, Rydholm A: Aspiration cytology of lipomatous tumors. *Diagn Cytol* 3:295–302, 1987.

32. Walaas L, Kindblom LG: Lipomatous tumors: A correlative cytologic and histologic study of 27 tumors examined by fine needle aspiration cytology. *Hum Pathol* 16:6–18, 1985.

33. Salej HA, Beydoun R, Masood S: Cytology of malignant schwannoma metastatic to the lung. *Acta Cytol* 37:409–412, 1993.

34. Kindblom LG: Light and electron microscopic examination of embedded fine needle aspiration specimens in the preoperative diagnosis of soft tissue and bone tumors. *Cancer* 51:2264–2277, 1983.

35. Pollock RE: Evaluation and treatment of soft-tissue sarcoma. *Cancer Bull* 44:268–274, 1992.

36. Shmookler BM, Lauer DH: Retroperitoneal leiomyosarcoma. *Am J Surg Pathol* 7:269–280, 1983.

37. Wile AG, Evans HL, Romsdahl MM: Leiomyosarcoma of soft tissue. *Cancer* 48:1022–1032, 1981.

38. Dahl I, Hagmar B, Angervall L: Leiomyosarcoma of the soft tissue. *Acta Pathol Microbiol Scand [A]* 89:285–291, 1981.

39. Allen PV: *Tumors and Proliferation of Adipose Tissue.* New York, Masson Publishing, 1981, pp 131–171.

40. Hood IC, Qizilbash AH, Young JEM, et al: Needle aspiration cytology of a benign and a malignant schwannoma. *Acta Cytol* 28:157–164, 1984.

41. Nash AD: *Soft Tissue Sarcomas: Histological Diagnosis.* New York, Raven Press, 1989, p 9.

42. Weiss SW, Enzinger FM: Malignant fibrous histiocytoma. An analysis of 200 cases. *Cancer* 41:2250–2266, 1978.

43. Wood GS, Beckstead JH, Turner RR, et al: Malignant fibrous histiocytoma tumor cells resemble fibroblasts. *Am J Surg Pathol* 10:323–335, 1986.

44. Walaas L, Angervall L, Hagman B, et al: A correlative cytologic and histologic study of malignant fibrous histiocytoma: An analysis of 40 cases examined by fine needle aspiration cytology. *Diagn Cytopathol* 2:46–55, 1986.

45. Hong IS: Cytologic findings in a case of malignant fibrous histiocytoma. *Acta Cytol* 22:519–522, 1978.

46. Lozowski MS, Mishriki YY, Epstein H: Metastatic malignant fibrous histiocytoma in lung examined by fine needle aspiration. *Acta Cytol* 24:350–354, 1980.

47. Seidal T, Kindblom LG, Angervall L: Rhabdomyosarcoma in middle-aged and elderly individuals. *APMIS* 97:236–248, 1989.

48. Cavazzana AO, Miser JS, Jefferson J, et al: Experimental evidence for a neural origin of Ewing's sarcoma of bone. *Am J Pathol* 127:507–518, 1987.

49. Mierau GW: Extraskeletal Ewing's sarcoma (peripheral neuroepithelioma). *Ultrastruct Pathol* 9:91–98, 1985.

50. Cavazzana AO, Magnani JL, Ross RA, et al: Ewing's sarcoma is an undifferentiated neuroectodermal tumor. *Proc Clin Biol Res* 271:487, 1988.

51. Kontozglou T, Krakauer K, Qizilbash AH: Ewing's sarcoma. Cytologic features in fine needle aspirates in two cases. *Acta Cytol* 30:513–517, 1986.

52. Brehaut LE, Anderson LH, Taylor DA: Extraskeletal Ewing's sarcoma. Diagnosis of a case by fine needle aspiration cytology. *Acta Cytol* 30:683–686, 1986.

53. Sclafani LM, Woodruff JM, Brennan MF: Extraadrenal retroperitoneal paragangliomas: Natural history and response to treatment. *Surgery* 108:1124–1130, 1990.

54. Linnoila RI, Keiser HR, Steinberg SM, et al: Histopathology of benign versus malignant sympathoadrenal paragangliomas. *Hum Pathol* 21:1168–1180, 1990.

55. Kontozoglou T, Qizibash AH, Sianos J, et al: Chordoma: Cytologic and immunocytochemical study of four cases. *Diagn Cytopathol* 2:55–59, 1986.

56. Perasole A, Infantolino D, Spigariol F: Aspiration cytology and immunocytochemistry of sacral chordoma with liver metastases: A case report. *Diagn Cytopathol* 7:277–281, 1991.

57. Walaas L, Kindblom LG: Fine needle aspiration biopsy in the preoperative diagnosis of chordoma. *Hum Pathol* 22:22–28, 1991.

58. Litzky LA, Brooks JJ: Cytokeratin immunoreactivity in malignant fibrous histiocytoma and spindle cell tumors: Comparison between frozen and paraffin-embedded tissues. *Mod Pathol* 5:30–34, 1992.

59. Miettinen M: Immunoreactivity for cytokeratin and epithelial membrane antigen in leio-myosarcoma. *Arch Pathol Lab Med* 112:637–640, 1988.

60. Akhtar M, Ali MA, Sabbah R, et al: Fine needle aspiration biopsy diagnosis of round cell malignant tumors of childhood. *Cancer* 55:1805–1817, 1985.

61. Howell LP, Russell LA, Howard PH, et al: The cytology of pediatric masses: A differential diagnostic approach. *Diagn Cytopathol* 8:107–115, 1992.

62. Perhoniemi V, Anttinen I, Kadri F, et al: Benign retroperitoneal schwannoma. *Scand J Urol Nephrol* 26:85–87, 1992.

63. Fletcher CDM, Davies SE, Mckee PH: Cellular schwannoma: A distinct pseudosarco-matous entity. *Histopathol* 11:21–35, 1987.

64. Allen PW: *Tumors and Proliferations of Adipose Tissue.* New York, Masson Publishing, 1981, p 166.

65. Jones JH, Ross E, Matz LR, et al: Retroperitoneal fibrosis. *Am J Med* 48:203–208, 1970.

66. Beahrs OH, Dockerty MB: Primary omental cysts of clinical importance. *Surg Clin North Am* 30:1073–1079, 1950.

67. Beahrs OH, Judd ES Jr, Dockerty MB: Chylous cysts of the abdomen. *Surg Clin North Am* 30:1081–1096, 1950.

68. Haaga JR, Weinstein AJ: CT-guided percutaneous aspiration and drainage of abscess. *AJR* 135:1187–1194, 1980.

69. Åkerman M, Rydholm A, Persson BM: Aspiration cytology of soft tissue tumors. The ten years experience at an Orthopedic Oncology Group. *Acta Orthop Scand* 56:407–412, 1985.

70. Layfield LJ, Anders KH, Glasgow BJ, et al: Fine-needle aspiration of primary soft-tissue lesions. *Arch Pathol Lab Med* 110:420–424, 1986.

71. Bennert K, Abdul-Karim FW: Comparison of fine needle aspirates and needle core biopsies in the diagnosis of soft tissue lesions (abstract). *Mod Pathol* 6:27A, 1993.

72. Barth RJ, Merino MJ, Solomon D, et al: A prospective study of the value of core needle biopsy and fine needle aspiration in the diagnosis of soft tissue masses. *Surgery* 112:536–543, 1992.

6

Retroperitoneum IV: Metastatic and Germ Cell Tumors

KEY FACTS

▶ Generally lymph node metastases first become apparent in the immediate regional lymphatic drainage of the primary tumor. To assess a nodal metastasis, the cytopathologist must know the location of the lymph node from which the aspirate has been taken, as well as the age and sex of the patient.

▶ Certain types of tumor may give rise to widespread metastases producing generalized lymphadenopathy, mimicking primary lymphoma. Examples are neuroblastoma in childhood, and anaplastic small cell carcinoma and melanoma in adults.

▶ Whenever feasible, the aspiration smears of the metastatic tumor should be compared with the original histology of the primary tumor to ensure diagnostic accuracy.

▶ It is particularly important to identify those tumors for which specific therapies are available, e.g., germ cell tumors, lymphoma, prostate cancer, breast cancer, and ovarian cancer.

▶ Germ cell tumors are among the most highly treatable cancers. The basis for the diagnosis is a combination of morphology and determination of the serum markers: α-fetoprotein, and β-human chorionic gonadotrophin.

▶ Malignant melanoma is a great masquerader. The best safeguard against misdiagnosis is for the cytopathologist to keep melanoma constantly in mind in the differential diagnosis of any undifferentiated neoplasm.

CLINICAL CONSIDERATIONS

Secondary tumors can involve the retroperitoneal space as a result of direct spread from adjacent organs or by metastasizing to the paraaortic and pelvic lymph nodes. Examples of direct tumor invasion include large gastric leiomyosarcoma, pancreatic carcinoma, uterine and ovarian tumors, and primary bone tumors, notably sacrococcygeal chordoma. On the other hand, cancer from more distant sites may metastasize to the abdominal and retroperitoneal lymph nodes. At times, a metastatic tumor can become so bulky as to suggest a primary retroperitoneal tumor.

To determine the possible site of origin of a nodal metastasis, the pathologist must know the age and sex of the patient and the location of the lymph node from which the aspirate was obtained. Generally, nodal metastases first become clinically manifest in the immediate regional lymphatic drainage of the primary tumor. Cancers arising from the pelvic organs—the prostate, testis, urinary bladder, uterine cervix, and endometrium—tend to spread to the lymph nodes in the pelvis and lower paraaortic lymph nodes in a sequential and rather predictable manner. Cancers of the stomach and pancreas characteristically spread to the celiac and upper paraaortic nodes. Cancers of the colon, gallbladder, and ovary frequently involve the mesentery and omentum as well. Carcinomas of the lung and breast initially involve the mediastinal and axillary lymph nodes respectively, but subsequent involvement of the paraaortic nodes and adrenal glands is also common. It is also important to be aware of the types of primary tumor that may give rise to widespread metastases producing generalized lymphadenopathy, mimicking primary lymph node disease. Examples are neuroblastoma in childhood,[1] and anaplastic small cell carcinoma and melanoma in adults.[2]

When a retroperitoneal malignancy with no obvious primary site is diagnosed, the cytopathologist must try to identify those tumors that will benefit from specific therapy.[3,4] Careful examination of the aspirate smears, together with judicious applications of immunocytochemical stains and electron microscopy, can often result in a more precise diagnosis. The adult tumors for which effective, or at least specific, therapy is available are listed in **Table 6.1.** Notably, highly effective therapy is available for the treatment of lymphoma and germ cell neoplasms.[3,5–7] Several tumors that occur in infants and young children, such as Wilms' tumor and neuroblastoma, can also be treated effectively even after they have become disseminated: their sites of origin can usually be identified with ease using a combination of histology and clinical findings.[8]

TABLE 6.1. Metastatic Tumors of Adults For Which Effective or Specific Treatment Is Available

Tumors that are potentially curable
Malignant lymphomas/leukemias
Germ cell tumors
Trophoblastic tumors

Tumors that respond to chemotherapy
Small cell carcinoma of lung
Ovarian carcinoma
Breast carcinoma

Tumors that respond to hormonal therapy
Breast carcinoma
Prostate carcinoma
Endometrial carcinoma

PATHOLOGY AND ASPIRATION BIOPSY CYTOLOGY

Metastatic cancer cells in a lymph node are usually easily recognized on ABC because the extrinsic tumor cells are quite different morphologically from the lymphocytes and histiocytes of the lymph node. Whenever feasible, the cytologic smears must be compared with the histologic sections of the primary tumor, as this will facilitate tumor typing.

Squamous Cell Carcinoma

Most of the squamous cell carcinomas metastatic to the retroperitoneum come from the uterine cervix, vagina, and lung. Less commonly, they may come from the renal pelvis, bladder, and anus. Although we separate squamous carcinoma into well-differentiated (keratinizing) and poorly differentiated (nonkeratinizing) categories for the purpose of discussion, in reality there is considerable overlap in morphology.

Aspirates from well-differentiated squamous carcinomas (**Fig. 6.1**) contain mainly dyshesive tumor cells that vary widely in size and shape, e.g., tadpole cells, fiber cells, and round cells. The nuclear chromatin is hyperchromatic and coarsely granular, and in many cells it is completely opaque. Nucleoli are generally not seen. The cell borders are distinct; cytoplasm is abundant and homogeneously dense. Keratinization is characterized by the glassy, brightly eosinophilic appearance of the cytoplasm. Squamous pearls are sometimes seen. Not all squamous cells show unequivocal features of malignancy; some only show cytologic atypia reminiscent of the dysplastic squamous cells seen in the uterine cervix (**Fig. 6.2**). One should look for more typical malignant cells to make a diagnosis.

In poorly differentiated squamous cell carcinoma (**Fig. 6.3**), the aspirates consist of ragged sheets of tumor cells in syncytial arrangement. The tissue fragments have frayed borders, in contrast to the smooth, community border so characteristic of adenocarcinoma (*vide infra*). The tumor cells are smaller and much more uniform in size and shape than those of keratinizing carcinomas. The cytoplasm is less dense or transparent. The nuclearcytoplasmic ratio is high. The nuclear chromatin is granular; opaque nuclei are uncommon. Nucleoli may be prominent. If not accompanied elsewhere in the smear by other cells with squamous features, the tumor may be confused with small cell anaplastic carcinoma or the small cell variant of adenocarcinoma. Occasionally, poorly differentiated squamous carcinoma may consist focally or entirely of spindle cells, mimicking spindle cell sarcoma (**Fig. 6.4**). Immunoperoxidase staining of these spindle cells shows them to be positive for cytokeratin.

Adenocarcinoma

These tumors arise from surface secreting epithelia or underlying glands and tend to organize themselves into acinar or tubular structures containing a central lumen into which secretion is discharged. Hence, they can be identified on ABC by one of the two features: glandular formation and mucin production. The tumor cells may be columnar, cuboidal, or rounded. The nuclei frequently show nuclear membrane irreg-

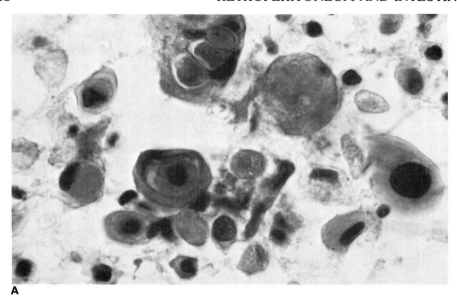

A

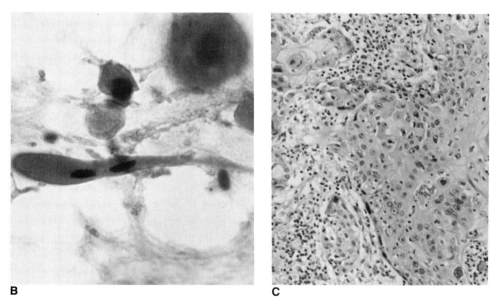

B   C

Fig. 6.1. Well-differentiated squamous cell carcinoma. **A.** ABC. Note marked variation in size and shape of the tumor cells, dense refractile cytoplasm, well-demarcated cell borders, and opaque nuclei. (H & E preparation; ×500). **B.** ABC. Note a tadpole cell. (H & E preparation; ×500). **C.** Histologic section showing keratinizing squamous cell carcinoma. (H & E preparation; ×160).

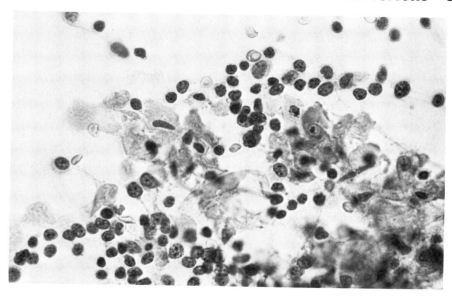

Fig. 6.2. Well-differentiated squamous cell carcinoma. ABC. The extremely differentiated tumor cells shown here resemble the dysplastic squamous cells of the uterine cervix. (H & E preparation; ×310).

ularities. The chromatin is finely to coarsely granular and unevenly distributed. Prominent nucleoli are usually present, and may be single or multiple. Cytoplasm is generally abundant and of a delicate, amphophilic, clear color, with occasional eosinophilia. Intracytoplasmic mucin may be observed as single vacuole or diffuse fine vacuolation **(Fig. 6.5)**. The most differentiated adenocarcinomas are exemplified by those originating from the bowel and show well-developed glands. The cells are columnar, arranged radially around a central lumen, with the nuclei located peripherally away from the luminal surface **(Fig. 6.6)**. When aspirated, some of the larger glands may be broken up and present as long strips of columnar cells in a characteristic side-by-side or picket-fence arrangement **(Fig. 6.7)**. In less well-differentiated tumors, there are merely clusters of epithelial cells with no attempt at lumen formation. The most undifferentiated adenocarcinomas may contain bizarre giant cells, simulating a pleomorphic sarcoma. These tumors are called giant cell adenocarcinomas and most commonly originate from the lung or pancreas. Identification of tumor cells with an epithelial pattern is a clue to the correct diagnosis **(Fig. 6.8)**.

Determination of the primary site of adenocarcinoma is often not feasible. When the patient has a previously documented cancer, it is important to review the histologic slides and compare them with the NAB specimen. Certain adenocarcinomas, however, show cytologic features that may be characteristic enough to suggest their origin. In prostatic adenocarcinomas, the microacinus is the most characteristic cellular structure. Unlike intestinal adenocarcinomas, in which the neoplastic cells are large and often columnar, the prostatic cells forming the microacinus are smaller and cuboidal, with minimal cellular pleomorphism **(Fig. 6.9)**. Metastatic mammary carcinomas have multiple patterns of cellular presentation, depending on the tumor type and cell size.

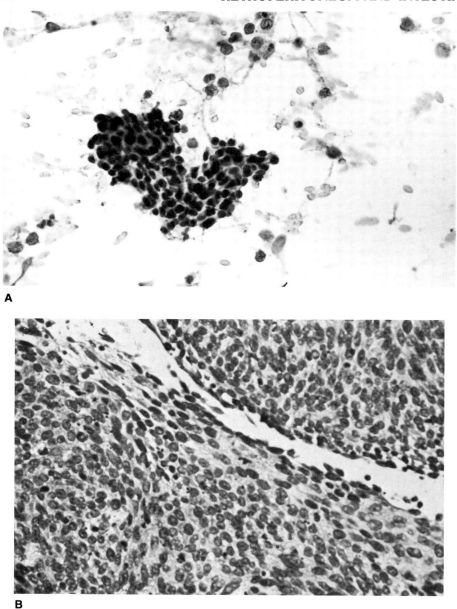

Fig. 6.3. Poorly differentiated squamous cell carcinoma in a lymph node, ABC. **A.** Note nonkeratinizing small squamous cells occurring as irregular, syncytial group. (H & E preparation; ×310). **B.** Histologic section of poorly differentiated squamous cell carcinoma with small oval cells. Keratinization is not seen in this field. (H & E preparation; ×310).

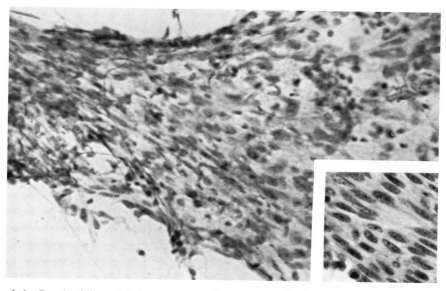

Fig. 6.4. Poorly differentiated squamous cell carcinoma, ABC. Note a syncytial tissue fragment consisting of densely packed spindle-shaped cells. *Inset:* Histology of the squamous cell carcinoma demonstrating the spindled squamous cells. (H & E preparation; ×310, inset ×500).

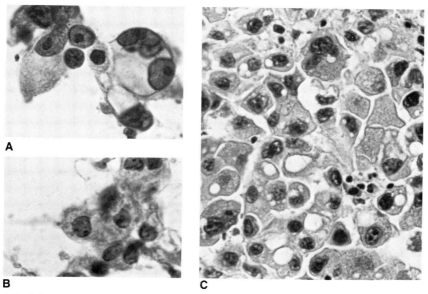

Fig. 6.5. Mucin-producing adenocarcinoma. **A,B.** ABC. Note rounded and columnar cells with cytoplasmic vacuolation and prominent nucleoli. **C.** Histologic section. Note cytoplasmic mucin vacuoles. (H & E preparation; A, B, C, ×500).

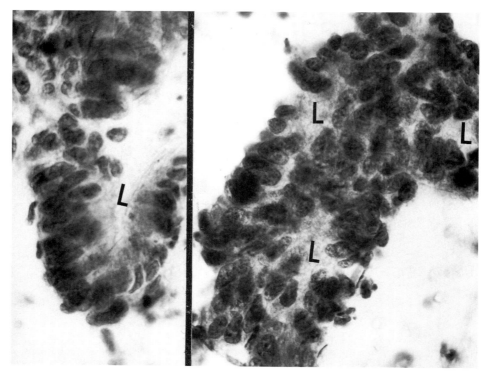

Fig. 6.6. Well-differentiated adenocarcinoma, gland-forming type, ABC. **A.** Note overlapping, columnar cells in side-by-side (picket-fence) arrangement. Nuclei are polarized away from the lumen (L). **B.** A complex tissue fragment consisting of three glandular units with lumina (L). Also note columnar cells in side-by-side arrangement (H & E preparation; A, B, ×500).

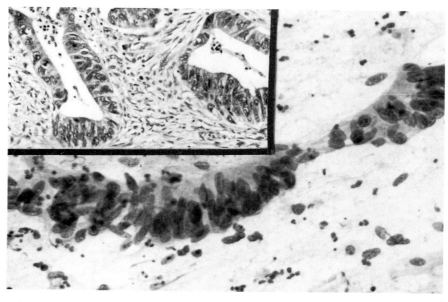

Fig. 6.7. Well-differentiated adenocarcinoma, ABC. A long strip of columnar cell epithelium, representing part of the wall from a large gland. *Inset:* Histologic section showing large malignant glands composed of palisading columnar cells. (H & E preparation; ×500, inset ×310).

142

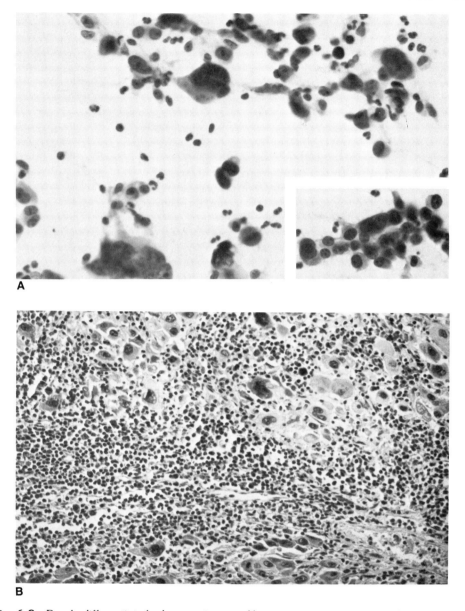

Fig. 6.8. Poorly differentiated adenocarcinoma of lung metastatic to paraaortic lymph nodes. **A.** ABC. Note large pleomorphic cells admixed with small lymphocytes. *Inset:* Note a cell cluster with attempted gland formation. (H & E preparation; ×310, inset ×310). **B.** Autopsy histologic section of metastatic poorly differentiated adenocarcinoma in a retroperitoneal lymph node. Note large malignant cells. (H & E preparation; ×310).

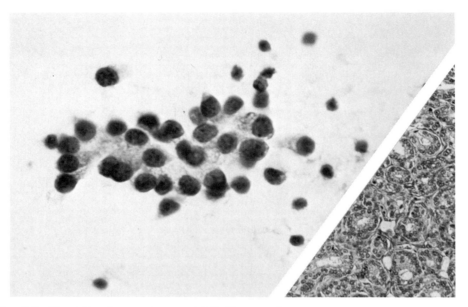

Fig. 6.9. Prostatic adenocarcinoma, ABC. Note small hyperchromatic cells arranged in a microacinar pattern. *Inset:* Histologic section of the primary prostatic adenocarcinoma. (H & E preparation; ×500, inset ×125).

When the aspirate shows dense clusters of overlapping tumor cells, it is not distinguishable from adenocarcinoma from other sites. There is, however, one pattern that is quite characteristic of metastatic breast carcinoma, but unfortunately it is not commonly encountered in NAB specimens. It consists of monolayered cells arranged in small loose groups or lying singly in a linear fashion, the so-called Indian-file pattern **(Fig. 6.10).** In ovarian adenocarcinomas, a frequently encountered pattern is that of papillary formations with psammoma bodies (*vide infra*).

Papillary Carcinoma

Papillary carcinomas are a variant of adenocarcinoma. When they are found as metastases in the retroperitoneum, the most likely primary sites are the gastrointestinal tract, ovary, and uterus, although they may also arise from other organs such as the lung and thyroid. The most characteristic feature of a papillary carcinoma is the presence of many finger-like processes, or fronds. These fronds are covered by a profuse neoplastic epithelium. Unlike a glandular structure, where the center is occupied by a lumen, the papillary core is made up of fibrovascular connective tissue. In histologic sections, the fibrous core is easily discernible when the plane of section passes through the middle of the frond **(Fig. 6.11A).** In aspirates, the fibrovascular core is only occasionally seen **(Fig. 6.11B);** instead, the papillae are often seen as three-dimensional, solid fronds, with peripheral cells forming a sharply defined, smooth community border **(Fig. 6.11C).** If there is adequate cytoplasm, one will notice that the orientation of the nuclei is opposite that of glandular structures. The basal ends

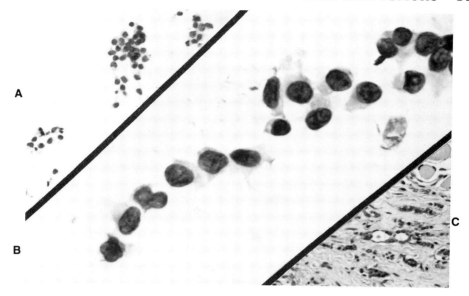

Fig. 6.10. Adenocarcinoma of the breast metastatic to the retroperitoneum. **A.** ABC. Low magnification view showing several clusters of loosely grouped tumor cells. **B.** High magnification view. Note polygonal cells with hyperchromatic nuclei, high nuclear–cytoplasmic (N:C) ratio, and an Indian file arrangement. **C.** Autopsy histologic section of a subdiaphragmatic metastatic nodule. Note tumor cells arranged in ductules and in linear arrangement. (H & E preparation; A ×125, B ×500, C ×125).

of the cells with their nuclei are identified toward the center of the papilla, whereas those of glandular cells are peripherally placed away from the central lumen. Another feature of papillary adenocarcinomas is the frequent presence of psammoma bodies, which are laminated, basophilic, calcified spherules measuring 30–100 μm in diameter **(Fig. 6.12)**. In about 15% of the ovarian adenocarcinomas in our file, psammoma bodies were identified in the NAB specimens.

Small Cell Anaplastic Carcinoma

Metastatic small cell anaplastic carcinoma of the lung is one of the tumors capable of producing a widespread lymphadenopathy, even though the primary tumor may be very small or undetectable. Although the majority arise in the bronchial epithelium, the possibility of other primary sites should be recognized. Small cell anaplastic carcinoma has been reported to occur in the esophagus, pancreas, cervix, salivary gland, and other organs.[9–11]

The ABC of small cell anaplastic carcinoma **(Fig. 6.13)** shows numerous small, pleomorphic cells with scanty basophilic cytoplasm and indistinct cytoplasmic borders. The nuclei are hyperchromatic, rounded or angulated, and show diffuse dispersion of coarse chromatin. Nucleoli are typically absent, but occasionally small multinucleoli

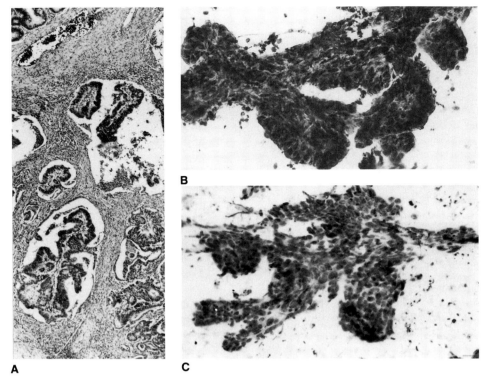

Fig. 6.11. Papillary adenocarcinoma of colon. **A.** Histologic section showing numerous papillary fronds with central fibrovascular cores. **B.** ABC. Retroperitoneal metastasis. Note papillary fronds with central fibrous cores and smooth outer community borders. **C.** ABC. Note solid papillae with no discernible fibrovascular cores. The centers of the fronds are occupied by *en face* tumor cells. (H & E preparation; A: ×125; B: ×180; C: ×160).

may be seen. The tumor cells are arranged single or in small aggregates with nuclear crowding and molding. The smear background often contains abundant necrotic nuclear debris, which may serve to distinguish this tumor from malignant lymphoma (see **Table 5.4**).

Malignant Melanoma

Malignant melanoma frequently involves multiple organs when it metastasizes.[2] In the abdominal cavity, the commonly affected organs are the lymph nodes, liver, spleen, adrenals, and intestinal tract. Malignant melanoma is notorious for masquerading as other tumors, and among the tumors with which it is often confused are lymphoma and poorly differentiated carcinoma. The best safeguard against failing to recognize a metastatic malignant melanoma is to keep melanoma constantly in mind in the differential diagnosis of a wide range of neoplasms.

Many investigators have described in detail the cytologic features of malignant melanoma as seen on fine needle aspirates.[12-15] The aspirates are cell-rich, with variably sized tumor cells lying singly. Cohesive cell sheets are distinctly uncommon.

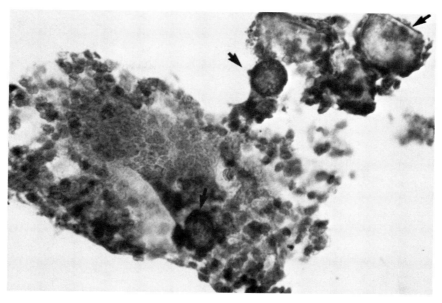

Fig. 6.12. Papillary serous adenocarcinoma of the ovary metastatic to the retroperitoneum. ABC. Note papillary tissue fragment showing *en face* cells. Psammoma bodies are indicated by arrows. (H & E preparation; ×310).

The prototypic cell **(Figs. 6.14–6.16)** is polygonal or round, and frequently has an eccentric nucleus, containing one or two macronucleoli. The nuclear eccentricity imparts a plasmacytoid appearance to some tumor cells. Intranuclear cytoplasmic inclusions can be seen in an occasional cell. Binucleation is fairly common. Cytoplasm varies from scanty to very abundant, often with a finely granulated texture. Kline and Kannan[12] divide the polygonal cells into three main groups according to their size: small cells (4 to 9 μm in diameter), medium-sized cells (10 to 20 μm), and giant cells (20 to 50 μm). These authors emphasize this characteristic triphasic-sized cell population **(Fig. 6.15),** which was observed in half of their cases. Although round or polygonal tumor cells predominate in most cases, fusiform or spindle cells **(Fig. 6.17)** may also be seen.

Melanin pigment, in the form of fine to coarse brown-black granules, may or may not be present. When present, it may be found in the cytoplasm of the neoplastic cells, in the macrophages, or extracellularly. Hemosiderin pigment is a potential source of confusion, particularly when the pigment granules are found within atypical macrophages. When needed, a Prussian blue stain for iron may be used to distinguish the two.

The ABC features of malignant melanoma are summarized in **Table 6.2.** When melanin pigment is sparse or absent, the polygonal melanoma cells may be mistaken for anaplastic carcinoma, large cell lymphoma, plasmacytoma, or seminoma. When the fusiform or spindle cells predominate, they may be mistaken for sarcoma or spindle cell variant of squamous carcinoma.

On immunostaining malignant melanoma is negative for leukocyte common antigen

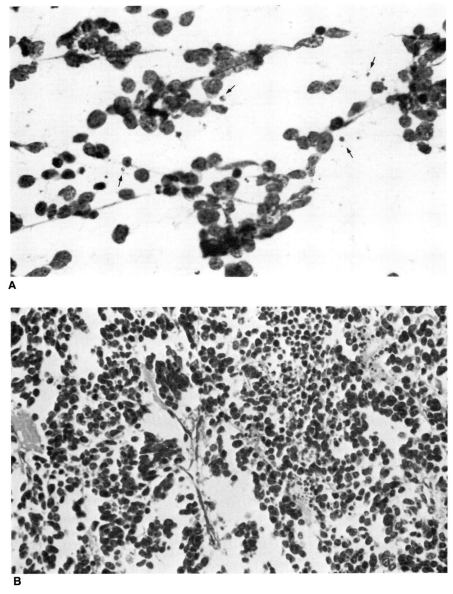

Fig. 6.13. Small cell anaplastic carcinoma of lung metastatic to the retroperitoneum. **A.** ABC. Note small cells with irregular nuclear membranes and nuclear molding. Arrows indicate necrotic nuclear debris in the background. (H & E preparation; ×500). **B.** Histologic section of the small cell anaplastic carcinoma at autopsy. Note extensive individual cell necrosis. (H & E preparation; ×310).

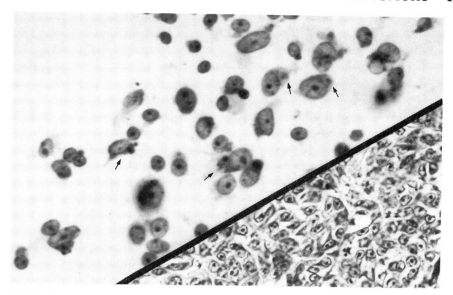

Fig. 6.14. Metastatic melanoma to retroperitoneal lymph nodes, ABC. Note the characteristic isolated cell pattern, prominent nucleoli, and cytoplasmic coarse pigment granules (*arrows*). *Inset:* Histologic section. (H & E preparation; ×500, inset: ×310).

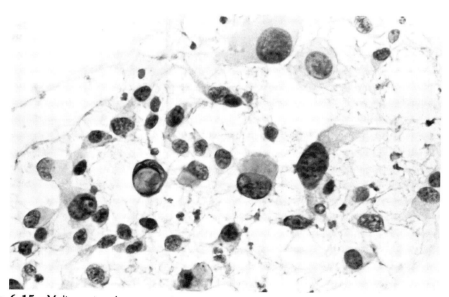

Fig. 6.15. Malignant melanoma metastatic to retroperitoneal lymph nodes, ABC. Note triphasic population of small, medium, and large tumor cells with eccentric nuclei and abundant granular cytoplasm. Also note dispersed cell pattern and a large intranuclear cytoplasmic inclusion. (H & E preparation; ×500).

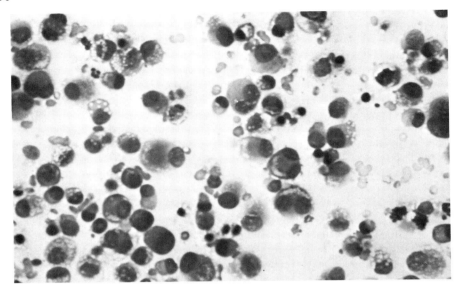

Fig. 6.16. Aspirate showing malignant melanoma cells with a plasmacytoid appearance misinterpreted as multiple myeloma by a pathology resident. This is an air-dried smear and the nuclear details are poorly preserved. Nucleolar prominence is not discernible. (May-Grünwald Giemsa preparation; ×500).

(LCA), cytokeratin, and epithelial membrane antigen. Positive reactions with antibodies to S100 protein and melanoma-cell antigen (HMB45) may be obtained in a large proportion of cases. Electron microscopy shows characteristic premelanosomes and melanosomes with diagnostic cross-striations **(Fig. 1.9).**

Carcinosarcoma

Although biphasic tumors composed of mesenchymal and epithelial tissues can arise in a variety of organs, such as the lung, breast, and pancreas, when found in the retroperitoneum or pelvis, one should seriously consider the possibility of metastases from malignant mixed mesodermal (müllerian) tumor of the uterus or ovary.[16,17] We have encountered two such cases of malignant mixed mesodermal tumor metastatic to the retroperitoneum. The aspirates were hypercellular and showed both malignant glandular cells and malignant spindle cells. The latter might represent fibrosarcoma, leiomyosarcoma, or endometrial stromal sarcoma, but characterization was not possible in the aspirates **(Fig. 6.18).** Not uncommonly, heterologous tissue elements such as rhabdomyosarcoma or chondrosarcoma are also present in the tumor.

Gynecologic Tumors

Although some workers have effectively used NAB to diagnose primary ovarian and uterine tumors,[18,19] this usage has remained controversial because of fear of causing intraperitoneal tumor dissemination.[20] However, NAB has become a powerful tool in

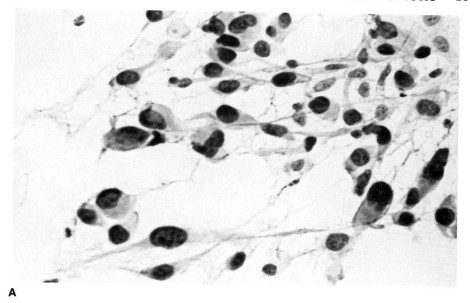

A

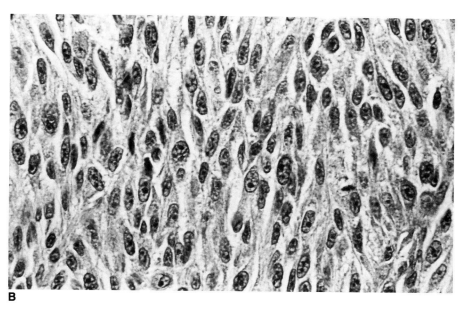

B

Fig. 6.17. Malignant melanoma, spindle cell variant. **A.** ABC. Note the predominant spindle cells, admixed with a few polygonal cells. (H & E preparation; ×500). **B.** Histologic section of spindle cell melanoma. The polygonal epithelioid cells are not present in this photomicrograph. (H & E preparation; ×500).

TABLE 6.2. Aspiration Biopsy Cytology of Malignant Melanoma

Dyshesive cell pattern (Cohesive cell sheets are distinctly uncommon)
Polygonal or oval and fusiform cells, sometimes bi- or multinucleated giant cells
Eccentric (plasmacytoid) nuclei with prominent nucleoli
Variable amounts of finely granular, brown melanin pigment
Special studies:
    a) Immunopositivity for S100 protein and HMB45
    b) Melanosomes and premelanosomes demonstrable by electron microscopy

evaluating patients with recurrent or metastatic gynecologic cancers. Many such patients have received prior radiation or chemotherapy, and further surgical intervention may result in significant complication.

The most commonly encountered ovarian carcinoma metastatic to the retroperitoneum is the adenocarcinoma, frequently of the papillary serous variety. The ABC of adenocarcinoma and its papillary variant has already been discussed in the earlier sections of this chapter. Neoplastic papillary fronds and psammoma bodies **(Fig. 6.12)** are characteristically seen in papillary serous adenocarcinoma of the ovary.

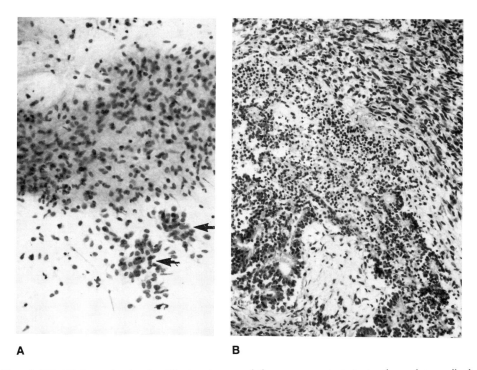

A   **B**

Fig. 6.18. Malignant mixed müllerian tumor of the ovary metastatic to the pelvic wall. **A.** ABC. Note primitive mesenchymal spindle cells in a mxyoid stroma and epithelial cells attempting to form small acinar structures (*arrows*). **B.** Autopsy histologic section. Note primitive spindle cells at upper right and gland formations at bottom. (H & E preparation; A ×160; B ×125).

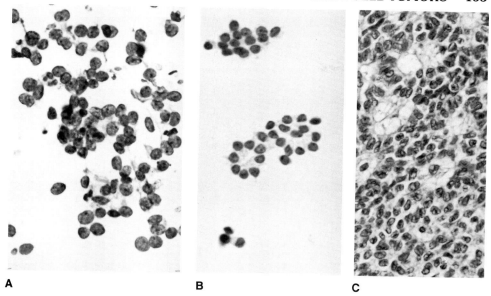

A   **B**   **C**

Fig.6.19. Granulosa cell tumor, recurrence in the pelvis 17 years after removal of the tumor in the left ovary. **A.** ABC. Note many small cells loosely arranged in poorly formed pseudorosettes. **B.** ABC. Note well-developed pseudorosettes, formed by radially oriented tumor cells. **C.** Histologic section from the originally resected granulosa cell tumor. Note many Call-Exner bodies.

Sarcomas of female organs also are encountered in needle aspirates. The most common ones are uterine leiomyosarcoma (see Chapter 5) and malignant mixed müllerian tumor of the ovary.

The common members of the sex cord-stromal tumors are the thecoma and granulosa cell tumor. Thecoma is seldom aspirated, because it is a benign tumor confined to the ovary. On the other hand, granulosa cell tumor, a low-grade malignancy, may present as bulky recurrence in the pelvis and lower abdomen, providing a suitable target for needle aspiration biopsy.[21-23] Unless the cytopathologist is familiar with the ABC of this tumor type, the diagnosis may not be easy. The tumor is well known for its late recurrence and it is not unusual that ten or more years elapse before recurrence occurs and the previous gynecologic surgery may be forgotten or considered irrelevant. The aspirates **(Figs. 6.19** and **6.20)** are generally quite cellular and consist of many single small cells as well as cell groups in a clean background. Granulosa cells have round, regular, uniform nuclei. The cytoplasm is indistinct and, when it is seen, most often faintly eosinophilic. In addition to the round cells, spindle cells, reminiscent of theca cells and fibroblasts, may be seen. The spindle cells have elongated or fusiform, bland nuclei and pale eosinophilic cytoplasm. These cells are generally not present in large numbers and may be easily overlooked. The round granulosa cells are arranged singly, in irregular groups, or in pseudorosettes. The latter correspond to the Call-Exner bodies seen in histologic sections. These are small follicular structures containing eosinophilic basement-membrane-like material with nuclear debris. On ABC, the Call-Exner pseudorosettes superficially resemble an acinus, containing inspissated secretion. Both consist of radially oriented cells; however, in con-

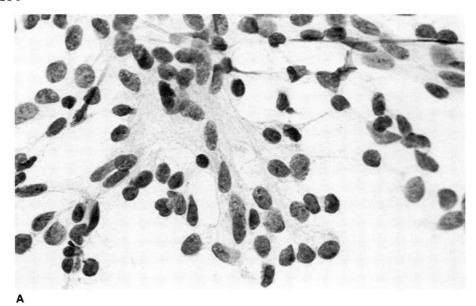

A

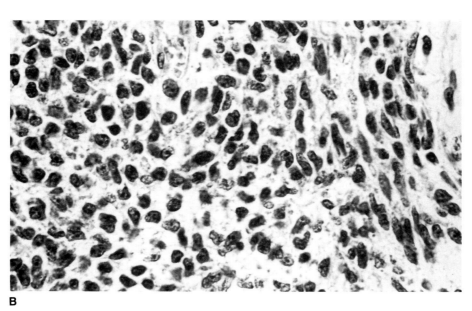

B

Fig. 6.20. Bulky recurrence of granulosa cell tumor in the lower abdomen. **A.** ABC. Note small round cells admixed with some spindle cells. Superficially, these cells resemble small cell anaplastic carcinoma, but note clean background with no necrotic debris. (H & E preparation; ×500). **B.** Histologic section of the recurrent granulosa cell tumor. (H & E preparation; ×500).

trast to glandular acini, Call-Exner bodies have a fuzzy or indefinite central margin. Granulosa cells do not contain glycogen or mucin, but they may contain lipid. Longitudinal nuclear grooves are a characteristic feature of granulosa cells in histologic sections; unfortunately they are difficult to see on aspirate smears.

The differential diagnosis of granulosa cell tumor includes small cell anaplastic carcinoma, carcinoid tumor, and lymphoma.[23] The nuclei of small cell anaplastic carcinoma are hyperchromatic, usually of unequal size and shape. Nuclear molding and cell necrosis are common findings. In the case of carcinoid tumor, the cells generally have more cytoplasm than granulosa cells. The cytoplasm is finely granulated and the border is distinct. The nuclei are more round and lack indentations or grooves. The acini of carcinoid tumors are more sharply outlined than the Call-Exner bodies. Carcinoid cells contain neurosecretory granules, which can be readily demonstrated by histochemistry, immunocytochemistry, or electron microscopy. Lymphomas are distinguished by a dispersed cell pattern. The smears do not contain spindle-shaped cells and lack epithelial groupings or the pseudorosettes of Call-Exner bodies. Immunostaining of the cells for LCA shows positive immunoreactivity.

Germ Cell Tumors

Germ cell tumors are not as rare as was once believed. They are among the most highly treatable tumors.[24] Many of the so-called retroperitoneal undifferentiated carcinomas of unknown primary site in young adult males are now believed to be germ cell tumors.[25] In a review of 49 retroperitoneal neoplasms, Parkinson and Chabrel[26] identified 20 germ cell tumors. In eight patients the retroperitoneum appeared to be the primary site. In 12 patients the retroperitoneal tumor was a metastasis from a primary testicular tumor, and in seven of these the gonad was not clinically suspected as the primary site until after biopsy or surgery had been performed. Interestingly, a recent study reported that in those patients with retroperitoneal germ cell tumors and no obvious primary site, only 21% showed normal testicular histology, others had premalignant carcinoma in situ or evidence of atrophy and hyaline change of the seminiferous tubules, suggesting a rejected primary tumor.[27]

The clinical extragonadal germ cell cancer syndrome was recognized and described as early as 1981 (Table 6.3).[28,29] Without a morphologic diagnosis, however, the clinical features are not unequivocal. The basis for the diagnosis is a combination of morphology[30–35] and determination of the serum markers: placental alkaline phosphatase (PLAP), α-fetoprotein (AFP), and β-human chorionic gonadotropin (β-HCG). Fine needle aspiration biopsy plays a useful role in the diagnosis of extragonadal and metastatic germ cell cancer.[36]

TABLE 6.3. The Extragonadal Germ Cell Cancer Syndrome*

Usually occurs in younger men (<50 yr). Women are rarely affected.
Tumor in the midline (mediastinum, retroperitoneum) or multiple pulmonary nodules.
Serum levels of β-HCG, AFP, or both are elevated.
Evidence of rapid tumor growth.
A good response to previously administered radiotherapy or chemotherapy.

*Adapted from Greco and Hainsworth.[29]
β-HCG = beta–human chorionic gonadotropin; AFP = α-fetoprotein.

Seminoma

Seminoma is the most common malignant germ cell tumor in males. In females the identical tumor in the ovary is called dysgerminoma and is rather uncommon. The ABC (**Fig. 6.21** and **Table 6.4**) of seminoma (dysgerminoma) consists of numerous dispersed, large round cells with abundant clear to vacuolated cytoplasm. A central, large, eosinophilic nucleus, giving rise to a bull's eye appearance, is characteristic. Multiple nucleoli can also sometimes be seen. The cytoplasmic border is well-defined, which is a useful feature in differentiating seminoma from embryonal carcinoma (*vide infra*). Large cell lymphoma can simulate seminoma, but the reniform or cleaved character of the lymphoma nuclei generally enables one to make the correct diagnosis.

Immunostains may be helpful in difficult cases. Seminoma cells are positive for PLAP.[37] However, PLAP is very sensitive to fixation, which often induces false negativity. Antibodies to PLAP, keratin, and leukocyte common antigen, when employed in combination, are helpful in distinguishing between seminoma, carcinoma, and lymphoma. Their immunophenotypic profiles are as follows: seminoma (PLAP +, keratin −, and LCA −), carcinoma (PLAP −, keratin +, LCA −) and lymphoma (PLAP −, keratin −, and LCA +).

Embryonal Carcinoma and Yolk Sac Tumor

Embryonal carcinoma and yolk sac tumor were considered together as one group in the older classification.[38] It is difficult to distinguish between the two on ABC (**Table 6.5**). Generally, cells of embryonal carcinoma are larger and more pleomorphic than those of yolk sac tumor (known also as endodermal sinus tumor). Unlike seminoma cells, which are uniform, round, and dispersed, cells in this group of tumors show more pleomorphism and tend to cluster like adenocarcinoma. The nuclei exhibit clumped chromatin, irregular nuclear contour, and prominent nucleoli, which may be single or multiple. Whereas the cytoplasmic borders of seminoma cells are well-defined, the cells of embryonal carcinoma and yolk sac tumor have indistinct cytoplasmic membranes, creating a syncytial appearance (**Fig. 6.22**). Brightly eosinophilic globules may sometimes be found within the cytoplasm of the tumor cells, particularly more often in yolk sac tumors (**Fig. 6.23**). These hyaline globules are PAS-positive and diastase-resistant. Immunostaining for α-fetoprotein is positive in the cytoplasm of the tumor cells and within some of these globules.[39] In addition, some giant cells are positive for β-HCG, indicating syncytiotrophoblastic differentiation. Although these tumors may mimic a poorly differentiated adenocarcinoma on light microscopic examination, they do not immunostain for epithelial membrane antigen as many adenocarcinomas do.

Choriocarcinoma

This tumor is a highly malignant germ cell tumor, and it may arise as a uterine tumor associated with a pregnancy or as a gonadal tumor. The nongestational choriocarcinoma seldom occurs as a pure tumor, but often contains other germ cell elements. At times the gonads are normal and the tumor may be considered as an extragonadal germ cell tumor. The morphologic diagnosis of choriocarcinoma is based on the

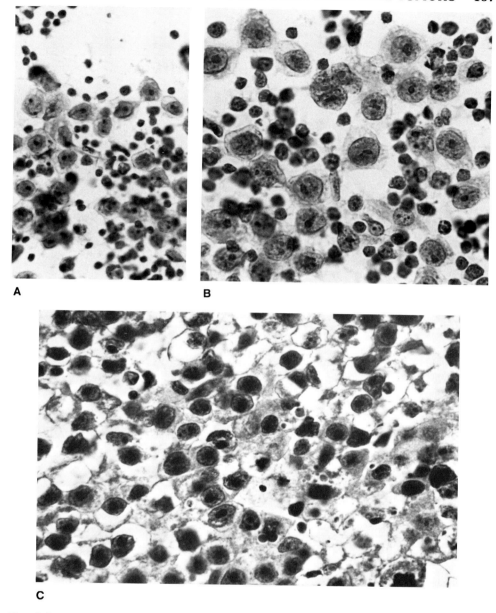

A

B

C

Fig. 6.21. Testicular seminoma manifesting first as a retroperitoneal mass. **A,B.** ABC. Note dispersed cells having large round uniform nuclei, eosinophilic macronucleoli, and pale or clear cytoplasm with well-defined margin. The small cells are lymphocytes. (H & E preparation; A ×310, B ×600). **C.** Histologic section of the primary testicular seminoma. (H & E preparation; ×500).

TABLE 6.4. Aspiration Biopsy Cytology of Seminoma (Dysgerminoma)

Homogeneous population of dispersed, large round cells
Uniform, round, vesicular nuclei
One or two central macronucleoli (bull's eye appearance)
Clear or vacuolated cytoplasm with distinct outline

TABLE 6.5. Aspiration Biopsy Cytology of Embryonal Carcinoma and Yolk Sac Tumor

Papillary syncytial clusters of anaplastic cells, simulating poorly differentiated adenocarcinoma (but true glandular formations are absent).

Single cells are infrequent.

Anaplastic nuclei with large, irregular nucleoli.

PAS-positive, diastase-resistant, hyaline globules in cytoplasm (particularly in yolk sac tumors).

Immunoperoxidase stains show α-fetoprotein in tumor cells and within some hyaline globules.

PAS = periodic acid-Schiff stain.

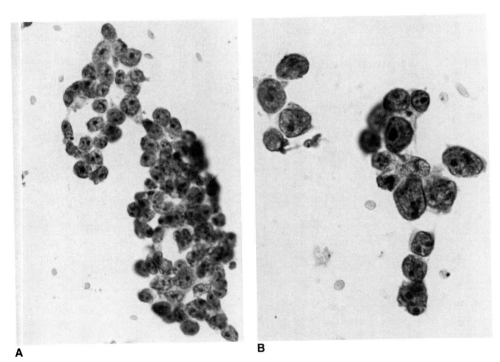

A   **B**

Fig. 6.22 Recurrent embryonal carcinoma in the retroperitoneum. **A,B.** ABC. Note clusters of tumor cells simulating adenocarcinoma, but true glandular formations are not seen. Generally, cells of embryonal carcinoma are much more pleomorphic than those of adenocarcinoma. Note macronucleoli similar to those seen in seminoma, but the cytoplasmic margins are indistinct resulting in syncytia. (H & E preparation; A ×310; B ×500).

158

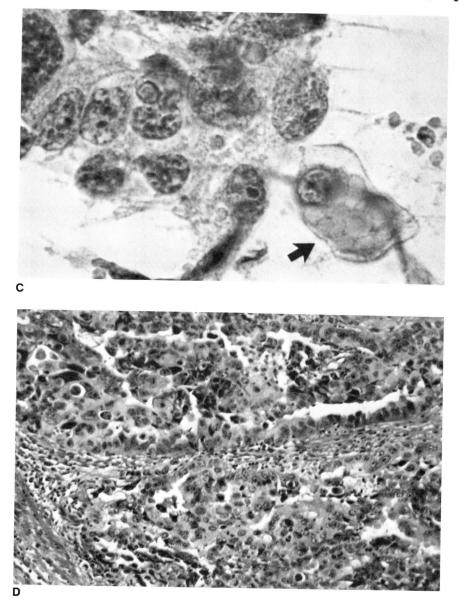

Fig. 6.22 C. ABC. Higher magnification of a syncytial group of tumor cells, one of which contains numerous eosinophilic hyaline globules in the cytoplasm (*arrow*). (H & E preparation; ×1,200). **D.** Histologic section of the original embryonal carcinoma of the testis. (H & E preparation; ×310).

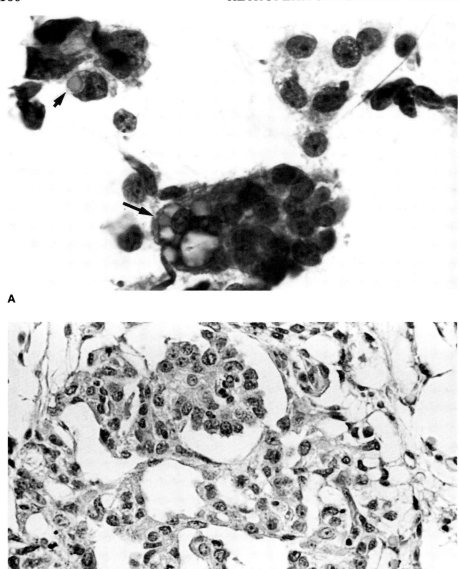

Fig. 6.23. Metastatic yolk sac tumor in the retroperitoneum. **A.** ABC. The tumor cells are arranged in small nests, and are more uniform and smaller than those of embryonal carcinoma. Arrows indicate cytoplasmic eosinophilic globules. (H & E preparation; ×500). **B.** Histologic section of yolk sac tumor showing multiple cleftlike spaces transversed by interconnecting cords of tumor cells. (H & E preparation; ×310).

TABLE 6.6. Aspiration Biopsy Cytology of Choriocarcinoma

An extensively necrotic and hemorrhagic aspirate.

Large pleomorphic multinucleated giant cells with abundant granular or vacuolated cytoplasm (syncytiotrophoblastic cells).

Large pleomorphic mononucleated or binucleated cells (intermediate trophoblasts).

Smaller, round, uniform mononucleate cells (cytotrophoblastic cells) in loose clusters.

In all cell types, nuclear hyperchromatism is often marked, and nucleoli are prominent.

Immunostaining for β-HCG is positive in the syncytiotrophoblast and the intermediate trophoblast cells.

β-HCG = beta–human chorionic gonadotropin.

identification of various types of trophoblast cells in a highly hemorrhagic and necrotic background **(Table 6.6)**. The cytotrophoblast cells **(Fig. 6.24A)** are uniform, round, medium-sized cells with distinct cell borders and a single malignant nucleus. They have a tendency to form loose sheets. The syncytiotrophoblast cells **(Plate 6.1A and Fig. 6.24C)** are large multinucleated cells containing bizarre, irregular, hyperchromatic nuclei. Cytoplasm is abundant and varies from homogeneous to vacuolated. The intermediate trophoblast cells have cytologic features that bridge those of cytotrophoblast and syncytiotrophoblast. The intermediate trophoblast cells **(Figs. 6.24B and 6.25)** differ from the cytotrophoblast cells by being larger in size and having greater nuclear pleomorphism. They are generally mononucleated, but binucleated and multinucleated forms are also present. They vary in shape, ranging from round to spindle-shaped, with abundant cytoplasm. Immunoperoxidase staining will show positive reactivity for β-HCG in the cytoplasm of the syncytiotrophoblast and the intermediate trophoblast cells **(Plate 6.1B)**, and absence of reactivity in the cytotrophoblast cells.[40] It should be noted that the presence of syncytiotrophoblast giant cells without accompanying cytotrophoblast cells is not sufficient to establish the diagnosis of choriocarcinoma, because the former can also be seen occasionally in other types of germ cell tumor.

Teratoma

Teratoma are neoplasms composed of elements derived from all three germ layers. Microscopically, a wide range of tissue in various stages of maturation may be seen, including neuroepithelium, epidermis, bronchial and intestinal epithelia, as well as mesenchymal tissues. The malignant potential of these tumors is related to the presence of immature or partially differentiated tissues. However, even perfectly mature teratomas have been known to metastasize from adult testes. In contrast, mature teratomas of the ovary are benign.

Not uncommonly, malignant components of other germ cell tumors, such as embryonal carcinoma or choriocarcinoma, may also be present in a teratoma (teratocarcinoma), and the presence of these elements should be specified in the diagnosis.

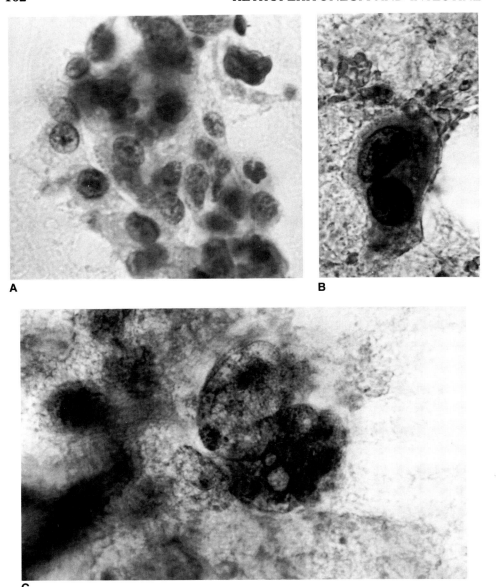

A   B

C

Fig. 6.24. Aspirate of a choriocarcinoma presenting as a large retroperitoneal mass in a 19-year-old man. The serum β-HCG was subsequently found to be markedly elevated. **A.** Note a loose cluster of cytotrophoblast cells with fairly round, uniform nuclei, prominent nucleoli, and demarcated cytoplasmic borders. There is a certain resemblance of cytotrophoblast cells to seminoma cells, except the former tend to occur in groups. **B.** Note an intermediate trophoblast cell containing two malignant nuclei. The background is markedly hemorrhagic. (H & E preparation; A ×500; B ×500). **C.** Note a multinucleate syncytiotrophoblast cell in a hemorrhagic necrotic background. (H & E preparation; ×500).

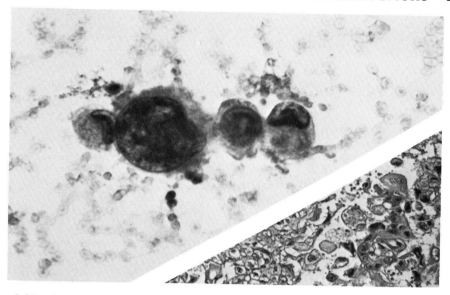

Fig. 6.25. Aspirate of metastatic choriocarcinoma in the retroperitoneum. The patient had a previous testicular teratocarcinoma. Note several intermediate trophoblastic cells with hyperchromatic coarse chromatin, prominent nucleoli, and granular cytoplasm with well-defined borders. It is not clear whether the largest cell shows genuine multinucleation or hyperlobation of the nucleus. Note hemorrhagic background. *Inset:* Cell block section. Note the characteristic admixture of different forms of malignant trophoblast. (H & E preparation; ×500, inset ×310).

ACCURACY OF FINE NEEDLE ASPIRATION BIOPSY

Diagnosis of metastatic disease of the retroperitoneal lymph nodes by NAB is highly accurate when adequate specimens are obtained.[41–46] Cochand-Priollet et al[41] reported a series of 228 patients with genitourinary tract cancer who underwent NABs of retroperitoneal lymph nodes as part of the staging evaluation. The overall diagnostic accuracy of the procedure was 93%. There were 5% false-negative results and no false-positive diagnoses. Bonfiglio et al[42] reported a series of 47 patients who underwent NABs of retroperitoneal lymph nodes for metastatic workup; the NAB was positive for metastasis in 11 patients. There were no false-positive examinations but two negative aspirations proved to have metastatic nodal disease during the follow-up procedures. Al-Mofleh[43] analyzed 37 cases and reported a diagnostic specificity of 100% and a sensitivity of 85%. In a series reported by Wajsman et al[44] 57 patients with genitourinary cancers had abdominal and/or pelvic node aspirations. Adequate specimens were obtained in 41 patients (72%). In 26 of the patients with adequate cytologic specimens, histologic findings of lymph node dissection were available for correlation. Cytologic-histologic concordance was found in 17 patients (65%), false-negative findings in seven patients (27%), and false-positive findings in two patients (8%). The seven patients with false-negative findings had microscopic involvement of the lymph nodes. The authors cautioned that a negative cytologic report should

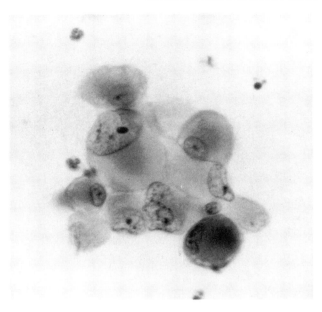

Fig. 6.26. Transabdominal NAB showing a cluster of highly atypical mesothelial cells which was misinterpreted as recurrent adenocarcinoma. The patient had undergone a colectomy for adenocarcinoma 5 months previously.

not always be viewed as definitive and if clinically indicated a repeat aspiration or surgery should be performed. In the case of unsatisfactory specimens, the aspiration should be repeated as well.

On the other hand, it is quite safe to assume that positive cytology can confirm the evidence of lymph node involvement and can spare the patient unnecessary radical surgery or staging lymphadenectomy. In the two patients with false-positive results in their study, one had invasive bladder cancer and received radiation to the pelvic nodes after NAB, with apparent sterilization of the nodes. While no nodal metastasis could be found at the time of subsequent surgical lymph node dissection, a metastasis in the liver was identified, providing support to the validity of this explanation. In the second case, review of the cytologic slides showed obvious malignant cells typical of prostatic cancer cells. The authors believed that more meticulous examination of the removed lymph nodes might have uncovered the metastasis, citing a study in which a 33% increase in positive identification of nodal metastases was achieved by serial sectioning of the apparently pathologically negative lymph nodes.[47]

We reviewed the NABs of abdominal, pelvic, and retroperitoneal lymph nodes, performed in a 3-year period, 1988 to 1990, from 103 patients who had previously documented carcinomas. Satisfactory material was obtained in 85 cases (83%). Positive metastatic cytology was reported in 62 cases and benign cytology in 23 cases. Clinical and/or histologic follow-up of these 85 cases revealed one false-positive report and six false-negative reports. The one false-positive report occurred in a 49-year-old woman who had had an adenocarcinoma of the colon resected 8 months earlier. The FNA showed groups of highly atypical mesothelial cells **(Fig. 6.26)** diagnosed erroneously as adenocarcinoma. The sensitivity of NAB in our series was 90%, specificity 94%, predictive value of a positive report 98%, and predictive value of a negative report 74%. The high predictive value of a positive report in our hands means that a positive cytologic diagnosis is reliable evidence of metastatic disease; however, one must be cautious in accepting a negative cytologic report because of its low predictive value.

REFERENCES

1. Bowman LC, Santana VM, Green AA, et al: Staging systems in neuroblastoma; which is best? *J Clin Oncol* 9:189–193, 1991.

2. Amer MH, Al-Sarraf M, Vaitkevicius VK: Clinical presentation, natural history and prognostic factors in advanced malignant melanoma. *Surg Gynecol Obstet* 149:687–692, 1979.

3. Kelly SL, Meyer TJ: Carcinomas of unknown primary site: A prudent approach. *Postgrad Med* 74:269–280, 1983.

4. Steckel RJ, Kagan AR: Metastatic tumors of unknown origin. *Cancer* 67:1242–1244, 1991.

5. Smith RB, Haskell CM: Testis. In Haskell CM: *Cancer Treatment.* Philadelphia, Saunders, 1990, pp 779–797.

6. Urba WJ, Longo DL: Lymphocytic lymphomas: Clinical course and management. In Moossa AR, Schimpff SC, Robson MC: *Comprehensive Textbook of Oncology.* Baltimore, Williams & Wilkins, 1991, pp 1277–1295.

7. Urba WJ, Longo DL: Burkitt's lymphoma. In Moossa AR, Schimpff SC, Robson MC: *Comprehensive Textbook of Oncology.* Baltimore, Williams & Wilkins, 1991, pp 1296–1301.

8. Kagan AR, Steckel RJ: Abdominal mass and cervical adenopathy in a child. *AJR* 132:643–645.

9. Sabanathan S, Graham GP, Salama FD: Primary oat cell carcinoma of the esophagus. *Thorax* 41:318–321, 1986.

10. Gnepp DR, Corio RL, Brannon RB: Small cell carcinoma of the major salivary glands. *Cancer* 58:705–714, 1986.

11. Groben P, Reddick R, Askin F: The pathologic spectrum of small cell carcinoma of the cervix. *Int J Gynecol Pathol* 4:42–57, 1985.

12. Kline TS, Kannan V: Aspiration biopsy cytology of melanoma. *Am J Clin Pathol* 77:597–601, 1982.

13. Gutpa SK, Rajwanshi AK, Das DK: Fine needle aspiration cytology smear patterns of malignant melanoma. *Acta Cytol* 29:983–988, 1985.

14. Woyke S, Domegala W, Czerniak B, et al: Fine needle aspiration cytology of malignant melanoma of skin. *Acta Cytol* 24:529–538, 1980.

15. Schwartz JG, Zollars PR: Fine needle aspiration cytology of malignant melanoma of soft parts. *Acta Cytol* 34:397–400, 1990.

16. Nguyen GK: Cytopathologic aspects of a metastatic malignant mixed müllerian tumor of the uterus. Report of a case with transabdominal fine needle aspiration biopsy. *Acta Cytol* 26:521–526, 1982.

17. Silverman JF, Gardner J, Larkin EW, et al: Ascitic fluid cytology in a case of metastatic malignant mixed mesodermal tumor of the ovary. *Acta Cytol* 30:173–176, 1986.

18. Kjellgren O, Angström T: Aspiration biopsy cytology of ovarian tumors. In Blaustein A (ed): *Pathology of Female Genital Tract.* New York, Springer-Verlag, 1982, pp 741–751.

19. Kohler MF, Clarke-Pearson DL: Fine-needle aspiration biopsy in gynecologic oncology. *Clin Obstet Gynecol* 35:73–88, 1992.

20. Trimbos JB, Hacker NF: The case against aspirating ovarian cysts. *Cancer* 72:828–831, 1993.

21. Fidler WJ: Recurrent granulosa-cell tumor: Aspiration cytology findings. *Acta Cytol* 26: 688–690, 1982.

22. Ehya H, Lang WR: Cytology of granulosa cell tumor of the ovary. *Am J Clin Pathol* 85:402–405, 1986.

23. Brenda JA, Zaleski S: Fine needle aspiration cytologic features of hepatic metastasis of granulosa cell tumor of the ovary. Differential diagnosis. *Acta Cytol* 32:527–532, 1988.

24. Roth BJ, Greist A, Kubilis PS, et al: Cisplatin-based combination chemotherapy for disseminated germ cell tumors: Long-term follow-up. *J Clin Oncol* 6:1239–1247, 1988.

25. Hainsworth JD, Greco FA: Poorly differentiated carcinoma and germ cell tumors. *Hematol Oncol Clin North Am* 5:1223–1231, 1991.

26. Parkinson MC, Chabrel CM: Clinicopathological features of retroperitoneal tumors. *Br J Urol* 56:17–23, 1984.

27. Daugaard G, Rorth M, Vondermaase H, et al: Management of extragonadal germ-cell tumors and the significance of bilateral testicular biopsies. *Ann Oncol* 3:283–289, 1992.

28. Richardson RL, Schoumacher RA, Fer MF, et al: The unrecognized extragonadal germ cell cancer syndrome. *Ann Intern Med* 94:181–186, 1981.

29. Greco FA, Hainsworth JD: Cancer of unknown primary site. In DeVita VJ, Hellman S, Rosenberg SA: *Cancer: Principles and Practice of Oncology.* Philadelphia, Lippincott, 1993, pp 2072–2092.

30. Akhtar M, Ali MA, Huq M, et al: Fine needle aspiration biopsy of seminoma and dysgerminoma: Cytologic, histologic and electron microscopy correlations. *Diagn Cytopathol* 6:99–105, 1990.

31. Akhtar M, Ali MA, Sackey K, et al: Fine needle aspiration biopsy diagnosis of endodermal sinus tumor: Histologic and ultrastructural correlations. *Diagn Cytopathol* 6:184–192, 1990.

32. Fleury-Feith J, Bellot-Besnard J: Criteria for aspiration cytology for the diagnosis of seminoma. *Diagn Cytopathol* 5:392–395, 1989.

33. Dominquez-Franjo P, Vargus J, Rodriguez-Peralto JL, et al: Fine needle aspiration biopsy findings in endodermal sinus tumors. *Acta Cytol* 37:209–215, 1993.

34. Sangalli G, Livraghi T, Giordano F, et al: Primary mediastinal embryonal carcinoma and choriocarcinoma. A case report. *Acta Cytol* 30:543–546, 1986.

35. Balslev E, Francis D, Jacobsen GK: Testicular germ cell tumors. Classification based on fine needle aspiration biopsy. *Acta Cytol* 34:690–694, 1990.

36. Oliver RTD, Highman WJ, Kellette MJ, et al. The value of fine needle aspiration cytology in the management of metastatic germ cell tumors. *Br J Urol* 57:200–203, 1985.

37. Manivel JC, Jessurun J, Wick MR, et al: Placental alkaline phosphatase immunoreactivity in testicular germ-cell neoplasms. *Am J Surg Pathol* 11:21–29, 1987.

38. Dixon FJ, Moore RA: *Tumors of the Male Sex Organs. Fascicles 31b and 32, Atlas of Tumor Pathology.* Washington, DC, Armed Forces Institute of Pathology, 1952, pp 48–104.

39. Kapila K, Hajdu SI, Whitmore WF, et al: Cytologic diagnosis of metastatic germ-cell tumors. *Acta Cytol* 27:245–251, 1983.

40. Hoover LA, Hafiz MA: Fine needle aspiration diagnosis of extragonadal choriocarcinoma with immunoperoxidase studies. *Diagn Cytopathol* 5:84–87, 1989.

41. Cochand-Priollet B, Roger B, Boccon-Gibod I, et al: Retroperitoneal lymph node aspiration biopsy in staging of pelvic cancer: A study of 228 consecutive cases. *Diagn Cytopathol* 3:102–107, 1987.

42. Bonfiglio TA, MacIntosh PK, Patten SF Jr, et al: Fine needle aspiration cytopathology of retroperitoneal lymph nodes in the evaluation of metastatic disease. *Acta Cytol* 23:126–130, 1979.

43. Al-Mofleh IA: Ultrasound-guided fine needle aspiration of retroperitoneal, abdominal and pelvic nodes: Diagnostic reliability. *Acta Cytol* 36:413–415, 1992.

44. Wajsman Z, Beckley SA, Gamarra M, et al: Fine needle aspiration of metastatic lesions and regional lymph nodes in genitourinary cancer. *Urol* 19:356–360, 1982.

45. Nagano T, Nakai Y, Taniguchi F, et al: Diagnosis of paraaortic and pelvic lymph node metastasis of gynecologic malignant tumors by ultrasound-guided percutaneous fine-needle aspiration biopsy. *Cancer* 68:2571–2574, 1991.

46. Mennemeyer R, Bartha M, Kidd CR: Diagnostic and electron microscopy of fine needle aspirates of retroperitoneal lymph nodes in the diagnosis of metastatic pelvic neoplasms. *Acta Cytol* 23:370–373, 1979.

47. Saphir O, Amromin GG: Obscure axillary lymph node metastases in carcinoma of the breast. *Cancer* 1:238–241, 1948.

7

Stomach and Intestine

KEY FACTS

▶ Percutaneous fine needle aspiration biopsy does not replace or compete with conventional endoscopic biopsy in the diagnosis of gastrointestinal malignancy.

▶ Percutaneous NAB is most useful in circumstances where endoscopic biopsy fails to provide a diagnosis, e.g. when there is extreme narrowing of the gut lumen or the disease process is predominantly submucosal.

▶ Although adenocarcinoma is the most common malignancy of the gastrointestinal tract, the pathologist must remember that other tumors also occur and each group requires a different management strategy and has a different prognosis.

▶ The gastrointestinal tract is the most common site of primary extranodal lymphomas. The majority are non-Hodgkin's lymphoma, usually of the large cell type with a diffuse growth pattern.

▶ Other gastrointestinal malignancies that may be targets for NAB include smooth muscle tumor (stromal tumor) and carcinoid tumor. Each of these neoplasms shows distinctive cytologic features on NAB.

EMBRYOLOGY AND ANATOMY

The alimentary tract is formed from part of the yolk sac that lies within the body of the embryo. The entoderm forms the epithelial lining, and the splanchnic mesenchyme forms the surrounding muscle and serous coats. The fully developed stomach comprises three histologically different zones: cardia, fundus, and pylorus. The cardia is composed of simple columnar mucous epithelial cells that extend into pits or glands. This cell type is also indigenous to the other two zones. The body, or fundus, is the largest portion of the stomach; there the gastric pits are lined with cuboidal or low columnar mucous cells at the isthmus, or neck, of the gland. Such undifferentiated cells give rise to daughter cells, which migrate, to the surface or lumen, where they mature into tall columnar mucus-secreting cells. Below the isthmus are the fundic glands, which are lined with chief, or zymogen, cells and parietal, or acid-secreting, cells. The mucous neck cells are believed to act as stem cells for these specialized cells. The endocrine polypeptide cells, which are thought to have a neural crest (neuroectoderm) origin, are interspersed among the mucous cells, but occur principally in the midzone of the gastric glands. The pyloric antrum has deeper gastric pits, which are primarily lined with a cell type similar to the mucous neck cells.

The mucous membrane of the small intestine is arranged in crypts and villi to increase the surface area for absorption. The epithelial cells present include columnar epithelial cells, globlet cells, enteroendocrine cells, and Paneth cells. Prominent lymphoid aggregates, known as Peyer's patches, are present in the lamina propria of the mucosa.

The mucous membrane of the large intestine has a comparatively smooth surface, for there are no villi as in the small bowel. Long, tubular glands extend from the surface down through the entire thickness of the mucosa. The epithelial cells include tall columnar cells and numerous goblet cells, but no Paneth cells. Enteroendocrine cells are sparse, as are lymphoid aggregates in the lamina propria.

ENDOSCOPIC BIOPSY VERSUS FINE NEEDLE ASPIRATION BIOPSY

In the past decade, the use of fiberoptic endoscopy has dramatically increased the accuracy with which gastrointestinal cancer has been diagnosed. Carcinomas of the esophagus, stomach, duodenum, colon, and rectum can now be diagnosed by a combination of endoscopic inspection, biopsy, and brush cytology in over 90% of the cases.[1]

The more recent use of percutaneous fine needle aspiration biopsy with ultrasound or computed tomography guidance has added another dimension to gastrointestinal tumor diagnosis. NAB does not replace or compete with the endoscopic techniques; rather its greatest contribution is in circumstances where endoscopic diagnosis is difficult. When a gastric tumor is mainly exoenteric or when it is infiltrative with a necrotic mucosal surface, the accuracy of endoscopic diagnosis falls to as low as 50%.[2,3] Other simple factors, such as excessive mucus secretion, regurgitation through the pylorus, inability of the instrument tip to pass through the cardia because of severe narrowing, and uncooperative patients, can all preclude a satisfactory endoscopic examination.

Since the publication of the first edition of this monograph, numerous studies[4–11] have documented the important role of percutaneous NAB in the diagnosis of stomach- and bowel-wall lesions when endoscopic biopsy has failed to provide a diagnosis. Torp-Pedersen et al.[8] used percutaneous NAB to diagnose gastrointestinal mass lesions that were visualized ultrasonically. Fifty of 61 gastrointestinal malignancies were correctly diagnosed with no false-positive reports. Interestingly, in 5 of the 18 gastric tumors, conventional endoscopic biopsy failed to provide sufficient material, despite repeated attempts in two of the cases. Of the 40 colonic cancers, seven were not disclosed by barium enema studies.

Other uses of percutaneous NAB include the diagnosis of recurrent or metastatic cancer of the gastrointestinal tract,[12] and differentiation between neoplasm and benign conditions such as hematoma and abscess.[13]

More recently, many investigators[14–17] have reported the use of fine needle aspiration biopsy under direct-vision endoscopy in the diagnosis of upper gastrointestinal carcinoma and lymphoma. Using this technique Iishi et al[14] were able to make a correct diagnosis in 11 of 11 patients who had diffusely infiltrative gastric carcinomas. In four of these patients diagnostic material could not be obtained by endoscopic forceps biopsy.

At the Vancouver Hospital, as in most other centers, primary gastrointestinal malignancies are traditionally investigated by radiologic methods, endoscopic biopsy, and brush cytology. With the advent of ultrasound and computed tomography, more cases are being investigated by percutaneous NAB. Review of our files from 1986 through 1992 shows that with NAB we were able to diagnose accurately 32 of the 37 gastric and bowel wall tumors, with no false-positive reports. The sensitivity of this technique was 87% and the predictive value of a positive result was 100%. The 37 tumors included 22 adenocarcinomas (with two false-negative results), six lymphomas (with one false-negative result), six smooth muscle tumors (with two false-negative results), and three carcinoid tumors.

ADENOCARCINOMA OF THE STOMACH

General Consideration

Among the malignant lesions of the stomach, adenocarcinomas are by far the most common, while other tumors, such as lymphoma and leiomyosarcoma, constitute less than 12% of the total.[18] Although the incidence of gastric cancer is decreasing in the United States, it still poses a significant health problem. The number of new cases of gastric carcinoma in 1992 in the U.S. was estimated to be 24,400 and the estimated cancer deaths due to gastric cancer in the same year were 13,300.[19] In other countries, such as Japan, Chile, Iceland, and Finland, the incidence of gastric cancer is much higher.

Pathology

Adenocarcinomas of the stomach arise from the mucous cells of the superficial zone, from the mucous neck cells, or from the metaplastic intestinal epithelium derived therefrom. The prognosis of gastric carcinoma is dependent on the gross and microscopic appearances of the tumor and, most important of all, the presence or absence of lymph node metastases.[20–23]

Four gross patterns of presentation are recognized:

1. *Ulcerating tumor* (75%): Prognosis is poor.
2. *Polypoid or papillary tumor* (10%): Prognosis tends to be more favorable because the tumor shows more differentiated glands and infiltrates the gastric wall relatively late.
3. *Scirrhous or infiltrative tumor* (10%): Prognosis is poor because the tumor is frequently diffuse and nonresectable. The thickening and stiffening of the stomach wall produces the classic leather-bottle, or linitis plastica, appearance.

4. *Superficial tumor* (5%): This type is more commonly found in Japan than in the United States. Generally the tumor is found at an early stage and is surgically curable; hence, it has the best prognosis.

Histologically, two main types of gastric adenocarcinoma have been described by Lauren.[24] They are designated intestinal (53%) and diffuse (33%); the remaining 14% are unclassified. The intestinal type adenocarcinoma is thought to arise from metaplastic epithelium. The tumor is composed of distinct glands, sometimes large and containing papillary infoldings, resembling a differentiated colonic adenocarcinoma. The diffuse type is characterized by diffuse infiltration of tumor cells individually or in small nests. The tumor cells are round and rather small, and they typically produce intracytoplasmic mucin, resulting in the characteristic signet ring appearance. Well-formed glands are uncommon and, if present, small and indefinite. In many cases, the tumor cells infiltrate throughout the stomach wall; the resultant desmoplasia and stiffening of the wall gives rise to a leather-bottle (linitis plastica) appearance.

Clinically, the intestinal type has a better survival rate than the diffuse type. In one study,[25] the age- and sex-adjusted 5-year survival rate for the former was 27.4% and for the latter 9.9%. Integration of Lauren's histologic types with the gross appearance showed that 60% of the intestinal type carcinomas were polypoid, 25% ulcerating, and 15% were infiltrative. The corresponding figures for diffuse type carcinomas were 31%, 26%, and 43%, respectively.[26]

Aspiration Biopsy Cytology

An aspirate from an intestinal type adenocarcinoma is generally cell-rich. The diagnostic malignant cells are larger than normal cells and have nuclei that may be either hyperchromatic or pale and vesicular. Other features of malignancy are also present, such as prominent nucleoli, nuclear membrane irregularity, and irregular distribution of chromatin. Many tumor cells retain a columnar configuration with a basally positioned nucleus, and the cytoplasm is relatively abundant **(Fig. 7.1)**. The tumor cells frequently form tissue fragments with a glandular pattern, characterized by polarized cells arranged side-by-side and radially around the lumina **(Fig. 7.2)**. In other cases, the predominant cell pattern is an alveolar or acinar arrangement **(Fig. 7.3)**.

In the diffuse type adenocarcinoma, the aspirate is less cellular because the tumor is often associated with marked desmoplasia. The ABC shows dispersed single cells and small clusters of cells **(Fig. 7.4)**. The cells are smaller and rounded, with little anisokaryosis. They may be mistaken for histiocytes, but the nuclei of the tumor cells are hyperchromatic with thickened nuclear membranes, and the nucleoli are frequently prominent. Not uncommonly, the nucleus is distorted and displaced to one side of the cell by a large cytoplasmic mucin vacuole. These cells are referred to as signet-ring cells.

Diagnostic Pitfalls

Cytologic diagnosis of gastric adenocarcinoma is relatively easy because the cellular features of malignancy are often apparent.[27–29] Theoretically, a false-positive result can occur in diseases such as pernicious anemia, atrophic gastritis, and peptic ulceration, which can give rise to atypical glandular cells that may mimic carcinoma.[28,30]

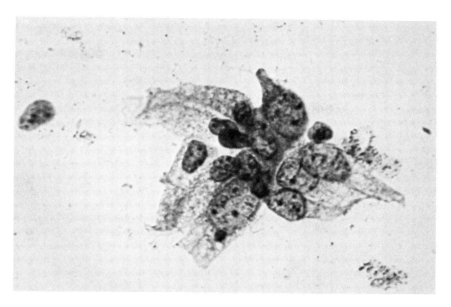

Fig. 7.1. Adenocarcinoma of stomach, intestinal type, ABC. Note a group of malignant columnar cells, with elongated basal nuclei and pale foamy cytoplasm. (Membrane filter, Papanicolaou preparation; ×500).

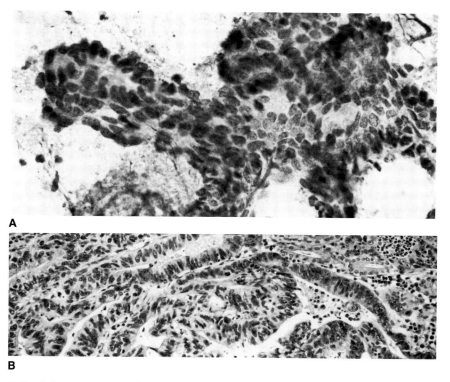

A

B

Fig. 7.2. Adenocarcinoma of stomach, intestinal type. **A.** ABC. A large tissue fragment showing a glandular pattern. Within the tissue fragment, clear spaces representing lumina are visible. **B.** Histologic section. (H & E preparation; A: ×310; B: ×125).

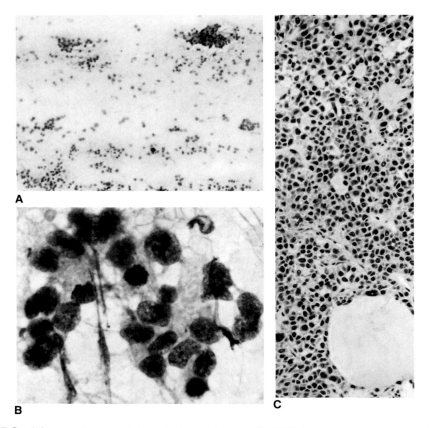

Fig. 7.3. Adenocarcinoma of stomach, intestinal type. **A.** ABC. Low magnification view showing many single cells and scattered acinous groups. **B.** ABC. Two acinous structures, formed by loosely grouped malignant cells. **C.** Histologic section showing many acini. (H & E preparation; A: ×80; B: ×500; C: ×125).

In practice, these conditions are unlikely targets for percutaneous NAB because they only occasionally present as a mass lesion on computed tomography or on ultrasound. **Figure 7.5A** is an example of chronic gastritis presenting as thickened stomach wall, investigated by percutaneous NAB. The reactive atypical glandular cells have prominent nucleoli, but the nuclear chromatin is evenly distributed and the nuclear membranes are smooth and round. In contrast, the cells of adenocarcinoma (**Fig. 7.5B**) are more dyshesive, nuclear chromatin is coarse and irregularly distributed, and the nuclear membranes are irregular in outline and thickness.

False-negative cytologic reports may occur in cases of linitis plastica as a result of the tumor cells being mistaken for histiocytes or because too few cells are present in the aspirate due to the desmoplastic nature of the tumor.

Because the management and prognosis are very different in patients having gastric adenocarcinomas than in those having lymphoma, the cytopathologist must be alert to the possibility that a malignant neoplasm in the stomach may not be an adenocarcinoma. If the lesion is so poorly differentiated that a definitive diagnosis cannot be

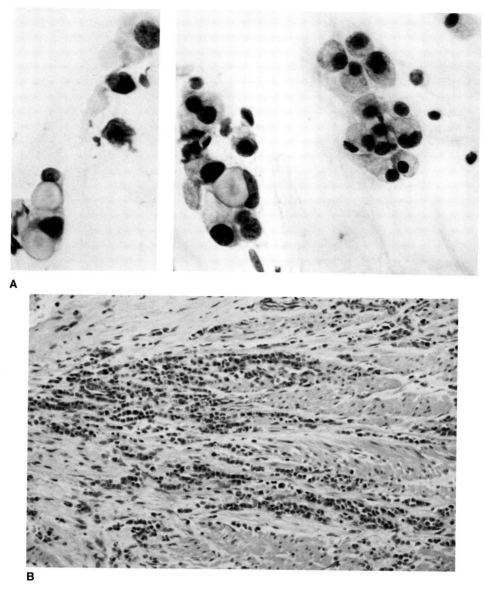

Fig. 7.4. Adenocarcinoma of stomach, diffuse type. **A.** ABC. Note signet-ring cells whose nuclei are displaced to one side by large mucin vacuoles. Superficially the malignant cells resemble histiocytes, but the former have hyperchromatic nuclei with coarse chromatin and irregular nuclear membranes. **B.** Histologic section of diffuse type adenocarcinoma of stomach. Note small hyperchromatic tumor cells infiltrating diffusely between muscle bundles of the stomach wall, resulting in a leather-bottle stomach. (H & E preparation; A: ×500; B: ×125).

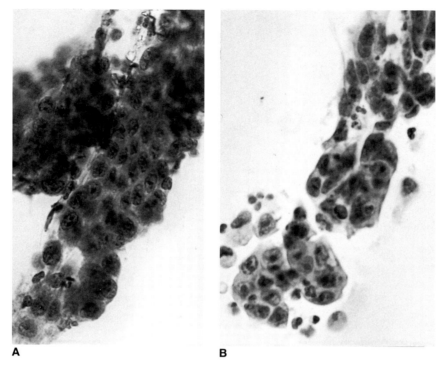

A   **B**

Fig. 7.5. Contrast ABC. **A.** Markedly atypical benign gastric epithelium from a case of chronic gastritis with thickened stomach wall. Note cellular cohesion and uniformity. **B.** Gastric adenocarcinoma. Note cellular dyshesion, nuclear pleomorphism, and prominent irregular nucleoli. (H & E preparation; A: ×500; B: ×500).

made on morphologic grounds alone, staining for mucin or epithelial markers and for leukocyte common antigen will make the distinction **(Fig. 7.6).**

ADENOCARCINOMA OF THE INTESTINE

Adenocarcinoma of the large intestine is a common neoplasm, exceeded in frequency only by cancer of the prostate and the lung in men and cancer of the breast in women.[19] About 65% occur in the rectosigmoid colon, 5% occur in the cecum, and the remainder are distributed about equally in the other parts of the colon.[31] Adenocarcinoma of the small bowel is rare. Perzin and associates reported only 130 cases of small bowel carcinoma compared with approximately 9,000 cases of colorectal carcinoma during the same period.[32] Adenocarcinomas of the small bowel are located most often in the duodenum and upper part of the jejunum.

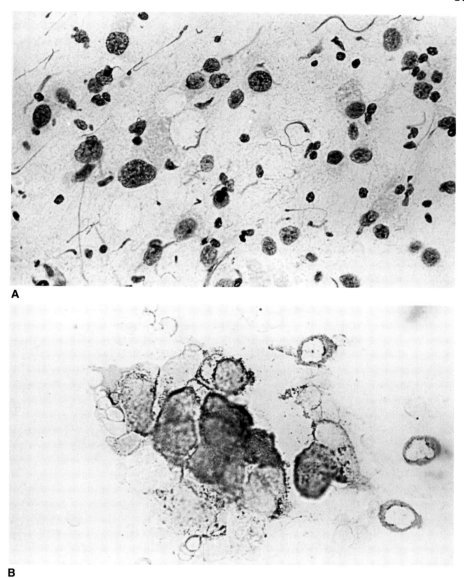

Fig. 7.6. Aspirate obtained from a thickened stomach wall of a 72-year-old man. A prior endoscopic biopsy showed necrotic debris only. **A.** Note many dispersed large malignant cells, quite consistent with a poorly differentiated adenocarcinoma. (H & E preparation; ×500). **B.** Tumor cells showing positive immunoreactivity for carcinoembryonic antigen, confirming the diagnosis of adenocarcinoma. The tumor cells do not stain for common leukocyte antigen (not shown). (Immunoperoxidase stain with Anti-CEA; ×500).

Pathology and Aspiration Biopsy Cytology

Primary intestinal adenocarcinomas demonstrate a broad histologic spectrum of differentiation, ranging from well to moderately to poorly differentiated. However, the majority are well to moderately differentiated, with glandular or tubular formation. In some cases, the tumor is characterized by abundant intracellular and extracellular mucin, giving rise to colloid or mucinous carcinoma.

The ABC shows features very similar to those of the intestinal-type carcinoma of the stomach discussed in the preceding section. Malignant cells are columnar or cuboidal, with hyperchromatic nuclei, single or multiple prominent nucleoli, and pale blue vacuolated cytoplasm. In the well-differentiated group, glandular and papillary structures can be recognized **(Figs. 7.7** and **7.8)**. Poorly differentiated adenocarcinomas lack a glandular pattern and often present as aggregates of dyshesive, polygonal, pleomorphic cells. The tinctorial characteristics of the cytoplasm and identification of mucin vacuoles aid in their proper classification as adenocarcinoma **(Fig. 7.9)**.

PSEUDOMYXOMA PERITONEI

Pseudomyxoma peritonei is a rare condition associated with a massive collection of mucinous material in the peritoneal cavity. The literature is somewhat confusing in that some authors have included both benign and malignant lesions as the causes of the condition. The current consensus regards the condition as a unique malignant presentation of peritoneal metastasis.[33] The condition is caused by rupture of a low-grade mucinous adenocarcinoma, usually of the ovary or appendix, but occasionally

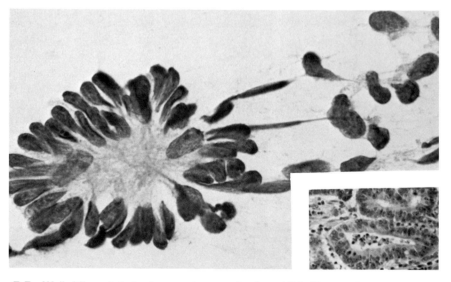

Fig. 7.7. Well-differentiated adenocarcinoma of colon, ABC. Note well-formed gland composed of palisading columnar cells around a lumen. A few isolated cells are seen on the right. *Inset:* Histologic section. (H & E preparation; ×500, inset ×125).

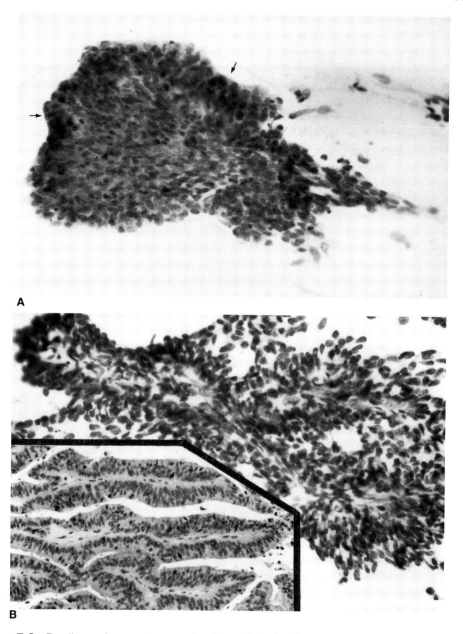

Fig. 7.8. Papillary adenocarcinoma of colon, ABC. **A.** Note a large solid papillary tissue fragment, with peripheral cells forming a sharp community border (indicated by arrows) and inner tumor cells viewed *en face*. The central fibrous core is not visible, being obscured by the *en face* cells. (H & E preparation; ×160). **B.** Note tissue fragment with well-formed papillary fronds. Central cores of fibrous connective tissue containing spindle cells are visible. *Inset:* Histologic section. (H & E preparation; B: ×125; inset ×125).

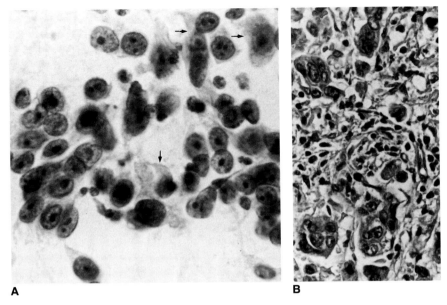

A   **B**

Fig. 7.9. Poorly differentiated adenocarcinoma of colon. **A.** ABC. Note macronucleoli and pale foamy cytoplasm (*arrows*). Some cells retain a columnar configuration, but no well-developed glands are seen. **B.** Histologic section. Note infiltrating small cell nests and absence of glandular lumina. (H & E preparation; A: ×500; B: ×310).

of the colon or pancreas. Unlike other forms of carcinomatosis, the disease is restricted to the peritoneal cavity, is not associated with lymph node metastases, and runs a protracted clinical course. The term "pseudomyxoma peritonei" should not be applied to the consequences of the rupture of a benign mucinous cystadenoma. In this condition the mucus collection is localized and is not associated with free epithelial cells, and the disease has a benign, self-limited course.[34]

Aspiration Biopsy Cytology

The cytopathology of pseudomyxoma peritonei has been reported in the literature.[35–37] and is essentially similar to the findings we observed in the three cases retrieved from our file. The most striking feature of pseudomyxoma peritonei on NAB is the presence of a large pool of thick mucus with scant cellularity **(Fig. 7.10).** Viable epithelial tumor cells must be identified to diagnose this condition. The epithelial cells are mucin-secreting, columnar cells, floating singly or in clusters within the mucus pool. The nuclear atypia is related to the degree of differentiation and the grade of the tumor. Usually the tumor cells exhibit only minimal nuclear atypia because the adenocarcinomas that give rise to pseudomyxoma peritonei are low-grade, well-differentiated neoplasms. The three cases in our file are two cystadenocarcinomas of the appendix and one cystadenocarcinoma of the ovary.

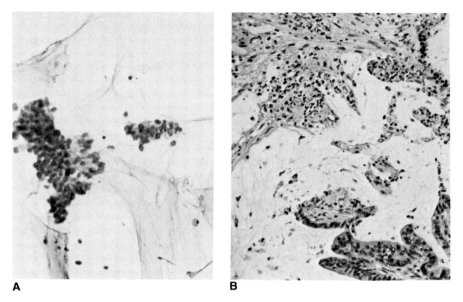

A   **B**

Fig. 7.10. Pseudomyxoma peritonei secondary to a ruptured, low-grade mucinous cystade-nocarcinoma of the appendix. **A.** ABC. Note scant aggregates of bland-looking tumor cells lying in a large pool of mucus. **B.** Histologic section of the primary appendiceal cystadenocarcinoma. (H & E preparation; A: ×160; B: ×120).

GASTROINTESTINAL LYMPHOMA

General Considerations

The most frequent site of primary extranodal lymphomas is the gastrointestinal tract, which accounts for 20% to 36%.[38,39] The majority of primary gastrointestinal lymphomas are non-Hodgkin's lymphoma (NHL); Hodgkin's lymphoma is exceedingly uncommon. With the exception of the small bowel, lymphomas of the gastrointestinal tract are far less common than carcinomas in the corresponding site. However, the incidence of NHL has been observed to be rising steadily and there has been a disproportionate increase in extranodal sites, particularly in the stomach, brain, and skin. The largest increases have occurred in the diffuse large cell and immunoblastic categories.[40]

Pathology

Stomach

The stomach is the most frequent site of malignant lymphoma of the gut, constituting 51% of all gastrointestinal lymphomas and 4% of primary gastric malignancy.[41,42] Gastric lymphomas are frequently ulcerated, and conventional endoscopic biopsy from the ulcerated area may show only degenerated or necrotic shadow cells such as may be seen in benign gastric ulcers as well as in ulceration secondary to lymphoma. Fine needle aspiration biopsy, performed percutaneously or endoscopically, has proved valuable in diagnosis. (Most primary gastric lymphomas are considered to arise from the mucosa-associated lymphoid tissue of the stomach.) Morphologically, gastric lymphomas are commonly of diffuse large cell type including the immunoblastic variety, but low-grade lymphomas are also seen.[43,44,45] In one study from Japan, 59% of gastric lymphomas were high-grade, as opposed to intestinal lymphomas in which 95% were high-grade tumors.[46]

Small Intestine

The small bowel is the second most common site of involvement by gastrointestinal lymphoma, accounting for 33% of the total gut lymphomas; most occur in the terminal ileum.[38,47,48] Small intestinal lymphomas represent one half or more of all primary malignant tumors of the small bowel.[49] Three distinct groups of lymphoma arise in the intestine. (1) In the Western countries, the commonest type of intestinal lymphoma seen in adult patients is the diffuse large cell lymphoma, followed by diffuse small cleaved cell lymphoma. (2) In children in Western countries, small non-cleaved cell lymphoma of the Burkitt's type is seen, frequently involving the ileocecal region. (3) In the Mediterranean basin and Middle East, a distinctive type of intestinal lymphoma has been described that is frequently associated with circulating alpha chains in the serum.[50] The Mediterranean type lymphoma is characterized by a pre-lymphomatous stage of intense benign-appearing lymphoplasmacytic infiltration of the intestinal mucosa. The lymphomatous stage is characterized by tumoral proliferation of large, pleomorphic immunoblasts with variable plasmacytic differentiation, best classified in the Working Formulation as an immunoblastic lymphoma.

Colon and Rectum

Lymphoma of the large bowel is uncommon; the cecum and rectum are the most frequent sites of involvement. Anorectal lymphoma is now increasing in frequency as a complication of immunosuppressive therapy following organ transplantation, or as a complication of the acquired immunodeficiency syndrome (AIDS).[51]

Needle Aspiration Cytology

The morphologies of gastrointestinal lymphomas, with the exception of the Mediterranean type lymphoma, are similar to those encountered in lymph nodes.[38] Like nodal lymphomas, the Working Formulation forms the basis for classification of gastrointestinal NHLs.[52] For a detailed description of the cytology of lymphoma, the reader is referred to Chapter 4.

Aspirates from lymphomas show a monomorphous population of lymphoid cells, displaying a ''lymphoma pattern'' characterized by dyshesive isolated cells rather than cohesive cell clusters. The cell morphology reflects the histologic type of the tumor. The most common is the diffuse large cell lymphoma, including the cleaved/non-cleaved type and the immunoblastic type **(Fig. 7.11).** The cells are large and cytologically dysplastic. Cytologic diagnosis is accurate. The small cleaved cell lymphomas are the second most common type and sometimes a nodular pattern may be seen on histologic sections. In children, the ileocecal area is the frequent site of involvement

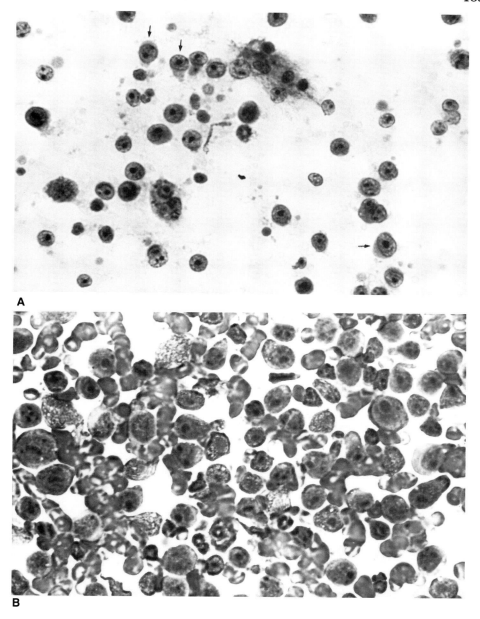

Fig. 7.11. Non-Hodgkin's lymphoma, large cell immunoblastic type, of the stomach, ABC. **A.** The dispersed single cell pattern is characteristic of, but by no means specific for, lymphoma. Note large round nuclei with a single, prominent, central nucleolus. Some cells show eccentric nuclei (*arrows*) characteristic of plasmacytic differentiation. (H & E preparation; ×500). **B.** Air-dried smear. Note large immunoblasts with large central nucleoli. Many red blood cells are present in the background. (May-Grünwald Giemsa preparation; ×500).

by small noncleaved cell lymphoma (Burkitt's lymphoma), of which accurate cytodiagnosis is possible. In HIV-infected patients, small noncleaved cell lymphoma and
immunoblastic lymphoma are the two most common types of lymphoma occurring
in this clinical setting and are readily recognized on NAB **(Fig. 7.12).**

Occasionally, lymphoma can be difficult for even the experienced cytopathologist
to diagnose on ABC. It must be distinguished from other lesions, such as lymphoid
hyperplasia, melanoma, nonepithelial tumors, and undifferentiated carcinoma. Immunocytologic marker studies, flow cytometry, and electron microscopy are most useful
in making the distinction (see Chapter 4).

CARCINOID TUMORS

Carcinoid tumors are derived from the neuroendocrine system. The cells of carcinoid
tumors contain amines, take up precursor amines, and are capable of decarboxy-
lation. The resulting acronym, APUD (for **A**mine **P**recursor **U**ptake, **D**ecarboxy-
lation), is used to describe the APUD concept, the APUD cells, and their tumors
(apudomas).[53] As these endocrine cells are present throughout the gastrointestinal
tract from the stomach to the anus (see section on Embryology and Anatomy), so
may be carcinoid tumors. The small intestine and appendix are the most frequent
sites. Carcinoids are the second most common form of small bowel malignancy in
the United States; between 20 and 40% of cancers of the small bowel are carcinoids.[54]

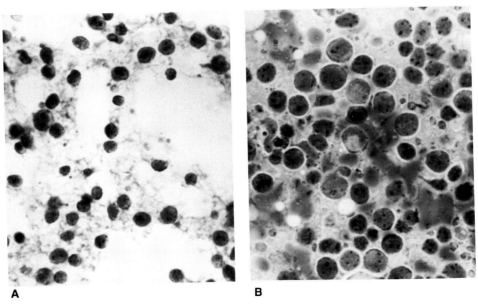

A   **B**

Fig. 7.12. Non-Hodgkin's lymphoma, small noncleaved cell type, in a patient with AIDS,
ABC. **A.** Note a fairly uniform cell population of small noncleaved cells. (H & E preparation;
×500). **B.** Air-dried smear. Note finely dispersed chromatin and multiple nucleoli. (May-
Grünwald Giemsa preparation; ×500).

Carcinoids of the stomach and large bowel are relatively rare. Morphologically identical neuroendocrine tumors may be seen in other organs, particularly in the lung and the pancreas (islet cell tumor).

Older reports divided carcinoid tumors into benign and malignant. The current consensus is to regard carcinoids as low-grade malignant tumors, with metastatic potential. Tumors of the APUD system are capable of elaborating many different types of amines and peptide hormones. Functionally, two major categories of carcinoid tumors have been defined: those associated with serotonin production and those associated with peptide secretion, primarily gastrin. The common symptoms of the carcinoid syndrome are flushing and diarrhea, presumably due to serotonin production.

Pathology and Aspiration Biopsy Cytology

Carcinoid tumor is usually a fairly well-demarcated yellow mass situated predominantly in the submucosa; less frequently, it may present as a yellow mural thickening that encircles the lumen. The tumor may be multicentric.

The histologic and cytologic aspects are similar and will be discussed together. The most striking feature is the overall impression of cellular uniformity, although nuclear pleomorphism may be seen to a varied extent in some tumors. The cells **(Fig. 7.13)** are polygonal and small to medium in size. The nuclei are round or oval, with finely stippled, evenly distributed chromatin. Chromocenters may be present, but nucleoli are absent or inconspicuous. There is a moderate amount of amphoteric, granular cytoplasm. The tumor cells are arranged in a variety of patterns, namely: insular (composed of solid sheets of cells), ribbon-like cords, and acinous units **(Figs. 7.14**

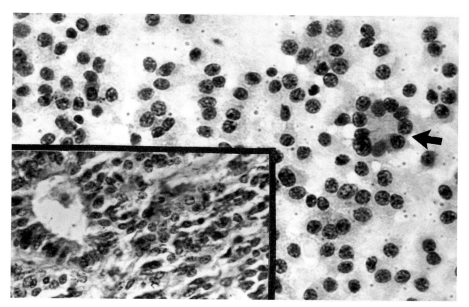

Fig. 7.13. Carcinoid tumor of duodenum, ABC. Note a monotonous population of uniform round cells and an acinous formation (*arrow*). *Inset:* Histologic section. (H & E preparation; ×500, inset ×310).

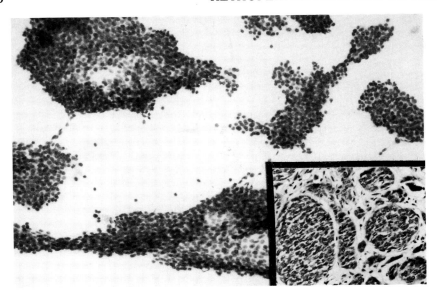

Fig. 7.14. Carcinoid tumor of ileum, ABC. A hypercellular aspirate with many solid sheets of small uniform cells (insular pattern). *Inset:* Histologic section showing similar insular pattern of tumor cells. (H & E preparation; ×125, inset ×125).

and **7.15).** These patterns can be seen alone or in various combinations. Many single cells are also present.

The diagnosis of carcinoid tumor can be confirmed by demonstration of cytoplasmic neuroendocrine granules, using the Grimelius silver stain **(Fig. 7.16).** The technical aspects of this procedure have been extensively reviewed by Ascoli et al.[55] Additionally, Wilander et al[56] have shown that fixation of smears in 10% buffered formalin gives persistently superior results compared with other types of fixative. With immunoperoxidase techniques, cells of carcinoid tumors can be shown to stain positively for neuron-specific enolase in virtually all cases, and for chromogranin and synaptophysin in the majority of cases.

Atypical Carcinoid

Although carcinoid tumors typically contain cells of the uniform polygonal type with finely granular cytoplasm, they may occasionally show cells with marked cellular pleomorphism, frequent mitoses, as well as tumor necrosis **(Fig. 7.17).** These tumors are referred to as atypical carcinoids and occur mostly in the stomach.[57] Clinically, like adenocarcinomas, they pursue an aggressive course.

Diagnostic Pitfalls

The acinous structures present in a carcinoid tumor may be mistaken for those of adenocarcinoma by the unwary. The latter are lined by malignant glandular cells that are variable in size and stratification, enclosing irregular lumina. The carcinoid acini, in contrast, are formed by orderly, uniform, polygonal cells.

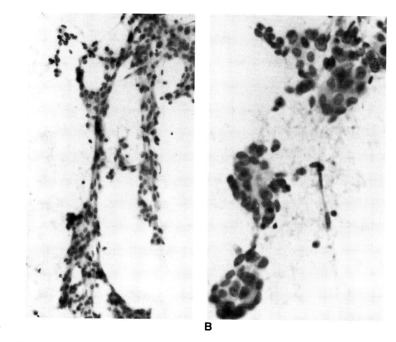

Fig. 7.15. Carcinoid tumor of stomach, ABC. **A.** Small uniform cells arranged in ribbons. **B.** Tumor cells in acinous formations. (H & E preparation; A: ×160; B: ×200).

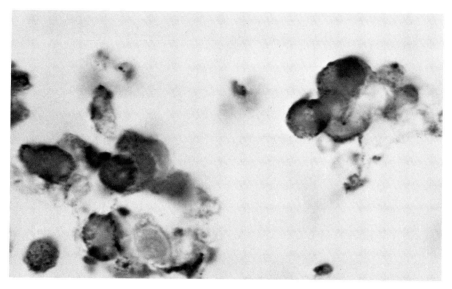

Fig. 7.16. Carcinoid tumor, ABC. Tumor cells with numerous cytoplasmic neurosecretory granules. (Grimelius silver preparation; ×1,250).

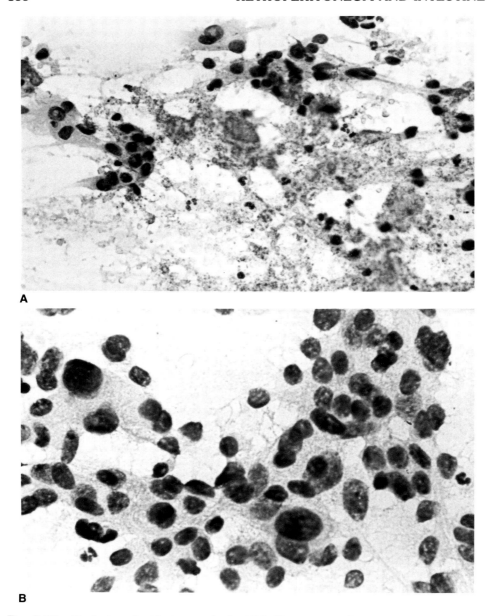

Fig. 7.17. Atypical carcinoid of stomach. **A.** ABC. Note tumor cells with massive necrosis in the background. Some tumor cells still retain the appearance of carcinoid with fairly regular nuclei and abundant cytoplasm. (H & E preparation; ×310). **B.** ABC. Note variability in nuclear size, hyperchromatism, and irregular coarse chromatin. Tumor cells retain abundant cytoplasm. (H & E preparation; ×600).

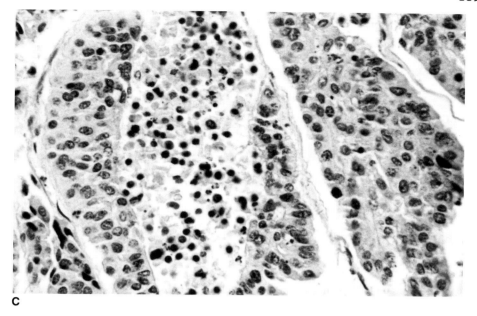

C

Fig. 7.17. C. Histologic section of atypical carcinoid. The individual cells are more pleomorphic than those of classic carcinoid and there is an area of tumor necrosis. (H & E preparation; ×310).

Diagnostic difficulties may arise when atypical carcinoid has to be distinguished from adenocarcinoma. Fortunately, atypical carcinoids of the gastrointestinal tract are not common. The reported cases contained tumor cells that ranged in appearance from uniform polygonal cells of the classic carcinoid type to large irregular cells. Sometimes the classic cell type can only be found after exhaustive examination; nevertheless, its presence should alert one to the possibility of carcinoid in the differential diagnosis. This should prompt further special studies, such as Grimelius silver stain, immunostains for neuron-specific enolase, synaptophysin, and chromogranin, or the search for dense core granules by electron microscopy.

SMOOTH MUSCLE TUMORS

Smooth muscle tumors of the gastrointestinal tract can arise from the smooth muscles of the muscularis propria, muscularis mucosae, or walls of the blood vessels. They are relatively rare, being fourth in occurrence after adenocarcinoma, lymphoma, and carcinoid tumor. Many leiomyomas are small and are often incidental findings at autopsy. Leiomyosarcomas are large and may present as a palpable abdominal mass, resulting in intestinal obstruction and pain. They can also cause mucosal ulceration and hemorrhage.

Pathology

Smooth muscle tumors are usually well-demarcated, with an expansile rather than an infiltrative border. The cut surface exhibits a smooth, lobulated, or whorled-silk appearance. Leiomyomas are generally smaller than leiomyosarcomas. Smooth muscle tumors of the stomach that are less than 5 cm in size and those of the small and large intestines that are less than 4 cm virtually never metastasize.[58,59] However, their behavior can be quite unpredictable and occasionally tumors as small as 1 cm may metastasize.[60]

It may be difficult to predict the malignant potential of gastrointestinal smooth muscle tumors on histologic grounds, because some low-grade leiomyosarcomas may not be histologically distinguishable from leiomyomas. While marked nuclear pleomorphism, dense cellularity, increased mitoses (a count of 5 or more mitoses/10 high-power fields) indicate malignancy, many well-differentiated leiomyosarcomas exhibit only mild nuclear atypia. Tumors with a maximal mitotic count as low as 1 per 10 high-power fields can metastasize.[60] Sagi and associates reported a histologically benign-appearing smooth muscle tumor of the small bowel that ran a rapid and malignant clinical course.[61]

Recent studies by immunocytochemical and electron microscopic techniques have demonstrated that some of these tumors diagnosed as smooth muscle tumors by light microscopy show Schwann cell differentiation in a few cases and total lack of differentiation in still others.[62] The noncommittal term "gastrointestinal stromal tumor" has been increasingly used to replace the conventional term "smooth muscle tumor."

Aspiration Biopsy Cytology

The aspirates of leiomyosarcomas (malignant stromal tumors) are cellular and consist of spindle-shaped cells arranged in parallel rows. If the tumor is poorly differentiated, there is no difficulty in recognizing it as malignant by its marked cytologic atypia. However, in well-differentiated leiomyosarcomas the nuclear changes may be subtle. The only clues to the malignant nature of the cells may be coarse nuclear chromatin and nuclear membrane irregularity. The finding of even one mitotic figure on ABC is strong presumptive evidence of malignancy (Fig. 7.18). In leiomyomas (benign stromal tumors), the spindle cells are more uniform and bland than their malignant counterparts. The nuclei are elongated, with blunted ends, described as cigar-shaped nuclei (Fig. 7.19).

Epithelioid Variant

Cells of smooth muscle tumors of the gastrointestinal tract, particularly of the stomach, not infrequently feature an epithelioid appearance. This is characterized by round rather than spindle-shaped cells, with centrally located nuclei and moderate to abundant eosinophilic cytoplasm (Fig. 7.20). The tumors are designated as epithelioid leiomyoma or epithelioid leiomyosarcoma depending on whether they are benign or malignant. At times they may be mistaken for epithelial tumors. In some cases, both round cells as well as spindle cells are present in the same aspirates (Fig. 7.21). The presence of spindle cells alerts one to the possibility of a stromal tumor rather than

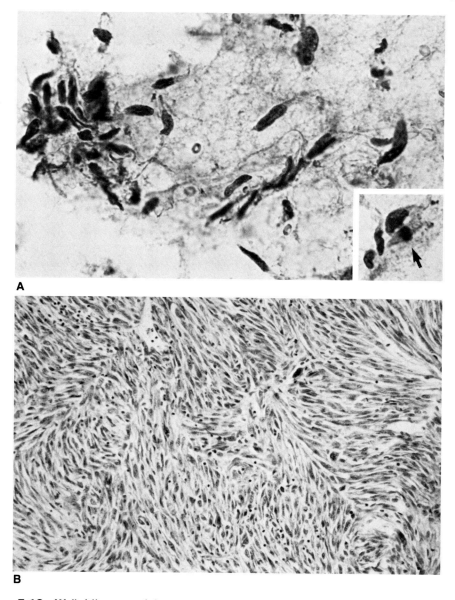

Fig. 7.18. Well-differentiated leiomyosarcoma of duodenum (malignant stromal tumor). **A.** ABC. Note spindle cells with nuclear membrane irregularities, uneven chromatin distribution, and a mitosis (*arrow*). (H & E preparation; ×310). **B.** Histologic section of leiomyosarcoma showing spindle cells arranged in herring bone pattern. (H & E preparation; ×125).

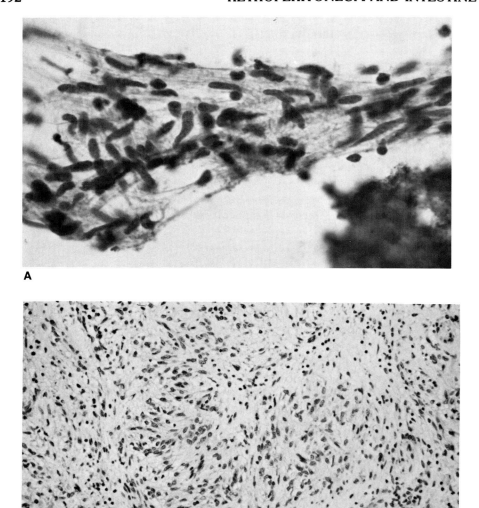

A

B

Fig. 7.19. Leiomyoma (benign stromal tumor) of stomach. **A.** ABC. The elongated nuclei show smooth nuclear membranes, and the nuclear chromatin is uniformly distributed. **B.** Histologic section of cellular leiomyoma. (H & E preparation; A: ×310; B: ×125).

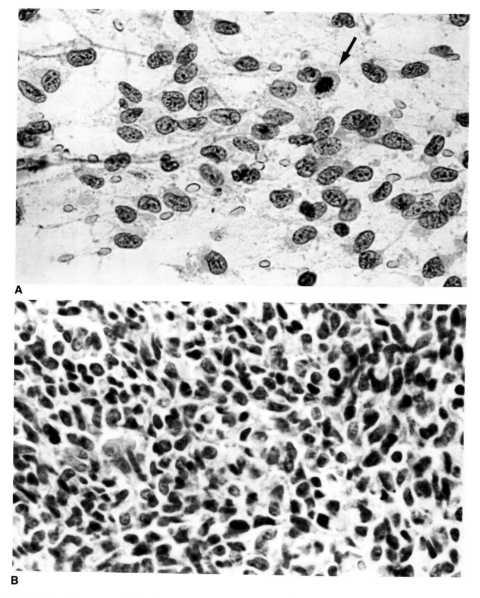

Fig. 7.20. A 9-cm, epithelioid leiomyosarcoma of stomach. **A.** ABC. Note dyshesive tumor cells with round to ovoid nuclei. The diagnosis of malignancy is suggested by the presence of a mitosis (*arrow*) and the size of the tumor. (H & E preparation; ×500). **B.** Histologic section of epithelioid leiomyosarcoma (H & E preparation; ×310).

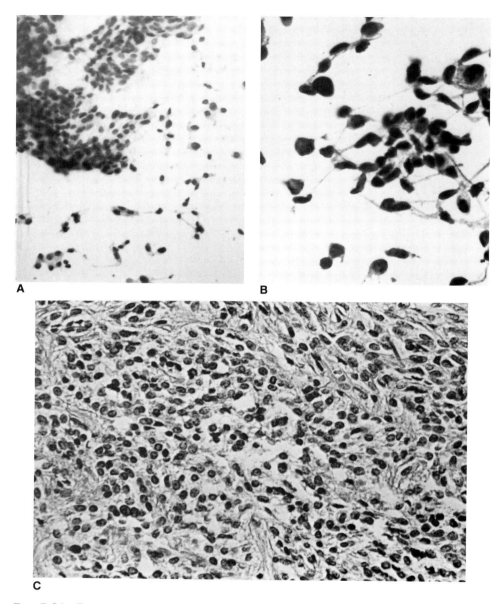

Fig. 7.21. Epithelioid leiomyoma of the duodenum. **A,B.** Note epithelioid round cells admixed with spindle cells. (H & E preparation; A: ×125, B: ×500). **C.** Histologic section of epithelioid leiomyoma. (H & E preparation; ×200).

an epithelial tumor. Furthermore, the immunocytologic profile of stromal tumors differs from that of epithelial tumors in that cells of the former typically stain for vimentin, many cases may stain for desmin, but they do not stain for cytokeratin.

REFERENCES

1. Benvenuti GA, Hattori K, Levin B, et al: Endoscopic sampling for tissue diagnosis in gastrointestinal malignancy. *Gastrointest Endosc* 21:159–161, 1975.

2. Winawer SJ, Sherlock P, Hadju SI: The role of upper gastrointestinal endoscopy in patients with cancer. *Cancer* 37:440–448, 1976.

3. Nelson RS, Lanza FL: The endoscopic diagnosis of gastric lymphoma. *Gastrointest Endosc* 21:66–71, 1974.

4. Carrera GF, Mascatello VJ, Holm HH, et al: Ultrasonically guided percutaneous biopsy of gastric lesions. *Wis Med J* 78:28–29, 1979.

5. Ennis MG, MacErlean DP: Biopsy of bowel wall pathology under ultrasound control. *Gastrointest Radiol* 6:17–20, 1981.

6. Owman T, Idvall I: Percutaneous fine needle aspiration biopsy guided by barium examination of the GI tract. *Gastrointest Radiol* 7:327–333, 1982.

7. Solbiati L, Montali G, Croce F, et al: Fine-needle aspiration biopsy of bowel lesions under ultrasound guidance: Indications and results. *Gastrointest Radiol* 11:172–176, 1986.

8. Torp-Pedersen S, Gronvall S, Holm HH: Ultrasonically guided fine-needle biopsy aspiration biopsy of gastrointestinal mass lesions. *J Ultrasound Med* 3:65–68, 1984.

9. Green J, Katz S, Phillips G, et al: Percutaneous sonographic needle aspiration biopsy of endoscopically negative gastric carcinoma. *Am J Gastroenterol* 83:1150–1153, 1988.

10. Abbitt PL: Percutaneous fine-needle aspiration of bowel wall abnormalities under ultrasonic guidance. *J Clin Ultrasound* 19:310–314, 1991.

11. Fornari F, Buscarini L: Ultrasonically-guided fine-needle biopsy of gastrointestinal organs: Indications, results and complications. *Dig Dis* 10:121–133, 1992.

12. van Overhagen H, Berger MY, Meijers H, et al: Influence of radiologically and cytologically assessed distant metastases on the survival of patients with esophageal and gastroesophageal junction carcinoma. *Cancer* 72:25–31, 1993.

13. Butch RJ, Wittenberg J, Mueller PR, et al: Presacral masses after abdominoperineal resection for colorectal carcinoma: The need for needle biopsy. *AJR* 144:309–312, 1985.

14. Iishi H, Yamamoto R, Tatsuta M, et al: Evaluation of fine-needle aspiration biopsy under direct vision gastrofiberscopy in diagnosis of diffusely infiltrative carcinoma of the stomach. *Cancer* 57:1365–1369, 1986.

15. Lange P, Kock K, Lausten J, et al: Endoscopic fine-needle aspiration cytology of the stomach. A new diagnostic procedure. *Endoscopy* 19:72, 1987.

16. Kochhar R, Gupta SK, Malik AK, et al: Endoscopic fine needle aspiration biopsy. *Acta Cytol* 31:481–484, 1987.

17. Layfield LJ, Reichman A, Weinstein WM: Endoscopically directed fine needle aspiration biopsy of gastric and esophageal lesions. *Acta Cytol* 36:69–74, 1991.

18. Ming SC: Adenocarcinoma and other malignant epithelial tumors of the stomach. In Ming SC, Goldman H: *Pathology of the Gastrointestinal Tract*. Philadelphia, WB Saunders, 1992, p 585.

19. Boring CC, Squires TS, Tong T: Cancer statistics, 1992. *CA* 42:19–38, 1992.

20. Ming SC: *Tumors of the Esophagus and Stomach. Atlas of Tumor Pathology.* Fascicle 7, Second Series. Washington, DC, Armed Forces Institute of Pathology, 1973, pp 162–205.

21. Ming SC: Gastric carcinoma. *Cancer* 39:2475–2485, 1977.

22. Correa P: Pathology of gastric cancer. *Clin Oncol* 3:251–257, 1984.

23. Ribeiro MM, Sarmento JA, Simoes MAS, et al: Prognostic significance of Lauren and Ming Classifications and other pathologic parameters in gastric carcinoma. *Cancer* 47:780–784, 1981.

24. Lauren P: The two histological main types of gastric carcinoma: Diffuse and so-called intestinal type carcinoma. *Acta Pathol Microbiol Scand* 64:31–49, 1965.

25. Stemmermann GN, Brown CA: Survival study of intestinal and diffuse types of gastric cancer. *Cancer* 33:1190–1195, 1974.

26. Fenoglio-Preiser CM, Lantz PE, Listrom MB, et al: *Gastrointestinal Pathology. An Atlas and Text.* New York, Raven Press, 1989, p 206.

27. Pilotti S, Rilke F, Clemente C, et al: The cytologic diagnosis of gastric carcinoma related to histologic type. *Acta Cytol* 21:48–59, 1977.

28. Hajdu SI: Cytopathology of human gastrointestinal cancers. In Lipkin M, Good RA: *Gastrointestinal Tract Cancer.* New York, Plenum, 1978, pp 489–508.

29. An-Foraker SH, Vise D: Cytodiagnosis of gastric carcinoma, linitis plastica type (diffuse, infiltrating, poorly differentiated adenocarcinoma). *Acta Cytol* 25:360–366, 1980.

30. Brandborg LL, Taniguchi L, Rubin CE: Exfoliative cytology in non-malignant conditions of the upper intestinal tract. *Acta Cytol* 5:187, 1961.

31. Correa P: Epidemiology of polyps and cancer. In Morson BC: *The Pathogenesis of Colorectal Cancer.* Philadelphia, WB Saunders, 1978, p 126.

32. Perzin KH, Fenoglio CM, Pascal RR: Neoplastic diseases of the small and large intestine. In Silverberg SG: *Principle and Practice of Surgical Pathology.* New York, Wiley, 1983, p 300.

33. Rosai J: *Ackerman's Surgical Pathology,* ed 7. St Louis, CV Mosby, 1989, pp 1645–1647.

34. Higa E, Rosai J, Pizzimbono CA, et al: Mucosal hyperplasia, mucinous cystadenoma, and mucinous cystadenocarcinoma of appendix. A re-evaluation of appendiceal "mucocele." *Cancer* 32:1325–1341, 1973.

35. Gustafson KD, Karnaze GC, Hattery RR, et al: Pseudomyxoma peritonei associated with mucinous adenocarcinoma of the pancreas: CT findings and CT-guided biopsy. *J Comput Assist Tomogr* 8:335–338, 1984.

36. Wood T, Hajdu SI: Cytopathology of pseudomyxoma peritonei. *Acta Cytol* 29:925–926, 1985.

37. Rammou-Kinia R, Sirmakechian-Karra T: Pseudomyxoma peritonei and malignant mucocele of the appendix. A case report. *Acta Cytol* 30:169–172, 1986.

38. Lewin KJ, Riddell RH, Weinstein WM: *Gastrointestinal Pathology and Its Clinical Implications.* New York, Igaku-Shoin, 1992, pp 151–196.

39. Freeman C, Berg JW, Cutler SJ: Occurrence and prognosis of extranodal lymphomas. *Cancer* 29:252–260, 1972.

40. Weisenburger DD: An epidemic of non-Hodgkin's lymphoma: Comments on time trends, possible etiologies, and the role of pathology. *Mod Pathol* 5:481–482, 1992.

41. Dragosics B, Bauer P, Radaszkiewicz T: Primary gastrointestinal non-Hodgkin's lymphomas: A retrospective clinicopathologic study of 150 cases. *Cancer* 55:1060–1073, 1985.

42. Lewin KJ, Ranchod M, Dorfman RF: Lymphomas of the gastrointestinal tract: A study of 117 cases presenting with gastrointestinal disease. *Cancer* 78:1587–1592, 1982.

43. Lim FE, Hartman AS, Tan EG, et al: Factors in the prognosis of gastric lymphoma. *Cancer* 39:1715–1720, 1977.

44. Isaacson P, Wright DH, Judd MA, et al: Primary gastrointestinal lymphomas. A classification of 66 cases. *Cancer* 43:1805–1819, 1979.

45. Harris NL: Low-grade B-cell lymphoma of mucosa-associated lymphoid tissue and monocytoid B-cell lymphoma: Relate entities that are distinct from other low-grade B-cell lymphomas. *Arch Pathol Lab Med* 117:771–775, 1993.

46. Aozasa K, Ueda T, Kurata A, et al: Prognostic value of histologic and clinical factors in 56 patients with gastrointestinal lymphomas. *Cancer* 61:309–315, 1988.

47. Dodd GD: Lymphoma of the hollow abdominal viscera. *Radiol Clin North Am* 28:771–783, 1990.

48. Haber DA, Mayer RJ: Primary gastrointestinal lymphoma. *Semin Oncol* 2:154–169, 1988.

49. McGovern VJ: Lymphomas of the gastrointestinal tract. In Yardley JH, Morson BC, Abell MR (eds): *The Gastrointestinal Tract*. Baltimore, Williams & Wilkins, 1977, pp 184–206.

50. Lewin KJ, Kahn LB, Novis BH: Primary intestinal lymphoma of "Western" and "Mediterranean" type, alpha chain disease and massive plasma cell infiltration: A comparative study of 37 cases. *Cancer* 38:2511–2528, 1976.

51. Ioachim HL, Weinstein MA, Robbins RD, et al: Primary anorectal lymphoma. A new manifestation of the acquired immune deficiency syndrome (AIDS). *Cancer* 60:1449–1453, 1987.

52. The Non-Hodgkin's lymphoma pathology classification project: National Cancer Institute sponsored study of classification of Non-Hodgkin's lymphomas: Summary and description of working formulation for clinical usage. *Cancer* 49:2112–2135, 1982.

53. Pearse AGE: The cytochemistry and ultrastructure of polypeptide hormone producing cells of APUD series and embryonic, physiologic and pathologic implications of the concept. *J Histochem Cytochem* 17:303–313, 1969.

54. Miles RM, Crawford D, Duras S: The small bowel tumor problem: An assessment based on a 20 year experience with 116 cases. *Ann Surg* 189:732–734, 1979.

55. Ascoli V, Newman GA, Kline TS: Grimelius stain for cytodiagnosis of carcinoid tumor. *Diagn Cytopathol* 2:157–159, 1986.

56. Wilander E, Norheim I, Oberg K: Application of silver stains to cytologic specimens of neuroendocrine tumors metastatic to liver. *Acta Cytol* 29:1053–1057, 1985.

57. Sweeney EC, McDonnell L: Atypical gastric carcinoids. *Histopathol* 4:215–224, 1980.

58. Shiu M, Farr GH, Papachristou DN, et al: Myosarcomas of the stomach: Natural history, prognostic factors, and management. *Cancer* 49:177–178, 1982.

59. Shiu M, Farr GH, Egeli RA, et al: Myosarcomas of the small and large intestine: A clinicopathological study. *J Surg Oncol* 24:67–72, 1983.

60. Evans HL: Smooth muscle tumors of the gastrointestinal tract. A study of 56 cases followed for a minimum of 10 years. *Cancer* 56:2242–2250, 1985.

61. Sagi A, Feuchtwanger MM, Yanai-Inbar I, et al: Smooth muscle tumors of the small bowel. *J Surg Oncol* 30:120–123, 1985.

62. Miettinen M: Gastrointestinal stromal tumors: An immunohistochemical study of cellular differentiation. *Am J Clin Pathol* 89:601–610, 1988.

8

Peritoneal Mesothelioma

KEY FACTS

▶ The value of cytology in the definitive diagnosis of malignant mesothelioma is controversial.

▶ To distinguish malignant mesothelioma from adenocarcinoma is less problematic today than it was in the past, due to ready availability of immunocytochemical stains and electron microscopy.

▶ An accurate cytologic diagnosis of malignant peritoneal mesothelioma is feasible, based on a combination of (1) a compatible clinical history, (2) characteristic radiologic findings, and (3) characteristic morphology, supported by special stains and/or electron microscopy.

▶ The pathologist must be aware of the conditions that may cause atypical mesothelial hyperplasia, such as cirrhosis associated with longstanding ascites and posttraumatic irritation of the peritoneum including that induced by surgical operation. If any of these conditions exist, the pathologist must exercise caution in making the cytologic diagnosis of malignant mesothelioma.

EMBRYOLOGY AND ANATOMY

During embryologic development, the lateral plate mesoderm splits into a somatic (parietal) layer and a splanchnic (visceral) layer, which ultimately become the tissues lining the celomic cavities of the body (see Chapter 3, section on Embryology and Anatomy). The mesothelial cells, which form a monolayer of simple cuboidal epithelium that lines the celomic cavities, are therefore of mesodermal origin. The subcelomic mesenchyme serves as the anchoring substratum for the mesothelium. The submesothelial stromal cells, having the characteristic structure of fibroblasts, are sometimes referred to as "multipotential subserosal cells" because they are thought to be a source of mesothelial cell renewal.[1] In the embryo the celomic epithelium gives rise to the mesonephros, metanephros, wolffian body, genital ridge, and the müllerian system. The embryologic development reflects the multipotentiality of the mesothelial cells and accounts for the different histologic patterns seen in mesotheliomas and their ability to mimic so many tumors. Furthermore, the enormous capacity for mesothelial cells to proliferate and undergo hyperplasia in response to inflammation or injury is well known. The hyperplasia may be so florid that it may histologically simulate neoplasm.

NORMAL CYTOLOGY

Normal and reactive mesothelial cells are commonly seen in abdominal aspirates. The individual cells are polygonal in shape with a round central nucleus and moderate to large amount of cytoplasm. The nuclei have finely granular chromatin and usually one or two, small or medium-sized nucleoli. The cytoplasm is optically dense and tends to become less dense at the periphery of the cell, as opposed to the usually diffusely pale and foamy cytoplasm of adenocarcinoma cells. Some mesothelial cells also display cytoplasmic vacuoles. In addition, the cytoplasmic borders often have a brushlike or ruffled appearance, due to the presence of numerous long, slender surface microvilli. The long microvilli constitute one of the characteristic ultrastructural features of mesothelioma.

On NAB, benign reactive mesothelial cells are frequently arranged in monolayered sheets or small cell groups **(Fig. 8.1)**. The cells are characteristically separated from each other by a narrow space or "window" created by the long, slender microvilli present on the cell surfaces.

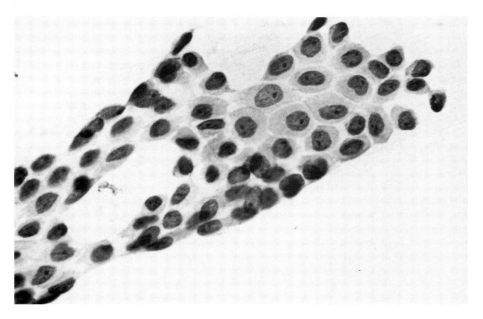

Fig. 8.1. Benign reactive mesothelial cells, ABC. Note a monolayered sheet of polygonal cells, having central round nuclei with small nucleoli, and distinct intercellular gaps. (H & E preparation; ×500).

BENIGN PERITONEAL MESOTHELIOMA

Peritoneal mesothelioma is a primary neoplasm of the mesothelial cells lining the peritoneal cavity. Benign mesotheliomas are very uncommon. They are circumscribed tumors and practically never produce effusion. The usual type is a papillary epithelial tumor whose papillae are covered by benign mesothelium. The fibrous mesothelioma, seen in the pleura, virtually does not occur in the peritoneum. A multicystic type also has been described.[2] The cysts, containing clear watery fluid, are lined by benign mesothelial cells.

Diagnosis of benign mesotheliomas is usually made after surgical excision in histologic sections or as an incidental finding at autopsy. They are rarely reported on NAB, due to their exceptional rarity and noninvasive nature. The cells obtained by NAB are indistinguishable from normal or reactive mesothelial cells (see **Fig. 8.1**).[3]

MALIGNANT PERITONEAL MESOTHELIOMA

General Considerations

Malignant peritoneal mesotheliomas occur in less frequency than their pleural counterparts, and constitute about 10–20% of the total mesotheliomas.[4,5] Like pleural mesothelioma, exposure to asbestos is the main etiologic factor.[6] The tumor covers the surface of the peritoneal cavity in the form of diffuse tumor plaques. The tumor also covers the serosal surface of the intestine, mesentery, and omentum. In one large series, 22 of the 83 malignant peritoneal mesotheliomas showed invasion of the wall of the gastrointestinal tract, with clinical evidence of subacute intestinal obstruction.[6] Ultrasound and computed tomography findings are characteristic, showing diffuse, mantle-like or nodular, soft-tissue thickening of the peritoneum, omentum, mesentery, and bowel wall, with small intraperitoneal nodules and ascites.[7,8] In some cases, a large localized mass may be encountered in addition to small nodules disseminated over both the visceral and parietal peritoneum. Most patients with malignant peritoneal mesotheliomas present with ascites, and effusion fluid is therefore readily available for cytologic examination.[9–11] Fine needle aspiration biopsy constitutes another method of cytologic appraisal and is especially useful for mass lesions and in cases where effusion is minimal or absent.[3,8,12–15]

Histopathology

Histologically, malignant peritoneal mesothelioma is composed of epithelial cells or spindle cells, or a mixture of the two cell types. The epithelial cells grow in sheets or are arranged in a tubulopapillary pattern, simulating an adenocarcinoma **(Fig. 8.2)**. The spindle cell component may resemble a fibrosarcoma **(Fig. 8.3)**. In the series reported by Kannerstein and Churg,[6] 75% of the 82 cases were designated as epithelial, 22% as mixed epithelial and sarcomatoid, and only 3% as purely sarcomatoid.

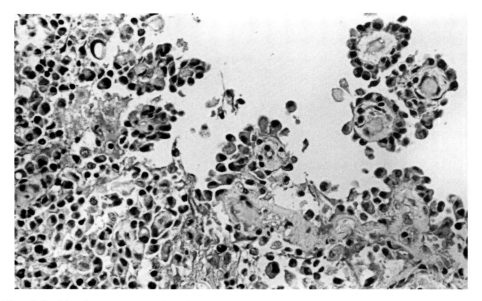

Fig. 8.2. Histologic section of malignant mesothelioma of the peritoneum, epithelial type. The peritoneum is replaced by a thick layer of neoplastic mesothelial cells, forming numerous papillary tufts. (H & E preparation; ×310).

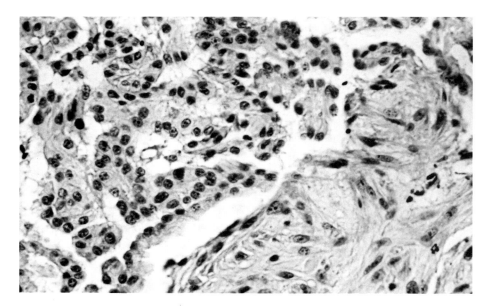

Fig. 8.3. Histologic section of malignant mesothelioma of the peritoneum, mixed epithelial and sarcomatoid type. Note epithelial cells forming a tubulopapillary growth pattern (*left*) and spindle cells resembling a fibrosarcoma (*right*). (H & E preparation; ×310).

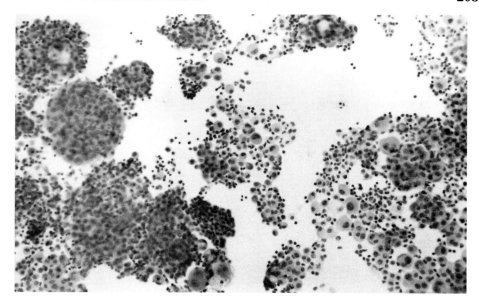

Fig. 8.4. Malignant mesothelioma of the peritoneum, epithelial type, ABC. Richly cellular smear showing large cell sheets and cell balls. (H & E preparation; ×125).

Aspiration Biopsy Cytology

Aspirates of malignant mesotheliomas are richly cellular. In almost all cases, the predominant cell type is the epithelial cell. The malignant epithelial cells are arranged singly, in cell sheets, and in large spherical clusters **(Fig. 8.4)**. Not uncommonly, a mixture of normal, reactive, and malignant mesothelial cells can be found in the same aspirated sample.

The malignant epithelial cells **(Fig. 8.5)** bear a strong resemblance to normal mesothelial cells, but they are larger. They show moderate variability in size, but are rarely pleomorphic. The cells are polygonal in shape and retain a round or oval nucleus, with a smooth nuclear membrane. The nuclei show a wide range of atypism, varying from mild to severe. The chromatin pattern is predominantly finely granular, but irregularly distributed and coarsely granular chromatin can also be seen in some nuclei. Some cells have small chromocenters while others have one or two eosinophilic macronucleoli. The nucleocytoplasmic ratio ranges from low to high. The cytoplasm of the cells is generally abundant, with a central dense homogenous area and a peripheral zone that is lightly stained. The cytoplasmic borders have a ruffled appearance **(Fig. 8.6)**, corresponding to the rich microvillous borders. A peripheral accumulation of small cytoplasmic vacuoles can sometimes be seen in the cells, and occasionally some larger vacuoles may be present. Presumably, these vacuoles represent cytoplasmic accumulation of hyaluronic acid or glycogen.[14] While binucleated cells may be seen in reactive mesothelial hyperplasia, multinucleated cells are common in malignant mesotheliomas.

In the epithelial cell sheets, the component cells may show a pavement-like arrangement, with a clear space between the cells **(Fig. 8.7)**. The intercellular spaces are

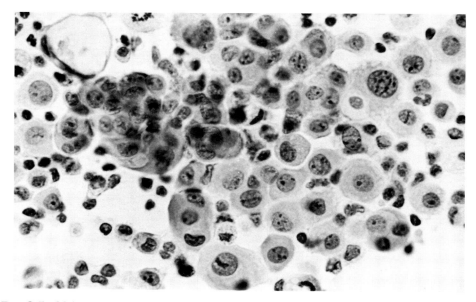

Fig. 8.5. Malignant peritoneal mesothelioma, epithelial type, ABC. The polygonal neoplastic cells retain mesothelial cell features. Note a wide range of cytologic atypia displayed by the cells. (H & E preparation; ×500).

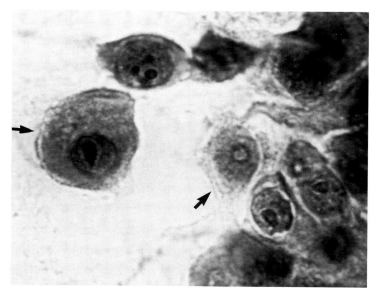

Fig. 8.6. Malignant mesothelioma, ABC. Note polygonal cells with prominent nucleoli, peripheral cytoplasmic vacuoles, and ruffled cell borders (*arrows*). (H & E preparation; ×1,250).

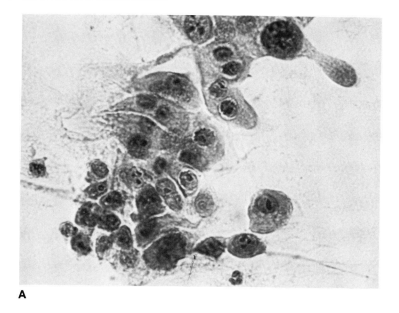

A

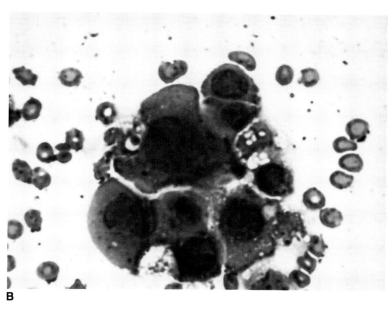

B

Fig. 8.7. Malignant mesothelioma, ABC. **A.** Note monolayer of malignant mesothelial cells showing characteristic cell-to-cell apposition, with a windowlike gap between cells. (H & E preparation; ×500). **B.** Air-dried smear showing a monolayered group of cells separated by prominent intercellular spaces. (May-Grünwald Giemsa preparation; ×500).

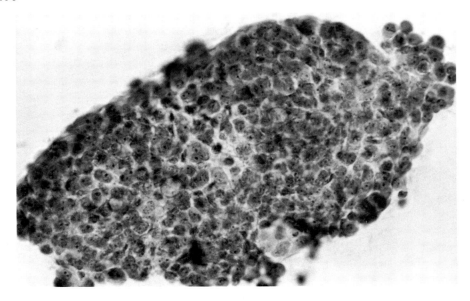

Fig. 8.8. Malignant mesothelioma, ABC. Large, three-dimensional cell ball, characteristic of malignant mesothelioma. It is worthy of note that reactive mesothelial proliferations seldom produce more than 15–20 cells in a cell ball. (H & E preparation; ×310).

attributed to the prominent microvillous borders between adjacent cells, pushing them apart.

The spherical cell clusters range from small round balls of four to five cells each to large three-dimensional structures with cellular crowding. The large cell balls are a characteristic feature of malignant mesotheliomas **(Fig. 8.8).** In these large clusters, the peripheral cells and their nuclei are generally flattened, and are oriented in a circular fashion around the core of the clusters. In some aspirates, large tissue fragments with distinct papillary fronds and fibrous cores can be seen **(Fig. 8.9).**

In the biphasic epithelial and sarcomatoid variant, fibroblastic spindle cells with slender pointed nuclei and scanty cytoplasm are seen **(Fig. 8.10),** but they are usually underrepresented in the aspirates because these cells are difficult to aspirate. More commonly, transitional forms are observed. These transitional forms are spindle-shaped but the nuclei are ovoid or fusiform and retain the nuclear characteristic of the epithelial mesothelial cells.

Histochemical and Immunocytochemical Stains, and Electron Microscopy

Once the possibility of mesothelioma is considered, the performance of histochemical, immunocytochemical and electron microscopic studies is very useful in confirming the diagnosis.[10,11,16–18] Mesothelial cells show negative reactions with the mucicarmine stain and periodic acid-Schiff diastase stain, indicating a lack of "epithelial" mucin. Immunostains for cytokeratin and vimentin usually show mesotheliomas to coexpress both antigens. In addition, malignant mesotheliomas immuostained with monoclonal

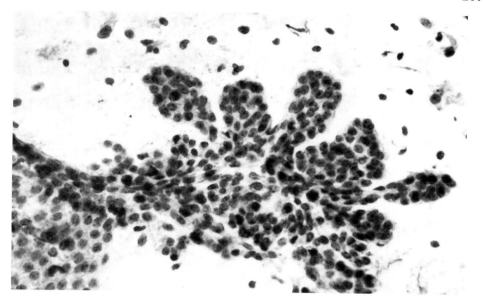

Fig. 8.9. Malignant mesothelioma, ABC. Note large tissue fragment with well-developed papillary fronds. (H & E preparation; ×200).

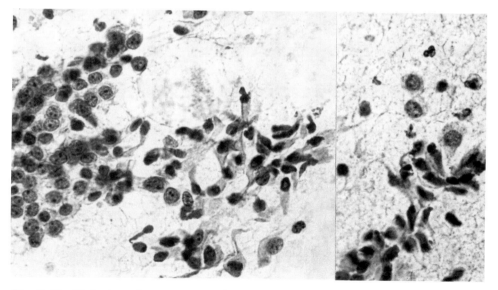

Fig. 8.10. Biphasic malignant peritoneal mesothelioma, ABC. Note admixture of polygonal epithelial cells and spindle cells. (H & E preparation; ×500).

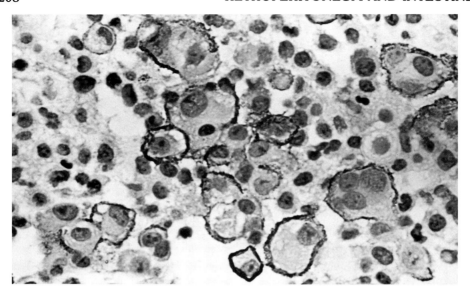

Fig. 8.11. Malignant mesothelioma, ABC. Malignant mesothelial cells, immunostained with monoclonal anti-EMA, showing characteristic thick, spiky, membranous staining pattern. (Immunoperoxidase stain; ×500).

antibody to epithelial membrane antigen (EMA) show a characteristic staining pattern.[11,19] The EMA-positive material is seen circumferentially on the villous borders of the mesothelial cells, resulting in a spiky, thick, membranous staining pattern **(Fig. 8.11).** While some metastatic adenocarcinomas may exhibit membranous staining, the thick, spiky pattern is not seen. In general, there is weak cytoplasmic staining of benign mesothelial cells and strong cytoplasmic staining of adenocarcinomas from diverse sites. Furthermore, adenocarcinomas frequently are positive for one or more of the following markers: carcinoembryonic antigen, Leu-M1, and B72.5.

Electron microscopic examination **(Fig. 8.12)** of mesothelial cells shows numerous long slender microvilli, well-formed desmosomes, and diffusely scattered bundles of tonofilaments with a perinuclear concentration.[11,20,21]

Diagnostic Pitfalls

One must differentiate malignant mesothelioma from reactive mesothelial hyperplasia. The aspirates from mesotheliomas are characteristically hypercellular and contain many cell sheets as well as three-dimensional cell balls of various sizes. Papillary clusters or spheres that contain up to several hundred cells are commonly seen in mesotheliomas. By contrast, reactive mesothelial hyperplasia seldom produces more than 15 to 20 cells in a cluster. Reactive mesothelial cells can show nuclear atypia as marked as malignant mesothelial cells, but they are not as numerous **(Fig. 6.26).** The pathologist must be aware of the conditions that may cause benign atypical mesothelial hyperplasia, such as hepatitis, cirrhosis, and chronic inflammation of the peritoneum including that induced by surgical operation. If such a condition is known to

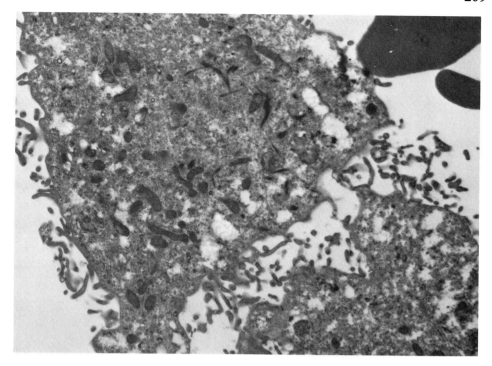

Fig. 8.12. Electron micrograph of a malignant mesothelioma, fine needle aspirate. Note long and tortuous surface microvilli and bundles of tonofilaments in the cytoplasm. (Uranyl acetate and lead citrate preparation; ×11,700).

exist, the pathologist must exercise caution in making the diagnosis of malignant mesothelioma on ABC.

Malignant peritoneal mesothelioma must be distinguished from diffuse peritoneal involvement by metastatic adenocarcinoma. Certain patterns of mesothelioma, such as the biphasic and the sarcomatoid, particularly when considered in conjunction with the gross and radiologic characteristics of the tumor, are almost diagnostic. Mesotheliomas with a pure tubulopapillary pattern may present a greater problem, but such a pattern may be quite distinctive when the tumor cells have the characteristic of mesothelial cells. The cells present in adenocarcinomas will exhibit more nuclear pleomorphism than malignant mesothelial cells, and their cytoplasm is paler and foamy. The cells may be arranged in glandular and acinous structures with central lumina. In contrast, smears of mesothelioma may contain sheets of cells showing characteristic cell-to-cell apposition with prominent intercellular gaps, resembling normal mesothelium and, although not entirely specific for mesothelioma, these cell sheets may be very helpful in tumor typing. To distinguish malignant mesothelioma from adenocarcinoma is less problematic today than it was in the past because of the easy availability of immunocytochemical stains and electron microscopy (*vide supra*). **Table 8.1** lists the differentiating features of malignant mesothelioma and adenocarcinoma.

An accurate cytologic diagnosis of malignant mesothelioma is feasible,[3,8,12,14,15,22]

**TABLE 8.1. Distinguishing Features of Malignant Mesothelioma
and Adenocarcinoma**

	Malignant Mesothelioma	*Adenocarcinoma*
Asbestos exposure	Often positive history	No
Radiologic findings	Diffuse thickening of perito- neum, bowel wall, mesen- tery, and omentum	Mass lesion or multiple nodules
Cytology		
Cells	Mesothelial-like and some spindle-shaped cells; Inter- cellular windows	Glandular cells with pale and foamy cytoplasm
Nuclei	Relatively uniform	More pleomorphic
Cell arrangement	Numerous cell balls	Glands, acini, cell balls
Mucicarmine	Negative	Frequently positive
PAS with diastase	Negative	Frequently positive
Immunostains for		
EMA	Thick, membranous staining	Diffuse staining
CEA, Leu M1, B72.5	Negative	Frequently positive
Electron microscopy	Long microvilli (1–3 µm) and perinuclear tonofila- ments	Short microvilli (< 1µm)

**TABLE 8.2. Combined Clinical/Radiologic/Morphologic Features of Malignant
Peritoneal Mesothelioma**

Clinical:	Male predominance, exposure to asbestos, abdominal pain, subacute intesti- nal obstruction, abdominal mass, and ascites.
US or CT:	Diffuse thickening of serosal and peritoneal surfaces, mantle-like soft-tissue nodules in omentum and mesentery.
ABC:	(1) Smear pattern: hypercellularity; large, three-dimensional cell clusters. (2) Cell morphology: resemblance to mesothelial cells, polygonal shape, ruf- fled cell borders, and cell-to-cell apposition with a prominent intercellular space. In biphasic tumors, fibroblastic spindle cells can be seen. (3) A wide range of cellular atypia seen even within the same aspirate. Fre- quent prominent nucleoli.
EM:	Well-developed desmosomes; abundant tonofilaments, often concentrated in perinuclear region; numerous long, thin, and branching microvilli.
IM:	Positive for EMA (thick membrane staining pattern); negative for Leu-M1, B72.5, and CEA.

US = ultrasound; CT = computed tomography; ABC = aspiration biopsy cytology; EM = electron
microscopy; IM = immunocytochemistry; EMA = epithelial membrane antigen; CEA = carcinoembryonic
antigen.

based on a combination of (1) a compatible clinical history, (2) characteristic radiologic findings, and (3) characteristic cytologic features, supported by special stains and/or electron microscopy **(Table 8.2).** Sterrett and associates,[12] who have had considerable experience in cytologic diagnosis of mesothelioma, believe that the relative ease of obtaining material by NAB and the low risk of tumor implantation make NAB worthy of consideration as a first-line diagnostic method in patients suspected of having mesothelioma, particularly in those cases without effusions that provide material for cytologic examination. In a series of 19 cases of malignant mesothelioma studied by NAB, these investigators were able to render a definite diagnosis of malignancy in 17 cases, a suggestive diagnosis of adenocarcinoma in one case, and unsatisfactory aspirate in one case. Of the 17 cases with a definite malignant diagnosis, eight were typed as definite mesothelioma, four were "consistent with mesothelioma," three were diagnosed as "mesothelioma versus carcinoma," one was called "malignant tumor not otherwise specified," and one "adenocarcinoma."

REFERENCES

1. Raftery AT: Regeneration of parietal and visceral peritoneum: An electron microscopical study. *J Anat* 115:375–392, 1984.

2. Miles JM, Hart WR, McMahon JT: Cystic mesothelioma of the peritoneum. *Cleveland Clin Quart* 53:109–114, 1986.

3. Tao LC: Aspiration biopsy cytology of mesothelioma. *Diagn Cytopathol* 5:14–21, 1989.

4. Chahinian AP, Pajak TF, Holand JF, et al: Diffuse malignant mesothelioma. Prospective evaluation of 69 patients. *Ann Intern Med* 96:746–755, 1982.

5. Musk AW, Dolin PJ, Armstrong BK, et al: The incidence of malignant mesothelioma in Australia, 1947–1980. *Med J Aust* 150:242–246, 1989.

6. Kannerstein M, Churg J: Peritoneal mesothelioma. *Hum Pathol* 8:83–94, 1977.

7. Yeh HC, Chahinian AP: Ultrasonography and computed tomography of peritoneal mesothelioma. *Radiology* 135:705–712, 1980.

8. Reuter K, Raptopoulos V, Reale F, et al: Diagnosis of peritoneal mesothelioma: Computed tomography, sonography and fine needle aspiration biopsy. *AJR* 140:1189–1194, 1983.

9. Triol JH, Conston AS, Chandler SV: Malignant mesothelioma. Cytopathology of 75 cases seen in a New Jersey Community Hospital. *Acta Cytol* 28:37–45, 1983.

10. Ehya H: The cytologic diagnosis of mesothelioma. *Semin Diagn Pathol* 3:196–203, 1986.

11. Leong ASY, Stevens MW, Mukherjee TM: Malignant mesotheliomas: Cytologic diagnosis with histologic, immunohistochemical, and ultrastructural correlation. *Semin Diagn Pathol* 9:141–150, 1992.

12. Sterrett GF, Whitaker D, Shilkin KB, et al: Fine needle aspiration cytology of malignant mesothelioma. *Acta Cytol* 31:185–193, 1987.

13. Jayaram G, Ashok S: Fine needle aspiration cytology of well-differentiated papillary peritoneal mesothelioma. Report of a case. *Acta Cytol* 32:563–566, 1988.

14. Whitaker D, Shilkin KB, Sterrett GF: Cytological appearances of malignant mesothelioma. In Henderson DW, Shilkin KB, Langlois SLP, et al (eds): *Malignant Mesothelioma.* New York, Hemisphere Publishing, 1992, pp 167–182.

15. Craig FE, Fishback NF, Schwartz JG, et al: Occult metastatic mesothelioma—Diagnosis by fine-needle aspiration. A case report. *Am J Clin Pathol* 97:493–497, 1992.

16. Lucas JG, Tuttle SE: Diagnostic histochemical and immunohistochemical studies in malignant mesothelioma. *J Surg Oncol* 35:30–34, 1987.

17. Bolen JW: Tumors of serosal tissue origin. *Clin Lab Med* 7:31–50, 1987.

18. van der Kwast TH, Versnel MA, Delahaye M, et al: Expression of epithelial membrane antigen on malignant mesothelioma cells. An immunocytochemical and immunoelectron microscopic study. *Acta Cytol* 32:169–174, 1988.

19. Leong ASY, Parkinson R, Milios J: "Thick" cell membranes revealed by immunocytochemical staining: A clue to the diagnosis of mesothelioma. *Diagn Cytol* 6:9–13, 1990.

20. Kobzik L, Antman KH, Warhol MJ: The distinction of mesothelioma from adenocarcinoma in malignant effusions by electron microscopy. *Acta Cytol* 29:219–225, 1985.

21. Weidner N: Malignant mesothelioma of peritoneum. *Ultrastruct Pathol* 15:515–520, 1991.

22. Sherman ME, Mark EJ: Effusion cytology in the diagnosis of malignant epithelioid and biphasic plueral mesothelioma. *Arch Pathol Lab Med* 114:845–851, 1990.

9

Adrenals

KEY POINTS

▶ Increase in the use of modern imaging technology has led to the incidental discovery of many small adrenal nodules, resulting in an increased demand for the interpretation of the cytologic specimens of these lesions.

▶ Percutaneous NAB of adrenal nodules can be used in staging patients with extraadrenal malignancies. A cytologic diagnosis is useful in therapeutic planning and in predicting prognosis.

▶ Primary adrenal tumors with benign cytology and under 5 cm in size can be safely managed conservatively, with follow-up scans.

▶ Adrenocortical carcinomas are almost always symptomatic and large. The chances of diagnosing an adrenocortical carcinoma in an incidentally discovered adrenal nodule are extremely low.

▶ Surgery should be considered for primary adrenal tumors that show atypical cytology or are greater than 5 cm.

▶ Adrenalectomy is the treatment of choice for any functioning adrenal tumors, irrespective of size or cytology.

EMBRYOLOGY AND ANATOMY

To understand the diversity of adrenal tumors, knowledge of the embryology and histology of the normal adrenal gland is necessary. Although the adrenal gland is an anatomic entity, it is made up of two distinct units that differ from each other in origin and function. The cortex originates from mesodermal cells on the posterior body wall near the urogenital ridge. The medulla is ectodermal in origin; cells from the neural crest invade the mass of mesenchymal fetal cortex and migrate to its center to form the medulla. These primitive cells mature in two directions to form either ganglion cells or pheochromocytes.

The two adrenal glands in humans are located in the retroperitoneum, resting on the superomedial borders of the kidneys. Each gland weighs 4–6 gm in a healthy adult. In cross-section, the glands are triangular. The cortex is bright yellow due to its high lipid content, and the medulla is pale gray. Microscopically, three zones of the cortex can be recognized. The outermost zone, the zona glomerulosa, is rarely prominent in the normal gland, being only focally present in the subcapsular areas of the cortex. It is composed of small, dark cells containing variable amounts of lipid. The middle zone, the zona fasciculata, is the broadest. Its cells are arranged in long straight columns or fascicles, and most have vacuolated cytoplasm because of their high lipid content. The innermost zone, the zona reticularis, has compacted cells that are arranged in nests, with granular, pink, lipid-poor cytoplasm. The medulla is composed of somewhat pleomorphic cells, which are ovoid, polygonal, or fusiform, and are grouped in nests and cords around sinusoidal vessels. The nuclei are frequently eccentrically placed within the cytoplasm, and prominent nucleoli are not uncommon. The cytoplasm is basophilic and finely granular. A few ganglion cells are interspersed.

Functionally, the zona glomerulosa synthesizes mineralocorticoids (e.g., aldosterone), which are responsible for the retention of salt and water and excretion of potassium. The zona fasciculata and zona reticularis function as one unit and are the site of production of glucocorticoids (e.g., cortisol) and androgens. The glucocorticoids accelerate glucose synthesis, increase protein catabolism, and influence fat mobilization. The adrenal medulla produces epinephrine and norepinephrine. These hormones cause a rise in blood pressure and redistribution of blood in response to stress and fear, facilitating better adaptation for "fight and flight."

OVERVIEW OF ADRENAL TUMORS

Structurally and functionally two main groups of primary tumors of the adrenal glands are recognized. One group originates in the adrenal cortex, and the other in the medulla.

Tissue origin	Corresponding neoplasm
Adrenal cortex	Adrenocortical adenoma
	Adrenocortical carcinoma
Adrenal medulla	Pheochromocytoma
	Neuroblastoma, ganglioneuroblastoma

Other primary neoplasms of the adrenal are very uncommon. Malignant melanomas arising primarily in the medulla are encountered occasionally.[1] Benign adrenal tumors and tumor-like lesions, such as lipomas, myelolipomas, fibromas, and cysts, are generally asymptomatic and discovered incidentally.[2]

Adrenocortical adenoma and carcinoma may be functioning or nonfunctioning. The most common features of functioning cortical tumors are those of Cushing's syndrome, caused by excessive production of glucocorticoids. The syndrome is characterized by central obesity, moon-face, muscle weakness, osteoporosis of the spine, hypertension, and diabetes. Less frequently, when a tumor secretes large quantities of androgenic hormones, virilization is the most conspicuous feature. A cortical tumor that secretes mineralocorticoids results in salt retention, hypokalemia, and hypertension (Conn's syndrome). The majority of patients manifesting Conn's syndrome have an adrenal adenoma rather than carcinoma. Since various steroid hormones are secreted by functioning tumors, measurements of levels of plasma hormones and urinary metabolites are diagnostically useful.

In cases of nonfunctioning adrenocortical carcinoma, signs and symptoms relate most frequently to local pain, abdominal mass, or the appearance of metastases. By contrast, nonfunctioning adrenocortical adenomas are frequently asymptomatic and discovered only during radiologic imaging or autopsy.

Pheochromocytomas and neuroblastomas arise in the adrenal medulla and are of neuroendocrine origin. About 90% of pheochromocytomas are benign and occur in adults, whereas neuroblastomas are highly malignant and occur in children. Both tumors secrete increased quantities of epinephrine, norepinephrine, and catechol metabolites. Measurements of these substances in the urine have been standardized.

NORMAL ADRENAL GLAND CYTOLOGY

The cells of the normal adrenal cortex **(Fig. 9.1)** appear in fine needle aspirates as small aggregates and cords of uniform polyhedral cells. Two main types of cortical cells are seen: vacuolated cells and compact cells. The former are mainly derived from the zona fasciculata and the latter from the zona reticularis. The vacuolated cells have abundant, pale cytoplasm that contains sharply delineated, honeycomb-type

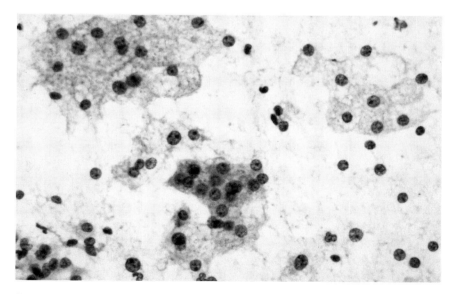

Fig. 9.1. Normal ABC of the adrenal cortex. Note two small sheets of vacuolated cells with uniform, round nuclei and a small sheet of nonvacuolated, compact cells (*lower center*). The dispersed single cells with stripped nuclei resemble lymphocytes. (H & E preparation; ×500).

vacuoles. The vacuolation is a result of extraction of the intracytoplasmic lipids by alcohol fixation. The nuclei are small to moderate in size, round, and centrally located, exhibiting fine chromatin and a single inconspicuous nucleolus. The nonvacuolated cells, also referred to as compact cells, lack cytoplasmic lipid and, thus, their cytoplasm stains homogeneously eosinophilic.

Cells of the adrenal medulla are scanty or absent in the aspirates. If present, the normal pheochromocytes **(Fig. 9.2)** are polygonal cells with finely granular, cyanophilic cytoplasm and distinct nucleoli. They exhibit more variation in size and shape than the cortical cells. Larger, irregular forms are occasionally seen.

Diagnostic Pitfalls

The cytopathologist must be familiar with the normal cytology of the adrenal gland, otherwise mistakes in interpretation may occur. For example, Mitchell et al[3] reported a case of adrenal aspiration in which the cells of a metastatic adenocarcinoma from the lung were mistaken for benign adrenal cortical cells. In general, cytologic features of malignancy in metastatic tumors are quite obvious. Careful scrutiny of the nuclear details can prevent confusion. In our experience, sampling errors as a result of misplacement of the needle are the main cause of false-negative diagnoses of adrenal aspirates. A false-negative report due to misinterpretation of metastatic cancer cells as normal adrenal cortical cells is uncommon.

Hoda et al[4] have pointed out the pitfall of mistaking normal medullary cells for cells of metastatic tumor. It is important to remember that some pheochromocytes can be large and have rather prominent nucleoli, and therefore constitute a potential source of false-positive diagnosis.

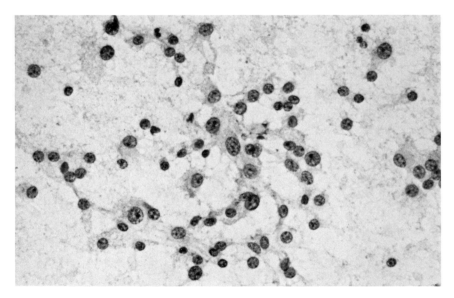

Fig. 9.2. Adrenal medulla, imprint preparation from a normal gland. The medullary cells, with finely granular cytoplasm, exhibit more variation in size and shape then the normal cortical cells. (H & E preparation; ×500).

ADRENOCORTICAL ADENOMA/ NODULES

Adrenocortical adenomas are discrete, solitary lesions of the adrenal cortex. They are usually small, 2–4 cm in diameter, although some are larger. Most cortical adenomas are nonfunctioning and are incidental findings during diagnostic imaging or autopsy. The clinical manifestations, if present, depend on the type of hormone secreted by the tumor. They may cause Cushing's syndrome, adrenogenital syndrome, Conn's syndrome, or a mixed syndrome. Multiple asymptomatic cortical nodules, regarded by most pathologists as a nodular form of cortical hyperplasia, are commonly seen at autopsy. Like adrenocortical tumors, nodular hyperplasia may be related to various clinical syndromes.

Histologically, adenomas typically, but not invariably, have capsules, whereas hyperplastic nodules do not. The adenoma/nodule consists of a mixture of lipid-laden vacuolated cells and compact cells with some intermediate forms, but for the most part the cell admixture is variable. The cells are arranged in sheets and in smaller alveolar nests. Occasionally there may be focal anisonucleosis. Some cells are large and hyperchromatic, and some are binucleated. One must be aware of these histologic features so as not to interpret them as malignant changes.[5]

Aspiration Biopsy Cytology

The ABC of cortical adenomas and hyperplastic nodules are indistinguishable and are therefore described together here. On an aspirate smear, the cells of cortical adenoma/nodule are arranged in small cords or in a vague nesting pattern. Lipid-rich vacuolated cells and compact cells are seen, either in combination or alone. The morphologic appearance of these cells is similar to the normal adrenal cortical cells **(Fig. 9.3)**. The nuclei are uniform, round or oval, with evenly distributed, finely granular chromatin. The process of aspiration and smearing often disrupts the cell membranes of the lipid-rich cells, resulting in dispersion of fat droplets in the smear background. In addition, because of cytoplasmic fragility, a large number of bare round nuclei, mimicking lymphocytes, may be seen.

In an occasional adenoma there may be cellular enlargement, anisonucleosis, nuclear hyperchromatism, and prominent nucleoli **(Fig. 9.4)**. One must remember that cellular atypia alone, especially when it is minimal, is not indicative of malignancy.

Diagnostic Pitfalls

Because the cells seen in the aspirates of many cases of adrenocortical adenoma/nodule may not be distinguishable from normal adrenal cortical cells, Heaston and colleagues[6] have stressed the importance of verifying the location of the aspiration needle by computed tomography to ensure its correct placement within the suspected mass. Without this placement verification, the pathologist may misinterpret the recovered normal cortical cells for cells from an adenoma/nodule, when in fact the needle has missed the target lesion and the normal part of the cortex has been aspirated. The role of a skilled and experienced aspirator cannot be overemphasized.

Cellular pleomorphism and anisonucleosis are seen in some adenomas. Familiarity

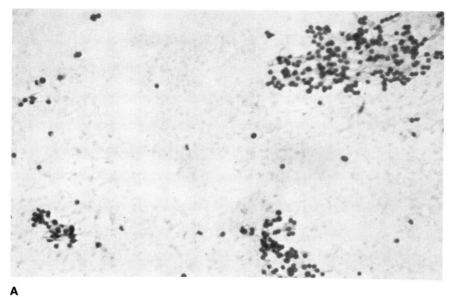

Fig. 9.3. Adrenocortical adenoma. **A.** ABC. Low magnification view showing monolayered sheets of vacuolated cells. (H & E preparation; ×125). **B.** ABC. Note smoothly contoured, round nuclei, uniformly distributed chromatin, and inconspicuous nucleoli. The cytoplasm is vacuolated with spilling of fat droplets onto the smear background. (H & E preparation; ×500).

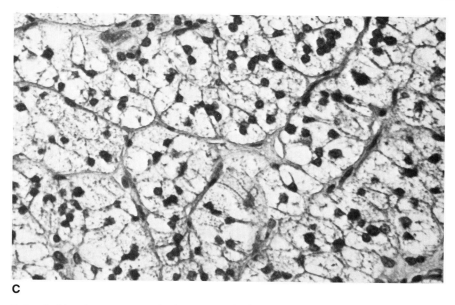

C

Fig. 9.3. C. Histologic section of adrenocortical adenoma. Note groups of lipid-laden tumor cells separated by thin fibrovascular septa. (H & E preparation; ×310).

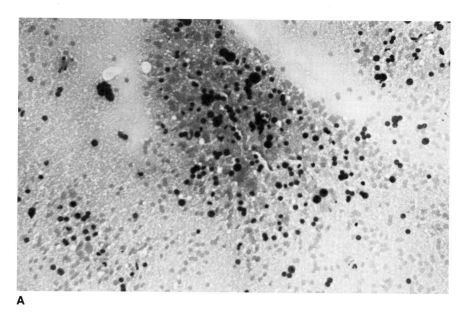

A

Fig. 9.4. Adrenocortical adenoma. **A.** ABC. Note anisonucleosis and hyerchromatism of nuclei. (H & E preparation; ×125).

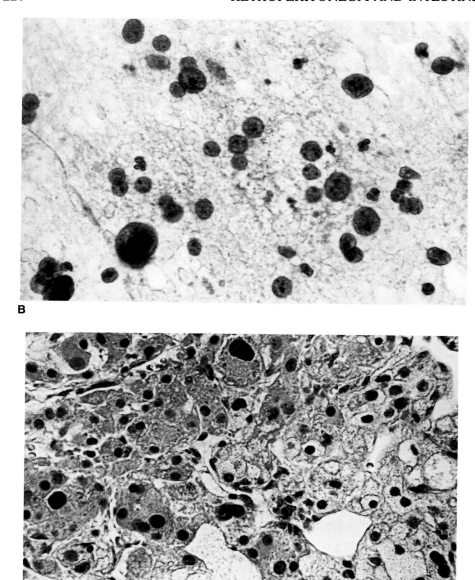

Fig. 9.4. B. ABC. Higher magnification view. Despite marked anisonucleosis and prominent nucleoli, the nuclear contour is smooth and round, and chromatin is evenly distributed. Note large amount of fat droplets in the background. (H & E preparation; ×500). **C.** Histologic section of adrenocortical adenoma showing marked variation in nuclear size and hyperchromatism. (H & E preparation; ×310).

with the nuclear features of these benign lesions aids in distinguishing them from cortical carcinomas. Generally in aspirates obtained from cortical adenomas, the cells show round and smoothly contoured nuclei, and chromatin is evenly distributed, despite anisonucleosis, nuclear hyperchromatism, and nucleolar prominence. In contrast, malignant cells show irregularity in nuclear contour, uneven thickness of nuclear membranes, and irregular chromatin distribution. Furthermore, atypia is usually focal in adenoma so that the enlarged atypical cells are seen often in association with many bland, benign-appearing cortical cells.

When the cortical cells are stripped of their cytoplasm during aspiration, they appear on the smears as naked round nuclei that may simulate lymphocytes. On occasion, these naked nuclei are present in such large numbers that they may suggest lymphoma. The presence of fat droplets in the background and their strong resemblance to the nuclei of the other cortical cells aid in identifying the true nature of these cells.

Finally, the naked nuclei of the adrenal cortical cells may be mistaken for metastatic small cell carcinoma **(Fig. 9.5)**.[7,8] This mistake can be avoided if one pays attention to the uniform chromatin distribution and smooth contour of the nuclei of the cortical cells. Common characteristics of small cell anaplastic carcinoma, such as nuclear molding, irregularity in nuclear membranes, cell necrosis, and cell smudging are conspicuously absent in aspirates containing the naked nuclei of benign adrenal cortical cells.

ADRENOCORTICAL CARCINOMA

Primary carcinoma of the adrenal cortex is rare, afflicting two per million in the general population and accounting for less than 0.2% of the deaths from cancer.[9–11] Although some adrenocortical carcinomas are nonfunctioning, the majority present with one of several endocrine abnormalities due to uncontrolled secretion of various hydroxycorticosteroids or their precursor substances.[2,12] At initial presentation, 40–60% of patients have clinical endocrine manifestations, and up to 80% of adrenocortical carcinomas may be found to be functioning when complete hormonal evaluation is performed.[13] Adrenocortical carcinomas are generally large—some exceed more than 20 cm in diameter when discovered.

Microscopically, they show wide histologic variability, ranging from well-differentiated areas in which the cells resemble those seen in adenomas, to less differentiated areas in which the cells are highly pleomorphic and exhibit numerous mitoses.[2,14] Most tumors have a morphologic appearance in between these two extremes. However, in the absence of vascular invasion or metastasis, there are no absolute histologic criteria to ascertain malignancy. Malignancy is highly likely when the following features are present:[15]

1. Widespread tumor necrosis
2. Numerous mitoses or atypical mitoses
3. Marked cellular pleomorphism
4. Diffuse architecture
5. Broad fibrous bands

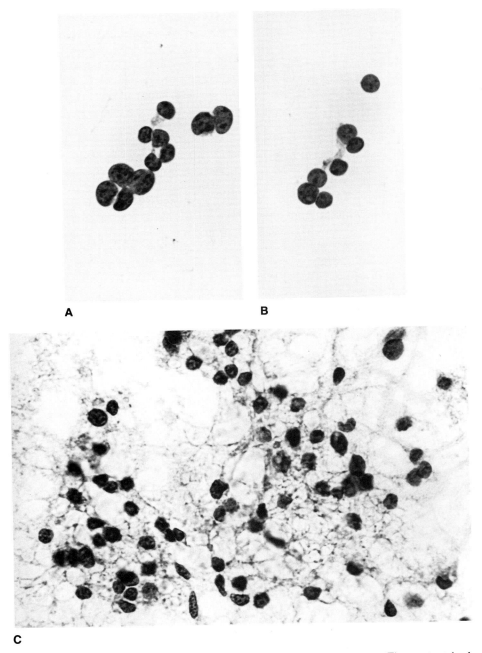

Fig. 9.5. Benign adrenocortical nodule mimicking small cell carcinoma. This patient had a pulmonary mass and underwent an abdominal computed tomography for staging workup. The computed tomography disclosed bilateral adrenal swellings. Fine needle aspiration biopsy of one of the adrenal masses was initially misinterpreted by a pathologist as metastatic small cell carcinoma of lung. Subsequent follow-up showed the pulmonary mass to be an adenocarci-

Another feature that favors malignancy is large tumor size. Rosai reported that, in his experience, most large tumors (over 5 cm or 50 gm) behaved in a malignant fashion.[16] Tang and Gray reported that all patients in their series whose tumors were less than 50 gm survived, and all tumors of 95 gm or more proved malignant.[17] Whether or not all adrenocortical neoplasms have the potential to metastasize and the smaller ones just have not had time to disseminate remains uncertain. This is a fairly common problem in the oncology of endocrine organs.

Aspiration Biopsy Cytology

Adrenocortical carcinomas are rare, and their cytologic features have seldom been reported. Most papers dealt only with single case reports.[18–21] Wadih et al[22] studied 50 NABs of the adrenal gland, which included only one case of adrenocortical carcinoma. Katz and associates[23,24] reported four cases in 1984, and subsequently gathered 12 cases which the authors called "cortical neoplasms/carcinomas," and published their preliminary findings in abstract form in 1992. We have retrieved seven cases from our files since 1978 and had the opportunity to see two additional cases (courtesy of Denise Hidvegi, M.D., Chicago).

All our cases showed extreme cellularity. The malignant cells showed loss of cellular cohesion and were lying singly or aggregated loosely in small clusters. Tumor necrosis was a frequent feature. The tumor cells were larger than normal cortical cells, but in one case the cells were smaller (Fig. 9.6). The degree of cellular atypia varied from case to case. Well-differentiated tumors were characterized by predominance of lipid-laden, vacuolated cells with somewhat enlarged nuclei, irregular nuclear membranes, and prominent nucleoli in some cells. Chromatin was coarsely clumped or diffusely hyperchromatic. Cytoplasm was fragile, and many naked nuclei were seen. The atypical stripped nuclei with loss of cell cohesion simulated the appearance of a malignant lymphoma. In the poorly differentiated carcinomas (Fig. 9.7), most of the tumor cells were lipid-poor, with eosinophilic granular cytoplasm. Cytologic criteria of malignancy were readily observed. There was extreme cellular pleomorphism, as evidenced by large, bizarre cells with multinucleation. Although we have described here well-differentiated and poorly differentiated tumors as though they were two distinct categories, in fact many adrenocortical carcinomas exhibit a broad range of cellular atypia, which varies from area to area within the same tumor.

Diagnostic Pitfalls

Adrenocortical carcinoma has to be distinguished from adenoma. Other than blood vessel invasion and evidence of metastasis, there is no one single morphologic criterion that can be used reliably to separate the two. Multiple criteria must be used—the

noma and the NAB represented a false-positive diagnosis. **A,B.** Aspirate smear showing naked nuclei of benign adrenal cortical cells simulating small cell anaplastic carcinoma. (H & E preparation; A, B: ×600). **C.** Another smear from the same specimen showing easily recognizable adrenal cortical cells with intact vacuolated cytoplasm. Had these cells been stripped of their cytoplasm, they could also mimic small cell carcinoma. (H & E preparation; ×500). (From Suen KC, McNeely TB: Adrenal cortical cells mimicking small cell anaplastic carcinoma in a fine needle aspirate. *Mod Pathol* 4:594–595, 1991, with permission.)

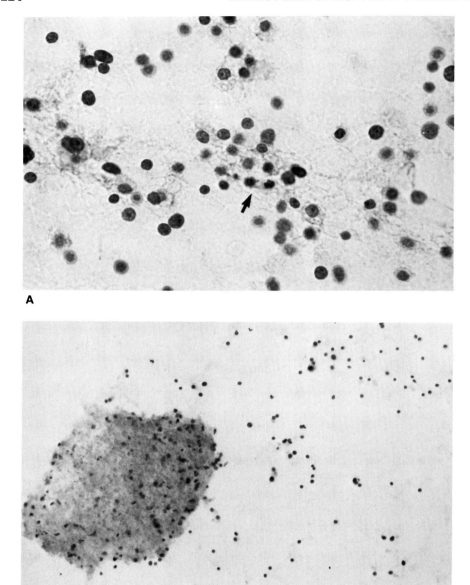

Fig. 9.6. Well-differentiated adrenocortical carcinoma, 10 cm in diameter. **A.** ABC. In this case, the tumor cells are smaller than normal adrenal cortical cells. Note subtle variability in nuclear shape (i.e., the nuclei are no longer smoothly contoured). Some cells show prominent nucleoli. Arrow indicates two mitoses. (H & E preparation; ×400). **B.** ABC. Note large fragment of eosinophilic necrotic tumor tissue. (H & E preparation; ×125).

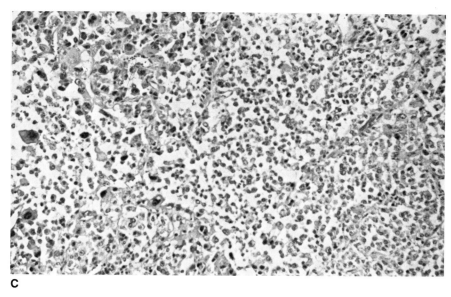

C

Fig. 9.6. C. Histologic section of adrenocortical carcinoma. Note tumor necrosis in center of the field. (H & E preparation; × 125).

more criteria that are observed, the more accurate will be the diagnosis. Features seen in NAB that are strongly in favor of malignancy include tumor necrosis, frequent mitoses, loss of intercellular cohesion, and marked cellular pleomorphism. Tumor size greater than 5 cm also suggests malignancy. Recent flow cytometric studies have shown that alterations in DNA content (aneuploidy) of the tumor cells correlate well with malignant behavior in adrenocortical tumors.[25]

Adrenocortical carcinomas with vacuolated cells may mimic renal cell carcinoma **(Table 9.1)**. In most cases, uroradiologic studies and urine and plasma hormonal measurements may clarify the origin of the tumor. In difficult cases, histochemical stains, immunostains, or electron microscopy, or a combination of any of these special procedures may be required for diagnosis. A characteristic, although by no means specific, feature of renal cell carcinoma is the presence of abundant cytoplasmic glycogen, demonstrable by a positive periodic acid-Schiff, diastase digestible reaction (see **Plate 10.2**) or by electron microscopy. Conversely, glycogen is rarely found in adrenocortical neoplasms. Adrenocortical carcinomas are immunopositive for vimentin but negative for keratin and epithelial membrane antigen (EMA),[26–28] although some investigators have also reported focal positivity for keratin and EMA in some adrenocortical carcinomas.[13,29] Using formalin-fixed, cell block sections prepared from the aspirates of four cases of adrenocortical carcinoma, we have failed to demonstrate immunoreactivity for EMA and keratin. Renal cell carcinomas, on the other hand, show positive immunostaining for epithelial markers, Lewis blood group antigens, as well as vimentin. More recently, some European investigators reported the use of D11 monoclonal antibody in identifying adrenocortical carcinomas. Nuclear D11 positivity appears to be highly specific and was demonstrated in 44–100% of adrenocortical carcinomas.[13,30] Electron microscopy may also provide diagnostic aid in difficult cases.

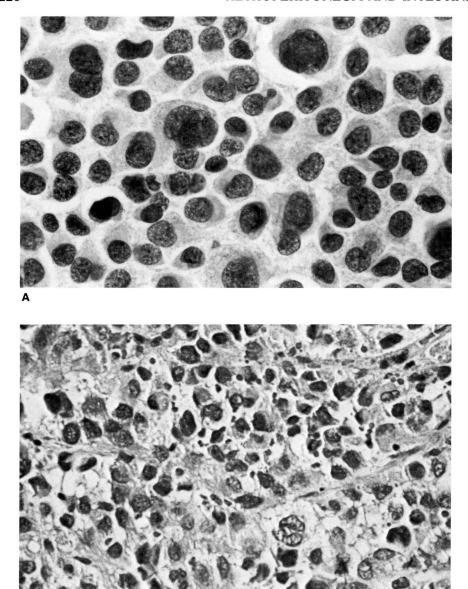

Fig. 9.7. Poorly differentiated adrenocortical carcinoma. **A.** ABC. Note large pleomorphic cells. They are lipid-poor cells with eosinophilic cytoplasm. (H & E preparation; ×500). **B.** Histologic section showing many necrotic pleomorphic tumor cells. (H & E preparation; ×500).

TABLE 9.1. Distinguishing Features of Adrenocortical Carcinoma and Renal Cell Carcinoma

	Adrenocortical Carcinoma	Renal Cell Carcinoma
Imaging	Tumor in adrenal gland	Tumor in kidney
Elevated hydroxycortico-steroids in urine/serum	Positive	Negative
Papillary fronds on ABC*	Negative	Positive
PAS stain for glycogen†	Negative	Positive
Immunostains		
EMA	Negative‡	Positive
Keratin	Negative‡	Positive
Vimentin	Positive	Positive
Lewis BGA	Negative	Positive
Electron microscopy	Abundant smooth ER, mitochondria with tubular cristae, lipid vacuoles	Microvilli, acinar formation, copious cytoplasmic glycogen, lipid vacuoles

*See Chapter 10, section on Renal Cell Carcinoma.

†See color plate 10.2.

‡Some authors reported focal positivity in occasional adrenocortical carcinomas.

BGA = blood group antigens; ER = endoplasmic reticulum.

The characteristic mitochondria with vesicular or tubulovesicular cristae, abundant smooth endoplasmic reticulum, and cytoplasmic lipid vacuoles are ultrastructural features of steroidogenic cells **(Fig. 9.8)**.[31–33] In renal cell carcinomas, evidence of tubular differentiation and microvilli may be seen.

Metastatic tumors such as malignant melanoma or large cell carcinoma of the lung can sometimes be confused with primary cortical carcinoma. Malignant melanomas often contain melanin pigment, may have spindle cells with macronucleoli, nearly always show positive immunostaining for S100 protein and HMB-45. Carcinoma cells from the lung may show a glandular arrangement with lumina, do not have any resemblance to normal adrenal cortical cells, and may contain cytoplasmic mucin droplets. Review of multiple smears may be necessary to identify these features.

Careful attention to the clinical setting and the patient's biochemical profiles also aids in resolving the diagnostic problem. Primary adrenal cancers may be clinically silent, but are rarely nonfunctional when appropriate biochemical tests are applied. The urine 17-ketosteroids are frequently markedly elevated in patients with adrenocortical carcinomas.[9]

PHEOCHROMOCYTOMA

Pheochromocytomas are neoplasms of the pheochromocytes. The pheochromocytes have their origin in the primitive neural crest and their tumors belong to the family of APUD tumors (see Chapter 7, section on Carcinoid Tumors). Besides occurring in the adrenal medulla, pheochromocytomas can be found in association with the

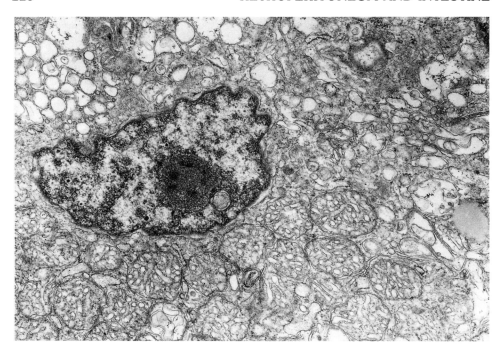

Fig. 9.8. Electron micrograph of adrenocortical carcinoma. Note cytoplasm containing abundant vesicular smooth endoplasmic reticulum and many mitochrondria with tubular and vesicular cristae. These features are typical of steroidogenic cells. (Uranyl acetate and lead citrate preparation; ×28,000).

sympathetic nerve chains and plexus. These extraadrenal pheochromocytomas are referred to as paragangliomas. Although not common, pheochromocytomas are by no means rare. In unselected autopsy populations, the prevalence of pheochromocytomas has been estimated as high as 0.1%.[34] These tumors secrete catecholamines and are responsible for about 0.5–1% of all cases of hypertension.[35] The hypertension can be dramatically relieved by surgical removal of the tumor; thus early diagnosis is of paramount importance. In 90% of cases diagnosis can be made by finding increased quantities of catecholamines or their metabolites such as vanillylmandelic acid in the patient's urine or plasma. If a biochemical diagnosis of pheochromocytoma has been established, NAB becomes superfluous. However, in the case of a clinically nonfunctional tumor or when the biochemical findings are equivocal, a correct preoperative diagnosis may be obtained using NAB.[36] Aspiration biopsy of a catecholamine-secreting tumor is not without risk—a case of fatality following the procedure has been reported.[37]

About 5–10% of pheochromocytomas are familial, and in up to 70% of these cases the tumors are bilateral. Pheochromocytomas may be part of the multiple endocrine neoplasia syndrome, type II (Sipple's syndrome). In this syndrome, the pheochromocytomas are associated with medullary thyroid carcinoma and parathyroid hyperplasia.[38] It is important that members of these kinships be monitored with periodic catecholamine or vanillylmandelic acid determinations to detect pheochromocytomas, and serum calcitonin estimations to detect medullary thyroid carcinomas.

Pathology and Aspiration Biopsy Cytology

Pheochromocytomas are generally well delineated, soft, red to yellow masses. Histologically, many tumors show a resemblance to the normal adrenal medulla, with cells arranged in ball-like nests, separated by thin connective tissue septa. The cells are polygonal, with moderate variation in size, and have round to oval nuclei with fairly prominent nucleoli. The cytoplasm is moderately abundant, finely granular and eosinophilic. Scattered bizarre cells may be seen, but they have no relationship to clinical malignancy. About 90% of these tumors have a benign clinical course. As with adrenocortical carcinoma, there are no reliable histologic features capable of predicting malignant behavior. Even when pheochromocytoma is metastatic, its histologic appearance is basically indistinguishable from that of the noninvasive, benign form.

The needle aspirates are usually cell-rich and contain much blood because of the rich vascularity of the neoplasms. The cells are lying singly, in loose alveolar groups which correspond to the cell nests in histologic sections, or in larger tissue fragments, some of which have festoons probably corresponding to the vacuolar spaces in tissue sections (**Figs. 9.9–9.11**).

The following three cell types are seen:

1. Small to medium-sized, uniform, polygonal cells with a moderate amount of finely granular cytoplasm. The nuclei are regular, round or oval, with evenly distributed granular chromatin, prominent chromocenters or nucleoli (**Fig. 9.9**). These cells

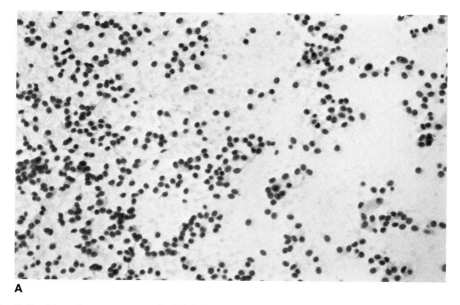

A

Fig. 9.9. Pheochromocytoma. **A.** ABC. Note small to medium-sized uniform cells, arranged in small alveolar groups. (H & E preparation; ×125).

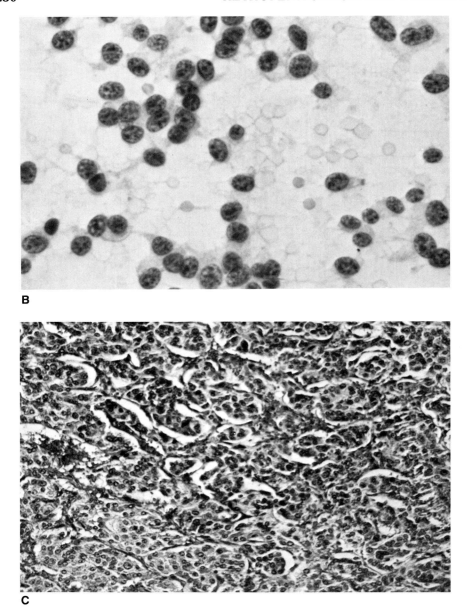

Fig. 9.9. B. ABC. Note uniform polygonal cells with eccentric nuclei and evenly dispersed, granular chromatin. These cells are the prototypic cells of neuroendocrine neoplasms. (H & E preparation; ×500). **C.** Histologic section of pheochromocytoma showing uniform polygonal cells arranged in ball-like nests separated by delicate fibrovascular tissue septa. (H & E preparation; ×310).

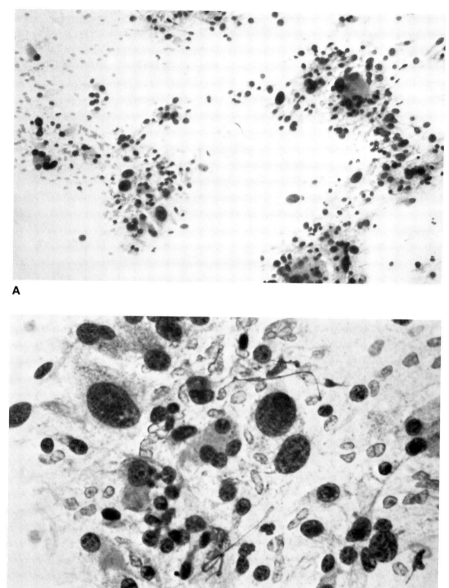

Fig. 9.10. Pheochromocytoma. **A.** ABC. Note marked cellular pheomorphism and nuclear gigantism. (H & E preparation; ×125). **B.** ABC. Note small uniform polygonal cells admixed with the large bizarre cells. (H & E preparation; ×500).

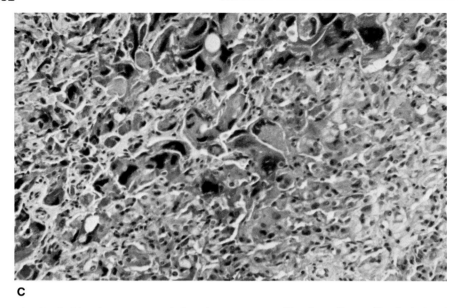

C

Fig. 9.10. C. Histologic section of pheochromocytoma. Note large "myoid" cells with voluminous eosinophilic granular cytoplasm. (H & E preparation; × 125).

are reminiscent of those seen in carcinoids and islet cell tumors, and are the prototypic cells of neuroendocrine tumors.

2. Large myoid-like cells often with eccentric large nuclei, prominent nucleoli, and abundant eosinophilic, finely granular cytoplasm **(Fig. 9.10).** Some of these large cells resemble ganglion cells, while others are multinucleated and have irregular shapes.

3. Fusiform or spindle cells with elongated, blunt-ended nuclei and eosinophilic cytoplasm **(Fig. 9.11).**

Most pheochromocytomas show a mixture of uniform polygonal cells, large myoidlike cells, and spindle cells. When the large irregular cells and spindle cells are present in large numbers, a polymorphic and pleomorphic cytologic picture emerges that may be mistaken for malignancy.

Diagnostic Pitfalls

Few reports on the cytology of pheochromocytomas are available because of their infrequent occurrence. Despite the fact that 90% of pheochromocytomas are benign, the literature and our own experience lead us to believe that a malignant diagnosis is almost always made when cytopathologists encounter such an uncommon tumor for the first time. Nguyen[39] diagnosed a case in which the tumor cells showed pleomorphic nuclei, chromatin clumping, and prominent nucleoli as an unclassified malignant epithelial tumor. Moussouris et al[40] made a diagnosis of malignant tumor, presumably of nonepithelial type, in a case of pheochromocytoma. The case reported by Lambert et al was interpreted initially as pancreatic carcinoma.[41] Even on frozen

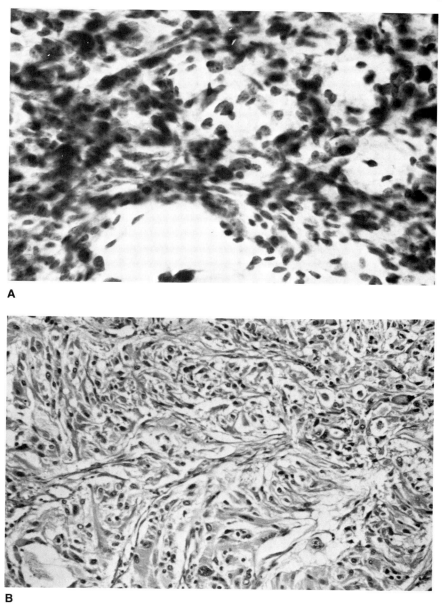

Fig. 9.11. Pheochromocytoma with a prominent spindle cell component. **A.** ABC. Tissue fragment composed of spindle cells. The festoons seen within the tissue fragment probably represent vascular channels. (H & E preparation; ×500). **B.** Histologic section of pheochromocytoma with many spindle cells. (H & E preparation; ×310).

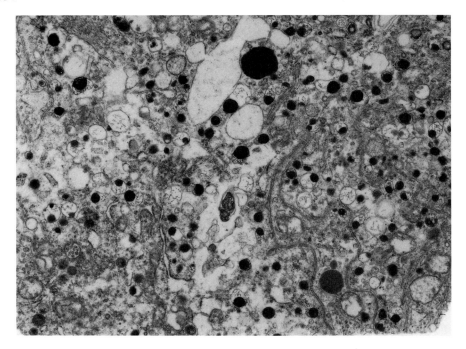

Fig. 9.12. Pheochromocytoma, electron micrograph. Note numerous membrane-bound neurosecretory granules with eccentric cores, consistent with nonepinephrine storage. The few larger granules are lysosomes. (Uranyl acetate and lead citrate preparation; ×12,000).

section examination, misdiagnosis as a malignancy is common because of cellular polymorphism and nuclear gigantism.[42] Our first case was also misinterpreted as malignant (it was called "probable sarcoma" because many spindle cells were present) and in our second case the tumor cells were called "highly atypical" by another pathologist. However, once the interpreters had been familiarized with the cytologic features, our subsequent cases were correctly diagnosed or suspected to be pheochromocytoma. Diagnostic mistakes can be prevented by recognizing the prototypic polygonal cells with fairly abundant finely granular cytoplasm that are always present in variable numbers in pheochromocytomas. If pheochromocytoma is suspected, the diagnosis can be confirmed by demonstrating neurosecretory granules in the cell cytoplasm, using electron microscopy **(Fig. 9.12)**, immunocytochemistry, or argyrophil staining technique.

NEUROBLASTOMA

Except for central nervous system tumors, neuroblastoma is the most common solid tumor of infancy and childhood. This highly malignant tumor originates from the primitive neuroblasts of the adrenal medulla or sympathetic ganglia. Hence the tumor can occur in a variety of paraspinal locations from neck to pelvis. Most commonly, the child presents with a large abdominal mass arising in the adrenal, and the mass may often cross the midline. In most cases, the provisional diagnosis of neuroblastoma can be confirmed by demonstrating abnormal quantities of catecholamines and their metabolites in the urine. About two-thirds of patients have metastases at the time of initial presentation.[43] The metastases are most common in the lymph nodes, liver, lung, and bones.[44] These sites are common targets for needle aspiration biopsy.[45-47]

Pathology and Aspiration Biopsy Cytology

Neuroblastoma is the prototypic "small, round, blue cell" tumor of childhood.[48] Histologically the tumor is composed of primitive small cells with diffuse growth pattern or ill-defined nests (lobules) separated by thin fibrovascular septa. Rosette formation is a common feature, although in some undifferentiated tumors, they may be absent. The rosettes are formed of one or two circular rows of tumor cells enclosing a central, pale-staining fibrillar matrix, which represents a tangled skein of neuritic cell processes.

The aspirates of neuroblastoma are highly cellular and consist of small uniform cells (neoplastic neuroblasts) that resemble, but are larger than, normal lymphocytes. They have dark-staining, round nuclei, with densely speckled chromatin, no obvious mitoses, and very little cytoplasm. In places the tumor cells tend to be arranged in a circular manner around a central area containing eosinophilic fibrils, reminiscent of the rosettes seen in tissue sections **(Fig. 9.13)**.

Immunostaining of neuroblastoma cells for neuron-specific enolase (NSE) and neurofilaments is consistently positive. However, one must be aware that NSE is not a specific marker for neuroblastoma, being positive in some Wilms' tumors that show neural differentiation.[49] NSE also shows cross reaction with differentiated myoblasts

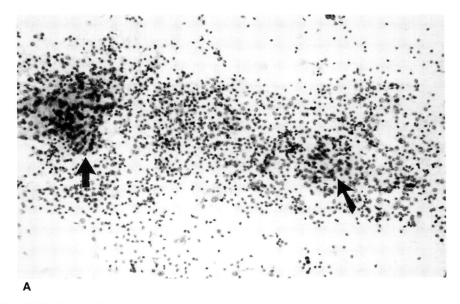

A

Fig. 9.13. Neuroblastoma, metastatic to a supraclavicular lymph node. **A.** ABC. Note clusters of dark-staining tumor cells forming rosettes (*arrows*) in a background of small lymphocytes. (H & E preparation; ×60).

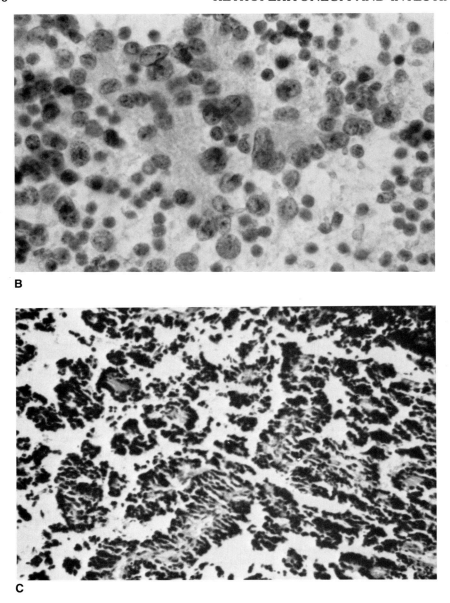

B

C

Fig. 9.13. B. ABC. Note radially arranged tumor cells with fine fibrillary cell processes. The smaller, uniform cells are lymphocytes. (H & E preparation; ×500). **C.** Histologic section of neuroblastoma with rosette formations. (H & E preparation; ×125).

in an embryonal rhabdomyosarcoma.[50] Electron microscopic examination shows neurosecretory dense-core granules and a large number of neuritic cell processes containing neurofilaments and microtubules.[48] The cell processes are particularly abundant in the center of the rosettes. These features serve to distinguish neuroblastoma from other small round cell tumors, such as Ewing's sarcoma, rhabdomyosarcoma, malignant lymphoma, and Wilms' tumor. Recently, cytogenetics for diagnostic purposes has gained increasing attention; neuroblastoma is characterized by a deletion on the short arm of chromosome 1 (1p-).[51] Interestingly, DNA hyperploidy and aneuploidy have been found to be associated with a favorable prognosis.[52] This favorable prognostic finding is contrary to the general rule in adult tumors, in which DNA aneuploidy is frequently a sign of a poor prognosis. Tumor cell ploidy, therefore, should be considered in the diagnostic workup of children with neuroblastoma.

Diagnostic Pitfalls

Thommesen et al[53] compared the fine needle aspirates of bone lesions of neuroblastoma with aspirates of Ewing's sarcoma, and concluded that the cytologic features of the two diseases were quite similar. Although in Miller's series,[46] the diagnoses in all four cases of neuroblastoma were made by NAB, the authors cautioned that the cytologic features alone may be insufficient to provide a definitive diagnosis. Rosette formations and eosinophilic fibrillary processes have been stressed by many investigators as very useful diagnostic features but rosettes may not be found if the neuroblastoma is too undifferentiated. Most authors indicate that it is feasible to make a correct diagnosis when NAB cytology, aided by immunocytochemistry or electron microscopy, is interpreted in the light of a complete clinical history, physical examination, radiologic and biochemical studies.[45–47]

Neuroblastoma is unique within the group of small round cell tumors of childhood in that a tumor marker is frequently present in the patient's urine or serum. More than 80% of patients have an increased urinary excretion of catecholamines, chiefly as vanillylmandelic acid. Serum neuron-specific enolase has been shown to be elevated in 96% of 122 children with metastatic neuroblastoma.[54] For further discussion of the differential diagnosis of small round cell tumors, see Chapter 5, section on Ewing's sarcoma.

GANGLIONEUROBLASTOMA AND GANGLIONEUROMA

Ganglioneuroblastomas are partly differentiated neuroblastomas. The biologic behavior of these uncommon tumors is intermediate between neuroblastomas and ganglioneuromas. The tumor shows all stages of neuroblast maturation, with variable mixtures of immature small dark-staining neuroblasts and variably mature ganglion cells **(Fig. 9.14).** The ganglion cells are larger than neuroblasts and have ample eosinophilic cytoplasm and prominent nucleoli.

Ganglioneuromas, representing the benign form of the clinical spectrum, are seen more often in the posterior mediastinum and are distinctly uncommon in the adrenal gland. Unlike neuroblastomas, they occur predominately in adults. Variable numbers of mature ganglion cells are seen in a background of nerve and fibrous tissues.

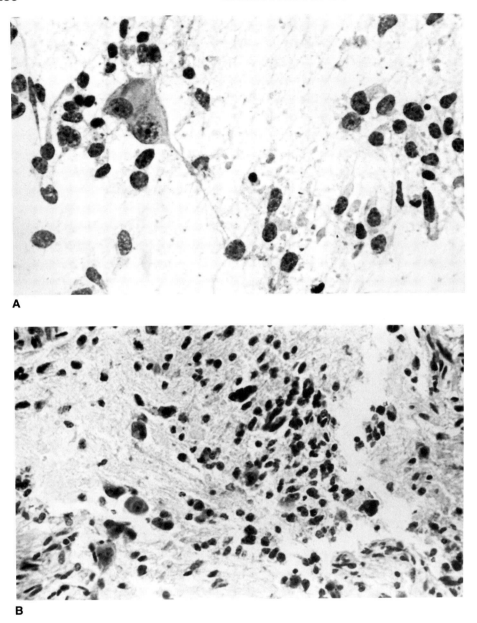

Fig. 9.14. Ganglioneuroblastoma. **A.** ABC. Note small neuroblasts and two large ganglionic cells with prominent nucleoli and abundant cytoplasm. (H & E preparation; ×500). **B.** Histologic section of ganglioneuroblastoma. Note admixture of small neuroblasts and variably mature ganglion cells in an eosinophilic fibrillary stroma. (H & E preparation; ×310).

MYELOLIPOMA

Myelolipoma is a benign, tumor-like lesion composed of fat cells and active bone marrow elements. The lesion is considered by most pathologists as a metaplastic rather than neoplastic condition. Generally it is small and asymptomatic, and found incidentally at autopsy. During life, myelolipoma is usually uncovered in the course of an evaluation of metastatic disease, hypertension, or hematuria.[55,56] The cut surface of the tumor-like lesion varies from yellow to gray, depending on the relative amounts of fat and myeloid tissue. The ABC features of the lesion have been reported.[55,56] The aspirates show a mixture of fat cells and normal hematopoietic cells, including megakaryocytes and granulocytic and erythrocytic cells at various stages of development (**Fig. 9.15**).

ADRENAL CYSTS

Adrenal cysts over several centimeters in diameter are uncommon. Ultrasound may demonstrate their cystic nature. Almost all adrenal cysts are really pseudocysts without an epithelial lining.[2] Most pseudocysts probably arise from an organization of an area of previous adrenal hemorrhage.[57,58] The cyst wall is composed of well-organized fibrous tissue with foci of hemosiderin deposition and collections of macrophages. The presence of calcification within the wall in a suprarenal location is a characteristic feature that can offer a diagnostic clue when seen on x-ray examination. The aspirates of pseudocysts contain bloody, pinkish or brownish fluid which may contain leukocytes and many hemosiderin-laden macrophages.[23] The cyst contents should always be sent to the laboratory for cytologic examination to rule out cystic degeneration of a malignant tumor.[59] The presence of abundant adrenocortical tissue in an aspirate should raise the possibility of previous hemorrhage into degeneration of an adenoma or carcinoma.

METASTASES TO THE ADRENAL GLAND

The adrenal glands provide fertile ground for the growth of metastases from tumors arising elsewhere, being the fourth most common site of metastatic cancer, following the lung, liver, and bone.[60] In one autopsy series 27% of 1,000 patients with malignant neoplasms had metastases to the adrenals.[61] In another series the adrenal gland was one of the sites of metastases in 60% of melanomas, 58% of breast carcinomas, 45% of renal cell carcinomas, and 36% of lung cancers.[10] In terms of actual numbers of cases, cancers of the lung, breast, colon, and rectum are the most frequently encountered metastatic malignancies found in the adrenal.

In the past, studies of adrenal metastases were carried out on autopsy material, but with the recent advances in imaging techniques adrenal metastases are being detected more frequently during life.[62,63] However, the radiologic findings of adrenal

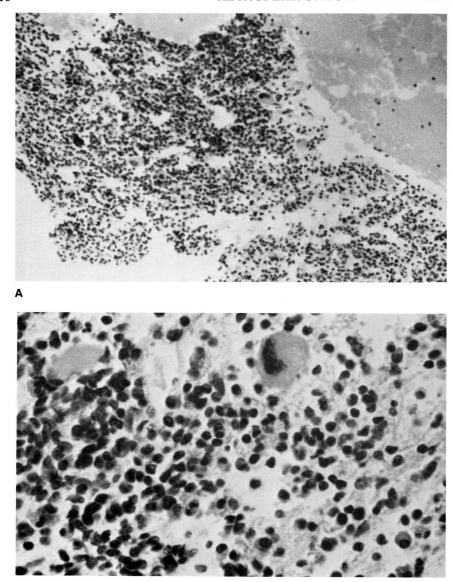

A

B

Fig. 9.15. A,B. Aspirate of myelolipoma (cell block) showing numerous hematopoietic cells and fatty spaces. The multinucleated giant cells are megakaryocytes. (H & E preparation; A: ×60; B: ×500). (Courtesy of Marguerite M. Pinto, M.D., Bridgeport Hospital, Bridgeport, CT).

metastases are nonspecific and can be confused with primary adrenal neoplasms. Computed tomography–directed NAB is a very useful method for distinguishing metastases from primary adrenal tumors.[64] For a description of the cytologic features of various metastatic tumors, the reader is referred to Chapter 6. Although the cytologic diagnosis of metastatic carcinomas is straightforward, sometimes renal cell carcinoma, melanoma, and metastatic undifferentiated carcinoma of lung can simulate a poorly differentiated adrenocortical carcinoma or pheochromocytoma (see sections on Adrenocortical Carcinoma and Pheochromocytoma, under Diagnostic Pitfalls).

INCIDENTALLY DISCOVERED ADRENAL MASSES AND THE ROLE OF NEEDLE ASPIRATION BIOPSY

Until recently, cortical adenomas/nodules, unless they were functioning, were rarely diagnosed during life, despite being found in 2–8% of the autopsy population.[65] The increasing use of modern imaging techniques for metastatic workup in cancer patients has led to the discovery of many incidental small adrenal masses.[66–68] O'Leary and Ooi[69] reviewed 95 cases of incidentally discovered adrenal masses reported in the medical literature up to 1986. Seventy-one of these had been surgically removed. A variety of conditions were identified: cortical adenoma (30 cases), metastases (17 cases), cysts (9), myelolipomas (5), and pheochromocytomas (4) but no adrenocortical carcinomas. On the basis of this extensive review, the authors recommended a conservative approach to the management of adrenal masses found incidentally during imaging procedures, using percutaneous needle aspiration biopsy and hormonal evaluation.

Patients With a Known Extraadrenal Malignancy

Metastases to the adrenal glands are common, but not all adrenal masses represent metastases. In one study, 73% of the adrenal masses were metastases and 27% had an unrelated adrenal lesion.[70] In another series 46% were metastases, and the rest represented a variety of other conditions.[71] Since the nature of the adrenal mass may determine the staging, therapy, and prognosis of the cancer, it is necessary to obtain a reliable morphologic diagnosis. NAB, performed and interpreted by experienced personnel, is ideally suited to the evaluation of these incidentally discovered nodules.[64,67,68,72] In this clinical setting, the main differential diagnosis is between an intrinsic benign adrenal lesion and a metastatic malignant nodule. Metastases generally have a morphologic appearance different from the normal cortical cells or cortical adenoma. It is highly unlikely that a cytologically benign cortical adenoma may, in fact, be a small, nonfunctioning cortical carcinoma in view of the extremely low prevalence of the latter (comprising only 0.02–0.04% of all cancers) and the fact that cortical carcinomas are large tumors (>5 cm).[73] Very rarely, a small cortical carcinoma has been reported in the literature,[74] but this serves only as an exception to the rule.

Patients Without an Extraadrenal Malignancy

When an adrenal mass is detected incidentally by abdominal imaging in a patient who has no evidence of an extraadrenal malignancy, the differential diagnosis is between a benign and a malignant primary adrenal lesion. Urinary and plasma hormonal profiles should be obtained to rule out a functioning tumor, such as cortical neoplasm, pheochromocytoma, or neuroblastoma. Adrenalectomy is the treatment of choice for any adrenal tumor associated with endocrine abnormalities, irrespective of whether it is benign or malignant. As for the nonfunctioning, asymptomatic adrenal masses, the great majority are benign adenomas or nodules of adrenal hyperplasia, because adrenocortical carcinoma is very uncommon. Based on our own experience[72] and literature review,[6,23,66,69] we believe that an incidentally discovered adrenal mass that is less than 5 cm in diameter and has a benign NAB cytology can be safely managed conservatively, provided subsequent scans do not show unabated growth. Surgery should be considered for those tumors that are larger than 5 cm and those that show atypical cytology.

DIAGNOSTIC ACCURACY

In a study of 22 patients who had undergone adrenal NAB, Katz and coworkers reported an overall sensitivity of 85% in detecting malignancy. The specificity was 100% for malignant lesions. Ninety percent of all adrenal masses were classified correctly.[23] Subsequently, in a larger series of 157 cases, these same authors reported an overall accuracy rate of 85%.[24] Heaston et al[6] performed percutaneous NAB of adrenal masses in 14 patients. Diagnostic material was recovered in 13 of 14 cases (93%). One false-negative diagnosis occurred, attributable to inadequate sampling. There were no false-positive diagnoses. In a study by Berkman and associates,[75] the success rate in obtaining diagnostic material was 94% (15 of 16 cases) and the diagnostic accuracy rate was 100%. There were no false-positive or false-negative reports.

We recently analyzed our experience of 57 cases of adrenal NAB, performed after 1986. (Our experience prior to 1986 was reported in the first edition of this monograph). All the cortical adenomas/nodules were discovered incidentally during diagnostic imaging in the investigation of other diseases or for metastatic staging. They varied from 1.5 to 4 cm in size. The adrenocortical carcinomas were all symptomatic masses, ranging from 6 to 14 cm in diameter. The three pheochromocytomas were not clinically suspected as such prior to NAB. Adequate material was obtained in 50 cases (88% success rate). These 50 cases included 27 (54%) metastatic tumors and 23 (46%) primary adrenal lesions. In the group of metastatic tumors there were no false-positive cytologic reports—all the diagnoses of metastatic malignancy were confirmed by clinical follow-up or autopsy. (One case of adrenocortical nodule was initially misinterpreted as metastatic small cell carcinoma from the lung, but the diagnosis was corrected in the final report; see **Fig. 9.5).** The 23 primary adrenal lesions included 13 cases of benign cortical adenomas or nodules, three adrenal cysts, three adrenocortical carcinomas (a fourth case of cytologically diagnosed adrenocortical carcinoma proved to be a renal cell carcinoma on subsequent laparotomy), and three pheochromocytomas (one of the pheochromocytomas was misdiagnosed as

TABLE 9.2. Differential Diagnostic Considerations of Adrenal Aspiration Biopsy

Adrenal Mass	Differential Diagnosis
Adrenocortical adenoma/nodule	Normal cortical cells
	Well-differentiated adrenocortical carcinoma
	Well-differentiated renal cell carcinoma
	Small cell anaplastic carcinoma
	Lymphocytes or lymphoma
Adrenocortical carcinoma	Adrenocortical adenoma
	Renal cell carcinoma
	Metastatic adenocarcinoma
	Melanoma
Pheochromocytoma	Undifferentiated large cell carcinoma
	Undifferentiated sarcoma
	Carcinoid tumor
Neuroblastoma	Ewing's sarcoma
	Embryonal rhabdomyosarcoma
	Malignant lymphoma
	Wilms' tumor
	Small cell carcinoma of lung

retroperitoneal epithelioid leiomyosarcoma). **Table 9.2** highlights the wide range of differential diagnostic possibilities commonly encountered in needle aspiration biopsy of adrenal masses.

REFERENCES

1. Das Gupta T, Brasfield RD, Paglia MA: Primary melanomas in unusual sites. *Surg Gynecol Obstet* 128:841–848, 1969.

2. Page DL, DeLellis RA, Hough AJ Jr: *Tumors of the Adrenal. Atlas of Tumor Pathology.* Second series, Fascicle 23. Washington, DC, Armed Forces Institute of Pathology, 1986, pp 115–149, 162–182.

3. Mitchell ML, Ryan FP Jr, Shermer RW: Pulmonary adenocarcinoma metastatic to the adrenal gland mimicking normal adrenal cortical epithelium on fine needle aspiration. *Acta Cytol* 29:994–998, 1985.

4. Hoda SA, Zaman MB, Burt M: Aspiration cytology in the evaluation of adrenal masses (abstract). *Acta Cytol* 35:594–595, 1991.

5. Schteingart DE, Oberman HA, Friedman BA, et al: Adrenal cortical neoplasms producing Cushing's syndrome. *Cancer* 22:1005–1013, 1968.

6. Heaston DK, Handel DB, Ashton PR, et al: Narrow gauge needle aspiration of solid adrenal masses. *AJR* 138:1143–1148, 1982.

7. Min KW, Song J, Boesenberg M, et al: Adrenal cortical nodule mimicking small round cell malignancy on fine needle aspiration. *Acta Cytol* 32:543–546, 1988.

8. Suen KC, McNeeley TB: Adrenal cortical cells mimicking small cell anaplastic carcinoma in a fine needle aspirate. *Mod Pathol* 4:594–595, 1991.

9. Lipsett MB, Hertz R, Ross GT: Clinical and pathophysiologic aspects of adrenocortical carcinoma. *Am J Med* 35:374–383, 1963.

10. Young JD, Karmi SA: Diagnosis and management of adrenal tumors. In Skinner DG, deKernion JB: *Genitourinary Cancer.* Philadelphia, WB Saunders, 1978, pp 166–178.

11. Schwartz RW, Sloan DA, Kenady DE: Diagnosis and treatment of primary adrenal tumors. *Curr Opin Oncol* 3:121–127, 1991.

12. Symington T: The adrenal cortex. In Bloodworth JMB Jr (ed): *Endocrine Pathology: General and Surgical.* Baltimore, Williams & Wilkins, 1982, pp 419–472.

13. Tartour E, Caillou B, Tenenbaum F, et al: Immunohistochemical study of adrenocortical carcinoma. *Cancer* 72:3296–3303, 1993.

14. Hajjar RA, Hickey RC, Samaan NA: Adrenal cortical carcinoma. A study of 32 patients. *Cancer* 35:549–554, 1975.

15. Weiss LM: Comparative histologic study of 43 metastasizing and non-metastasizing adrenocortical tumors. *Am J Surg Pathol* 8:163–169, 1984.

16. Rosai J: *Ackerman's Surgical Pathology,* ed 7. St. Louis, CV Mosby, 1989, p 791.

17. Tang CK, Gray GF: Adrenocortical neoplasms. *Urology* 5:691–695, 1975.

18. Levin NP: Fine needle aspiration and histology of adrenal cortical carcinoma. A case report. *Acta Cytol* 25:421–424, 1981.

19. Cochand-Priollet B, Jacquenod P, Warnet A, et al: Adrenal cortical carcinoma: A case diagnosed by fine needle aspiration cytology. *Acta Cytol* 32:128–130, 1988.

20. Elwood LJ: Fine-needle aspiration cytology of selected primary adrenal neoplasms. *Cytopathology Check Sample (C-198),* 12, 1989.

21. Varma S, Amy RW: Adrenal cortical carcinoma metastatic to the lung: Report of a case diagnosed by fine needle aspiration biopsy. *Acta Cytol* 34:104–105, 1990.

22. Wadih GE, Nance KV, Silverman JF: Fine-needle aspiration cytology of the adrenal gland. Fifty biopsies in 48 patients. *Arch Pathol Lab Med* 116:841–846, 1992.

23. Katz RL, Patel S, Mackay B, et al: Fine needle aspiration cytology of the adrenal gland. *Acta Cytol* 28:269–282, 1984.

24. Saboorian H, Katz R, Boyd D, et al: Fine needle aspiration cytology of primary and metastatic lesions of adrenal gland. *Mod Pathol* 5:28A, 1992.

25. Suzuki T, Sasano H, Nisikawa T, et al: Discerning malignancy in human adrenocortical neoplasms. Utility of DNA flow cytometry and immunohistochemistry. *Mod Pathol* 5:224–231, 1992.

26. Wick RC, Cherwitz DL, McGlennen RC, et al: Adrenocortical carcinoma. An immunohistochemical comparison with renal cell carcinoma. *Am J Pathol* 122:343–352, 1986.

27. Pinkus GS, Etheridge CL, O'Connor EM: Are keratin proteins a better tumor marker than epithelial membrane antigen? *Am J Clin Pathol* 85:269–277, 1986.

28. Cote RJ, Cordon-Cardo C, Reutor VE, et al: Immunopathology of adrenal and renal cortical tumors. *Am J Pathol* 136:1077–1084, 1990.

29. Miettinen M, Pekka V, Virtanen I: Immunofluorescence microscopic evaluation of the intermediate filament expression of the adrenal cortex and medulla and their tumors. *Am J Pathol* 118:360–366, 1985.

30. Schröder S, Padberg BC, Achilles E, et al: Immunocytochemical differential diagnosis of adrenocortical neoplasms using the monoclonal antibody D11. *Virchows Arch A Pathol Anat* 417:89–96, 1990.

31. Tannenbaum M: Ultrastructural pathology of the adrenal cortex. *Pathol Annu* 8:109–156, 1973.

32. Silva EG, MacKay B, Samann NA, et al: Adrenocortical carcinomas: An ultrastructural study of 22 cases. *Ultrastruct Pathol* 3:1–7, 1982.

33. Henderson DW, Papadimitriou JM: *Ultrastructural Appearances of Tumors. A Diagnostic Atlas.* Edinburgh; Churchill Livingstone, 1982, pp 87–88.

34. Harrison TS: Endocrine neoplasms: Pheochromocytoma. In Santen RJ, Manni A: *Diagnosis and Management of Endocrine-related Tumors.* Boston, Martinus Nijfoff, 1984, pp 409–418.

35. Van Way CW, III, Scott WH Jr, Page DL, et al: Pheochromocytoma. In Ratvitch MM: *Current Problems in Surgery.* Chicago, Year Book Publishers, 1974, p 27.

36. Montali G, Solbiati L, Bossi MC, et al: Sonographically guided fine-needle aspiration biopsy of adrenal masses. *AJR* 143:1081–1084, 1984.

37. McCorkell SJ, Niles NL: Fine needle aspiration of catecholamine-producing adrenal masses: A possibly fatal mistake. *AJR* 145:113–114, 1985.

38. Steiner AI, Goodman AD, Powers SR: Study of a kindred with pheochromocytoma, medullary thyroid carcinoma, hyperparathyroidism and Cushing's disease: multiple endocrine neoplasia, type II. *Medicine* 47:371–409, 1968.

39. Nguyen GK: Cytopathologic aspects of adrenal pheochromocytoma in a fine needle aspiration biopsy. *Acta Cytol* 26:354–358, 1982.

40. Moussouris HF, Koss LG, Rosenblatt R, et al: Thin needle aspiration biopsy of abdominal organs. In Koss LG, Coleman DV: *Advances in Clinical Cytology,* Vol 2. New York, Masson Publishing, 1984, pp 226–228.

41. Lambert MA, Hirschowitz L, Russell RCG: Fine needle aspiration biopsy: A cautionary tale. *Br J Surg* 72:364–366, 1985.

42. Phillips JG, Orr JW Jr, Grizzle W, et al: An extra-adrenal pheochromocytoma mimicking lymph node metastasis from a cervical cancer. *Gynecol Oncol* 13:416–420, 1982.

43. Kretschmar CS: Neuroblastoma. In Moossa AR, Schimpff SC, Robson MC: *Comprehensive Textbook of Oncology.* Baltimore, Williams & Wilkins, 1991, pp 1499–1513.

44. Evans AE, D'Angio GJ, Koop CE: Diagnosis and treatment of neuroblastoma. *Pediatr Clin North Am* 23:161–170, 1976.

45. Akhtar M, Ali A, Sabbah RS, et al: Aspiration cytology of neuroblastoma. Light and electron microscopic correlation. *Cancer* 57:797–803, 1986.

46. Miller TR, Bottles K, Abele JS, et al: Neuroblastoma diagnosed by fine needle aspiration biopsy. *Acta Cytol* 29:461–468, 1985.

47. Silverman JF, Dabbs DJ, Ganick DJ, et al: Fine needle aspiration cytology of neuroblastoma, including peripheral neuroectodermal tumor, with immunocytochemical and ultrastructural confirmation. *Acta Cytol* 32:367–375, 1988.

48. Triche T, Askin FB: Neuroblastoma and the differential diagnosis of small-, round-, blue-cell tumors. *Hum Pathol* 14:569–595, 1983.

49. Magee F, Mah RG, Taylor GP, et al: Neural differentiation in Wilms' tumor. *Hum Pathol* 18:33–37, 1987.

50. Tsokos M, Linnoila RI, Chandra RS, et al: Neuron-specific enolase in the diagnosis of neuroblastoma and other small, round cell tumors of childhood. *Hum Pathol* 15:575–584, 1984.

51. Fetcher JA. Cytogenetic observations in malignant soft tissue tumors. *Adv Pathol Lab Med* 4:235–246, 1991.

52. Gansler T, Chatten J, Varello M, et al: Flow cytometric DNA analysis of neuroblastoma. Correlation with histology and clinical outcome. *Cancer* 58:2453–2458, 1986.

53. Thommesen P, Frederiksen P, Lowhagen T, et al: Needle aspiration biopsy in the diagnosis of lytic bone lesions in Histiocytosis X, Ewing's sarcoma and neuroblastoma. *Acta Radiol Oncol* 17:145–149, 1977.

54. Zeltzer PM, Marangos PJ, Parma AM: Raised neuron-specific enolase in serum of children with metastatic neuroblastoma. *Lancet* 2:361–363, 1983.

55. Pinto MM: Fine needle aspiration of myelolipoma of the adrenal gland. *Acta Cyto* 29:863–866, 1985.

56. DeBlois G, DeMay RM: Adrenal myelolipoma diagnosis by computed-tomography guided fine-needle aspiration. *Cancer* 55:848–850, 1985.

57. Incze JS, Lui PS Merriam JC, et al: Morphology and pathogenesis of adrenal cysts. *Am J Pathol* 95:423–432, 1979.

58. Abeshouse GA, Goldstein RB, Abeshouse BS: Adrenal cysts: Review of the literature and report of three cases. *J Urol* 81:711–719, 1959.

59. Scheible W, Coel M, Siemers PT, et al: Percutaneous aspiration of adrenal cysts. *AJR* 128:1013–1016, 1977.

60. Travis WD, Oertel JE, Lack EE: Miscellaneous tumors and tumefactive lesions of the adrenal gland. In Lack EE: *Pathology of the Adrenal Glands.* New York, Churchill Livingstone, 1990, pp 351–378.

61. Abrams HL, Spiro R, Goldstein N: Metastases in carcinoma: Analysis of 1000 autopsied cases. *Cancer* 4:74–85, 1950.

62. Seidenwurm DJ, Elmer EB, Kaplan LM, et al: Metastases to the adrenal glands and the development of Addison's disease. *Cancer* 54:552–557, 1984.

63. Redman BG, Pazdur R, Zingas AP, et al: Prospective evaluation of adrenal insufficiency in patients with adrenal metastasis. *Cancer* 60:103–107, 1987.

64. Pagani JJ: Non-small cell lung carcinoma adrenal metastases. Computed tomography and percutaneous needle biopsy in their diagnosis. *Cancer* 53:1058–1060, 1984.

65. Mostofi FK, Davis CJ: Pathology of urologic cancer. In Javadpour N: *Principles and Management of Urologic Cancer.* Baltimore, Williams & Wilkins, 1983, pp 55–59.

66. Mitnick JS, Bosniak MA, Megebow AJ, et al: Non-functioning adrenal adenomas discovered incidentally on computed tomography. *Radiology* 148:495–499, 1983.

67. Lunning M, Neuser D, Kursawe R, et al: CT guided percutaneous fine needle biopsy in the diagnosis of small adrenal tumors. *Europ J Radiol* 3:358–364, 1983.

68. Katz RL, Shirkhoda A: Diagnostic approach to incidental adrenal nodules in the cancer patient. *Cancer* 55:1995–2000, 1985.

69. O'Leary TJ, Ooi TC: The adrenal incidentaloma. *Can J Surg* 29:6–8, 1986.

70. Belldegrun A, Hussain S, Seltzer SE, et al: Incidentally discovered mass of the adrenal gland. *Surg Gynecol Obstet* 163:203–208, 1986.

71. Bernardino ME, Walther MM, Phillips VM, et al: CT-guided adrenal biopsy: Accuracy, safety, and indications. *AJR* 144:67–69, 1985.

72. Suen KC, Chan NH: Fine needle aspiration biopsy of the adrenal gland: Cytological features and clinical applications. *Endocr Pathol* 3:173–181, 1992.

73. Herrera MF, Grant CS, van Heerden JA: Incidentally discovered adrenal tumors: An institutional perspective. *Surgery* 110:1014–1021, 1991.

74. Gandour MJ, Grizzle WE: A small adrenocortical carcinoma with aggressive behavior. *Arch Pathol Lab Med* 110:1076–1079, 1986.

75. Berkman WA, Bernardino ME, Sewell CW, et al: The computed tomography-guided adrenal biopsy. An alternative to surgery in adrenal mass diagnosis. *Cancer* 53:2098–2103, 1984.

10

Kidneys and Urinary Tract

KEY FACTS

▶ The role of percutaneous NAB in diagnosing primary kidney tumors remains controversial.

▶ In North America, the demonstration of a solid renal mass by ultrasound or computed tomography is considered sufficient indication for surgery and the aspiration technique is mostly reserved for identification and evacuation of renal cysts.

▶ In patients who are not candidates for surgery, because of poor risk or advanced tumor, NAB can be performed to establish a diagnosis and to determine treatment, e.g., embolization therapy.

▶ NAB can be used to differentiate a primary renal tumor from a metastatic tumor, and to differentiate a primary renal tumor from a retroperitoneal tumor.

▶ Patients on chronic hemodialysis are more prone than the general population to develop renal masses. NAB can be used in the differential diagnosis of renal masses in these patients.

▶ A preoperative diagnosis of Wilms' tumor by NAB increases the attractiveness of initiating preoperative chemotherapy or radiotherapy.

▶ A preoperative NAB diagnosis of benign renal neoplasms (e.g., renal oncocytoma and angiomyolipoma) can reinforce the urologist's decision to perform conservative rather than radical surgery.

EMBRYOLOGY

The development of the definitive kidneys is preceded by two primitive organs, the pronephros and the mesonephros. Although these are transitory structures, portions of their ducts are incorporated in the formation of the definitive urinary and reproductive systems. The permanent kidney (metanephros) is derived from two sources in the intermediate mesoderm. The secretory portion, which is composed of nephrons— including the glomeruli, proximal and distal tubules, and Henle's loops—is derived from a solid mass of tissue known as the metanephric blastema in the intermediate mesoderm. The collecting portion—including the collecting tubules, calyces, renal

247

pelvis, and ureter—is derived from the ureteric bud, which is an outgrowth from the earlier mesonephric duct. After the secretory and collecting parts have united, the kidney migrates along the posterior wall to its paravertebral, retroperitoneal position in the upper portion of the abdomen. The nephrons and proximal portion of the duct system lie within the adult kidney; the distal portion of the duct system (the ureter) communicates with the exterior via the urinary bladder and urethra.

To understand the histopathology of kidney tumors, it is important to remember that the kidney is a true metanephros. Although the lining cells of the renal tubules show epithelial characteristics, they are of mesodermal origin. Thus it is not surprising that some renal neoplasms, such as Wilms' tumor and renal cell carcinoma, may contain both epithelial and nonepithelial (mesenchymal) components.

ROLE OF NEEDLE ASPIRATION BIOPSY

Renal pathology can be divided into two broad groups: (1) mass lesions and (2) diffuse or medical renal diseases. A thick-needle core biopsy is required for the diagnosis of medical renal diseases, such as the glomerulitides and vasculitides. When a patient is found to have a solid mass lesion and has no other contributing medical history, the conventional approach is to perform a surgical excision of the mass. If the patient has any contraindications to surgery, such as severe cardiovascular or pulmonary disease, then percutaneous fine needle aspiration becomes a viable option. In Europe, NAB has been widely used for the preoperative diagnosis of renal neoplasm, its soft tissue extension, and its metastases.[1-8] In North America the aspiration technique has been used primarily for identification and evacuation of benign cysts.[9] More recently, workers in North America have also utilized NAB for the investigation of solid renal masses.[10-14] Nunez et al[15] reported the successful use of NAB in the differential diagnosis of various mass lesions of the kidney in patients on chronic hemodialysis. These patients have been shown to be more prone to develop renal cysts and neoplasms than the general population.[15,16] Bray et al instituted preoperative chemotherapy in the treatment of Wilms' tumor after the diagnosis had been established by NAB.[17] NAB has been effectively used in differentiating metastases causing ureteral obstruction from thickening of the ureteral wall due to irradiation, chemotherapy, or surgery in patients with known cancer.[18,19] Positive malignant cytology is helpful in the patient's management, although a negative aspirate is inconclusive. The sensitivity of NAB in identifying malignancy causing ureteral obstruction has been very high—100% in one study and four out of five cases in another.[18,19] The indications for NAB of renal masses are summarized in **Table 10.1**.

NORMAL HISTOLOGIC AND CYTOLOGIC CORRELATES

A normal kidney contains about 1.25 million nephrons. Each nephron is essentially a renal tubule into the proximal end of which is invaginated a capillary tuft called a glomerulus **(Fig. 10.1A)**. The glomerulus acts as a filter: as blood flows through its

TABLE 10.1. Indications for NAB of the Kidney

1. Evaluating a renal mass in a patient who is not a surgical candidate
2. Confirming a recurrent renal cancer in the renal fossa after nephrectomy
3. Evaluating a renal mass in a patient with a history of primary cancer elsewhere
4. Evaluating bilateral renal masses
5. Evaluating a renal mass in a patient on chronic hemodialysis
6. Providing a diagnosis in a patient for whom preoperative chemotherapy or irradiation is contemplated
7. Evaluating and evacuating renal cysts

capillaries, a protein-free filtrate of plasma collects in the glomerular space and flows down the tubule. During this tubular passage, there is resorption and secretion of water and electrolytes. In tissue sections and aspirated material **(Figs. 10.1A and B)**, the lining cells of the proximal tubules are represented by large polygonal cells with abundant eosinophilic granular cytoplasm. The nuclei are round or oval, and the nucleoli are small but distinct. The cells of the distal convoluted tubules are fewer in number. They are smaller, cuboidal, and compact, with darker nuclei and clear, pale cytoplasm. The cells of the collecting tubules are of similar size and also pale staining, but the intercellular margins are sharply defined. The glomeruli are seldom aspirated. When present in an aspirated smear **(Fig. 10.1C)**, they appear as large, lobulated, ball-like structures with irregularly arranged endothelial cells and mesangial cells.

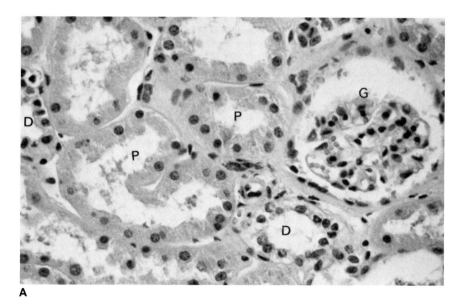

A

Fig. 10.1. Morphology of the normal kidney. **A.** Histologic section. Note proximal tubules (P) lined by large polygonal cells with granular eosinophilic cytoplasm, distal tubules (D) lined by smaller compact cells with pale cytoplasm, and a glomerulus (G). (H & E preparation; ×310).

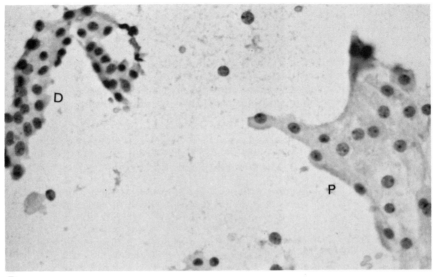

B

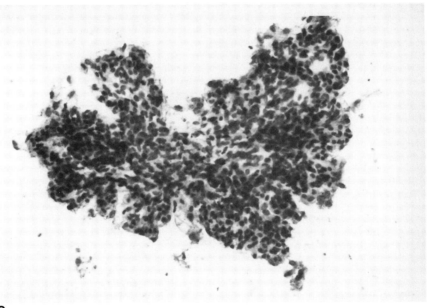

C

Fig. 10.1. B. ABC of normal kidney showing a monolayered sheet of proximal tubular cells (*P*) and a sheet of distal tubular cells (*D*). The proximal tubular cells are larger and show eosinophilic granular cytoplasm. The distal tubular cells are smaller and compact with dark nuclei. (H & E preparation; ×310). **C.** ABC of a normal glomerulus, characterized by a three-dimensional, multilobulated tissue fragment with hypercellularity consisting of mesangial cells and capillary endothelial cells. (H & E preparation; ×310).

RENAL CELL CARCINOMA

Renal cell carcinoma, also known as clear cell carcinoma, hypernephroma, or renal adenocarcinoma, is the most common neoplasm of the kidney. These tumors, constituting 80% of all renal neoplasms, occur twice as often in men as in women. The average age at diagnosis is 55 years. They metastasize mainly through the bloodstream to the lungs and bones, consequent upon renal vein invasion, but metastases may occur in any part of the body. About one-third of patients have distant metastases at the time of initial presentation. Some metastases occur before the primary lesion is discovered, while others appear many years after the primary tumor has been removed.[20] These metastases are good targets for NAB.[21–23]

Histopathology

Renal cell carcinoma arises from the epithelial cells of the proximal convoluted tubules. Histologically, the tumor exhibits many growth patterns, including solid, cystic, tubular, papillary, and sarcomatoid. These histologic patterns, depicted in **Figs. 10.2–10.5,** may be present alone or in various combinations. Necrosis and hemorrhage are often common and may be prominent features of the tumor.

Two types of tumor cells are generally recognized: clear cells rich in cytoplasmic lipid and glycogen, and granular cells containing many mitochondria that produce the effect of a granular eosinophilic cytoplasm. The majority of the neoplasms consist of both clear and granular cells, but about 30% are composed predominantly of clear cells and 12% are composed predominantly of granular cells.[24] An occasional tumor may show pleomorphic spindle cells and rhabdoid cells, mimicking a sarcoma.

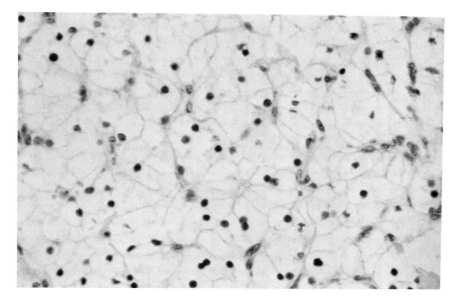

Fig. 10.2. Histology of grade I renal cell carcinoma with a solid pattern. Note clear cells with small uniform nuclei and sharply defined cytoplasmic borders. (H & E preparation; ×310).

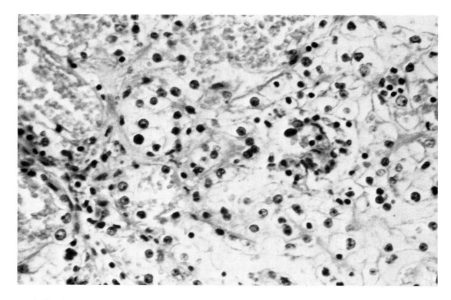

Fig. 10.3. Histology of grade II renal cell carcinoma with a cystic pattern. There is more nuclear pleomorphism than the tumor shown in Fig. 10.2. Note nuclear enlargement, increased nuclear-cytoplasmic ratio, and prominent nucleoli. (H & E preparation; ×310).

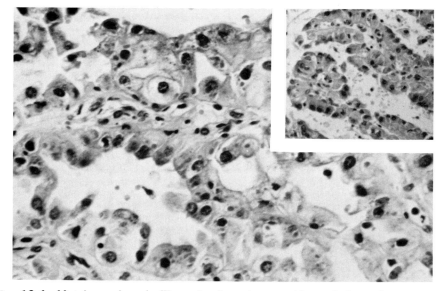

Fig. 10.4. Histology of grade III renal cell carcinoma with a tubulopapillary pattern. The tumor is composed of granular cells and some clear cells. *Inset:* Note two papillary fronds. (H & E preparation; ×500, inset ×125).

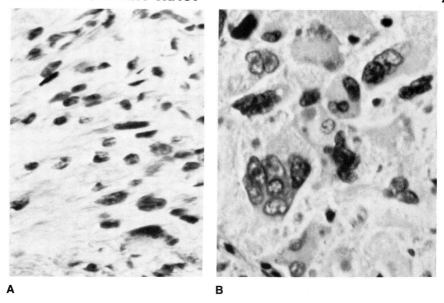

A   B

Fig. 10.5. Histology of grade III renal cell carcinoma, sarcomatoid variant. **A.** Fibrosarcoma-toid pattern. **B.** Note many large irregular rhabdoid cells. (H & E preparation; ×500).

Aspiration Biopsy Cytology

The aspirates of renal cell carcinomas show variable cellularity. They are usually moderately cellular, but because of marked vascularity of the lesion the aspirates may contain much blood, diluting the tumor cells and yielding hypocellular samples. The tumor cells are usually arranged singly, in small irregular groups, or in large solid sheets; others may form tubular structures and papillary fronds **(Figs. 10.6–10.8).**

The clear cells **(Plate 10.1, Figs. 10.6** and **10.7)** are large, polygonal or columnar, with fairly abundant clear or coarsely vacuolated cytoplasm and distinct cell borders. The clear or vacuolated cytoplasm reflects the presence of lipid and glycogen. The clear cytoplasm is readily apparent on paraffin sections as a result of histologic pro-cessing, but in aspirates the cytoplasm may appear translucent, ground glass–like rather than clear or vacuolated **(Fig. 10.9).** The degree of nuclear atypia varies from case to case depending on the tumor grade, but in general the nuclei are round and uniform, and there is minimal nuclear pleomorphism **(Table 10.2).** The chromatin is finely granular and shows some clumping under the nuclear membrane, and the nucleoli are frequently prominent. The granular cells **(Figs. 10.8, 10.9)** are usually more compact, with a higher nuclear–cytoplasmic ratio and homogeneous or granular eosinophilic cytoplasm. Other cell types, though uncommon, are also seen, including the spindle cells **(Fig. 10.10),** and the pleomorphic large rhabdoid cells **(Fig. 10.11).**

Cytologic grading of renal cell carcinoma based on the degree of nuclear anaplasia has been described by a number of investigators.[1,14,25,26] In well-differentiated (grade I) renal cell carcinomas the nuclei show only minimal deviation from those of normal tubular cells. In poorly differentiated (grade III) carcinomas there is marked nuclear anaplasia. The grade III tumors also encompass the sarcomatoid variant, characterized

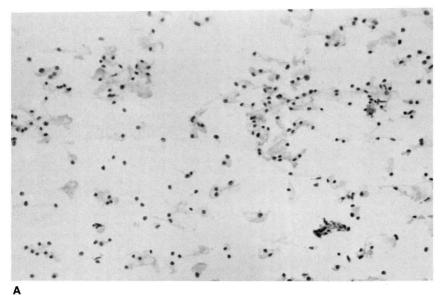

A

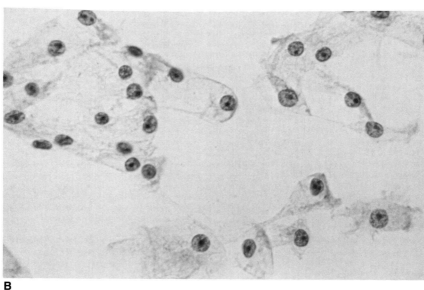

B

Fig. 10.6. Renal cell carcinoma, grade I, ABC. **A.** Low magnification view showing a cell-rich aspirate with many single clear cells and groups of clear cells. (H & E preparation; ×125). **B.** Higher magnification view of the clear cells. Note presence of nucleoli and thickened nuclear membranes. (H & E preparation; ×500).

Fig. 10.7. Renal cell carcinoma, grade II, ABC. **A.** Note tumor cells arranged in large tissue fragments with no recognizable pattern. (H & E preparation; ×80). **B.** Note tumor cells arranged in small tubular units (*arrows*). (H & E preparation; ×125). **C.** Note attempt in tubule formations, characterized by radial arrangement of tumor cells around lumina. (H & E preparation; ×500).

254

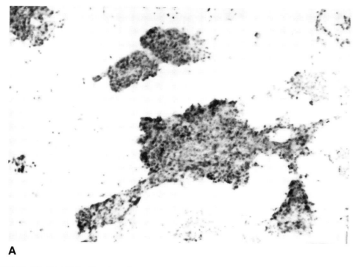

A

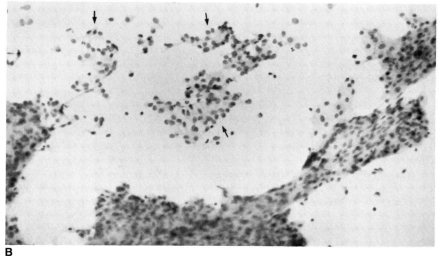

B

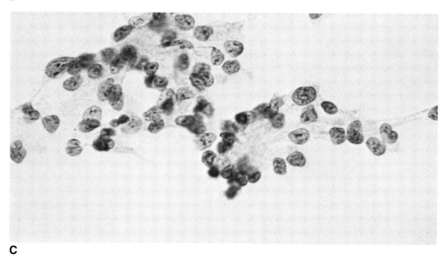

C

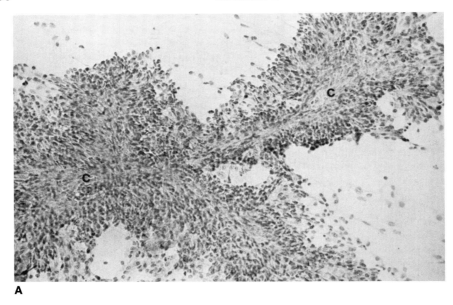

A

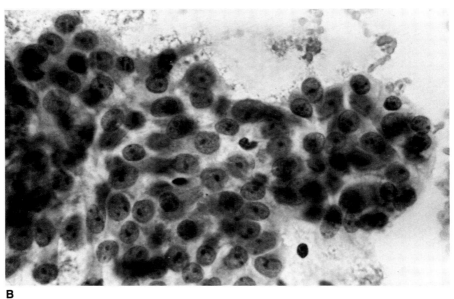

B

Fig. 10.8. Renal cell carcinoma, grade II, ABC. **A.** Low magnification view showing tumor cells forming papillary configuration. Note central fibrous connective tissue core (*C*). (H & E preparation; ×125). **B.** Higher magnification of the granular cells. Note prominent nucleoli, a characteristic feature of renal cell carcinoma. (H & E preparation; ×500).

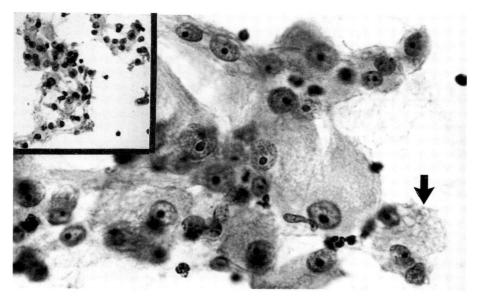

Fig. 10.9. Renal cell carcinoma, grade III, ABC. Note large polygonal cells with prominent nucleoli. Cytoplasm varies from granular to ground glasslike to vacuolated (arrow). (H & E preparation; ×500, inset ×125).

by spindle and pleomorphic large cells. In grade II carcinomas the nuclear atypia is intermediate between the two extremes. A good correlation between cytologic grading and prognosis was reported by Nurmi et al.[26] These authors found that the 5-year survival rate for grade I renal cell carcinoma was 72.2%, for grade II carcinoma it was 49.9%, and for grade III carcinoma it was 22.2%. In some Scandinavian centers, patients with grade III renal cell carcinoma are given preoperative irradiation as an integral part of the treatment.[1,27] Cajulis and associates[14] recently reported that cytologic grading of renal cell carcinoma had a high concordance rate with histology and with flow cytometric data.

Although many investigators have found nuclear grading to be of prognostic value, attempts to apply grading by others have not uniformly resulted in reproducibility.[28] Cytologic grading is most reliable for high-grade tumors and less accurate when the tumor is well-differentiated. This is because a more poorly differentiated area in the latter may be missed by NAB. It is the general consensus that multiple samples are necessary for accurate grading.

TABLE 10.2. Salient NAB features of Renal Cell Carcinoma

Pleomorphism	Minimal
Nucleoli	Prominent
Cytoplasm	Varies from granular to ground glasslike to vacuolated, moderate to abundant in amount, well-defined cell border
Other features	Polygonal cells, tubulopapillary pattern, hemorrhagic background

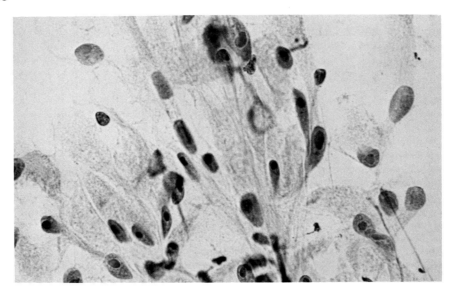

Fig. 10.10. Grade III renal cell carcinoma, fibrosarcomatoid variant, ABC. Note spindle cells with macronucleoli. The cytoplasm is neither clear nor granular but has a translucent, ground-glass appearance. (H & E preparation; ×500).

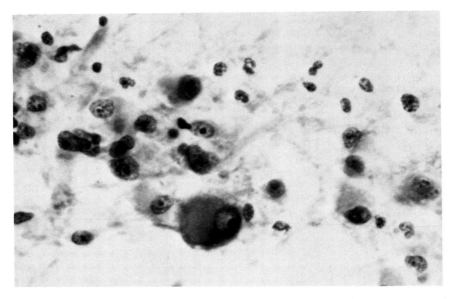

Fig. 10.11. Grade III renal cell carcinoma, sarcomatoid variant, ABC. Note pleomorphic, rhabdomyosarcoma-like cells with prominent nucleoli and abundant eosinophilic granular cyto-plasm. (H & E preparation; ×500).

TABLE 10.3. Pitfalls in ABC Interpretation of Renal Cell Carcinoma

Sampling Problems
1. Vascular tumor—bloody and hypocellular specimens
2. Deep-seated location—misplacement of needle

Interpretive Problems
1. Well-differentiated renal cell carcinoma
   - vs. benign neoplasms (renal cell adenoma, renal oncocytoma, and adrenocortical adenoma) and renal cyst
   - vs. normal tubular cells, hepatocytes, and histiocytes (xanthogranulomatous pyelonephritis)
2. Poorly differentiated renal cell carcinoma
   - vs. adrenocortical carcinoma, malignant fibrous histiocytoma, fibrosarcoma, spindle-cell squamous carcinoma, and poorly differentiated metastatic carcinoma

Diagnostic Pitfalls

Table 10.3 lists the potential pitfalls in diagnosing renal cell carcinoma on ABC. Most diagnostic difficulties center around grade I renal cell carcinomas, because of their well-differentiated cytologic features. A false-negative diagnosis may occur in the following circumstances:

1. Many renal cell carcinomas are vascular, resulting in bloody aspiration and a hypocellular specimen.
2. In the absence of clinical and radiologic data, one may not be able to separate a grade I renal cell carcinoma from a renal cell adenoma (see discussion later).
3. The clear cells of grade I renal cell carcinoma may be mistaken for foamy histiocytes.
4. Grade I clear cell carcinoma may be mistaken for adrenocortical adenoma.
5. Renal cell carcinoma of the granular cell type may be misinterpreted as benign oncocytoma (see section on Renal Oncocytoma).
6. The granular cells of grade I carcinoma may be confused with normal tubular cells of the convoluted tubules (see **Fig. 10.1B**). To avoid this confusion, the diagnosis of carcinoma should be made on the general picture of a cellular smear showing only one cell type and thus lacking the heterogenous population which characterizes aspirates obtained from normal renal parenchyma.
7. The granular cells of grade I renal cell carcinoma may be mistaken for normal hepatocytes (see **Fig. 3.1E**). The latter cells, however, often contain yellowish-brown pigment granules in their cytoplasm, and are arranged in uniform small monolayers or cords rather than in overcrowded cellular fragments.

A false-positive diagnosis may occur in the following circumstances:

1. Foamy histiocytes may simulate renal cell carcinoma of the clear cell type. Zajicek[27] stressed that diagnosis of renal cell carcinoma should be based on cells in clusters or in sheets, rather than based on single cells, as is the case with histiocytes. Prominent nucleoli are a reliable marker for renal cell carcinoma but are absent in histiocytes. In properly fixed and properly stained smears the benign nature of the histiocytes is more readily apparent (compare **Fig. 10.6** and **Fig. 10.28**).

2. Benign renal cysts have been misdiagnosed as renal cell carcinoma because of the reactive atypia of the epithelial lining cells of the cyst simulating malignancy.[2,29,30] Cells are usually few in number in the aspirates of benign cysts; the large tissue fragments seen in carcinomas are not present. Ultrasonography will demonstrate the cystic nature of the lesion and a double-contrast study will show a smooth lining of the cystic cavity.[31]

3. Adrenocortical adenomas may be mistaken for grade I renal cell carcinoma (*vide infra*).

4. Benign renal tubular cells, reactive hepatocytes, and oncocytes from renal oncocytoma are other potential sources of false-positive diagnosis.

Difficulties may arise in classifying a malignant tumor as renal in origin. The sarcomatoid variant of renal cell carcinoma may mimic malignant fibrous histiocytoma, fibrosarcoma, or spindle cell squamous carcinoma. Grade III renal cell carcinoma and poorly differentiated metastatic carcinoma to the kidney may resemble one another morphologically. Careful examination of the smears may show other cell types, such as the clear cells, which are more characteristic of renal cell carcinoma. Immunostaining of renal cell carcinoma shows positivity for both epithelial markers (e.g., cytokeratin, epithelial membrane antigen) and vimentin. These immunostaining findings aid in distinguishing renal cell carcinoma from most metastatic carcinomas, adrenocortical carcinomas, and sarcomas.

Adrenocortical neoplasms producing vacuolated and granular cells may be confused with renal cell carcinoma. Adrenocortical adenoma may simulate grade I renal cell carcinoma and poorly differentiated adrenocortical carcinoma may simulate grade III renal cell carcinoma. Readers are referred to **Table 9.1** for the distinguishing characteristics of renal cell carcinoma and adrenocortical carcinoma. A prominent tubulopapillary pattern on ABC has not been described for adrenocortical tumor and therefore its presence favors the diagnosis of renal cell carcinoma. Cytoplasmic lipid is present in both tumors. However, a large quantity of glycogen, demonstrable by the periodic acid-Schiff reaction followed by diastase digestion **(Plate 10.2)**, is characteristically found in the clear cells of renal carcinomas. Although cytoplasmic glycogen can also be present in few adrenocortical carcinomas, this is an exception rather than the rule. Uroradiographic and/or angiographic studies may clarify the topographic relationship of the tumor to the kidney. If an adrenocortical tumor is suspected, assessment of adrenocortical hormones and their metabolites in the patient's plasma and urine will be helpful.

Controversy in Diagnosing Renal Adenoma

There has been much controversy concerning the diagnostic criteria used to separate renal cell carcinoma from adenoma. It is customary to regard renal cell tumors larger than 3 cm as malignant and those less than 3 cm as most likely benign. However, there have been reports of tumors smaller than 3 cm producing widespread metastases[32] and larger tumors remaining localized.[33] Mostofi et al[34] suggested that, irrespective of size, tumors that produce clinical symptoms and those that show cellular anaplasia or evidence of aggressive behavior should be considered malignant. On the other hand, an asymptomatic tumor found incidentally at autopsy or in a kidney removed for other reasons should be classified as benign, unless the tumor shows nuclear anaplasia or evidence of invasion. Bennington[35] demonstrated a linear relationship between the diameter of renal cell tumors and their propensity to metastasize, thus providing evidence that renal adenoma and carcinoma represent different stages of the same tumor, whose metastatic potential increases proportionally with tumor size.

WILMS' TUMOR (NEPHROBLASTOMA)

Wilms' tumor is a malignant embryonal neoplasm that develops from the metanephrogenic mesoderm. It is the most common renal malignancy of infancy and childhood, but is very rare in adults. In the recent past, Wilms' tumors were rarely investigated by NAB. In many medical centers, the demonstration of a solid renal mass in a child has been considered sufficient indication for surgery. However, since the publication of the first edition of this monograph, many papers on NAB of Wilms' tumor have appeared in the literature and the results have been most promising.[17,36–39] Bray et al[17] used NAB to establish a preoperative diagnosis of Wilms' tumor in three of four cases, in the context of a classical clinical setting. These authors believe that NAB can assume a pivotal role in diagnosing a greater number of Wilms' tumors in the future. In particular, establishing the correct pathologic diagnosis in a relatively noninvasive manner will increase the attractiveness of preoperative radiation and chemotherapy in the management of those patients with bulky tumors and significant intravascular invasion. In addition to providing a primary diagnosis, NAB can document tumor recurrence and metastases. With modern aggressive multimodal therapy, the occurrence of pulmonary metastases does not necessarily indicate a dismal prognosis.[40] Confirmation of metastases by NAB will facilitate treatment decisions.

Histopathology

The histologic appearance of Wilms' tumor is more readily appreciated when the normal process of nephrogenesis is understood. Nephrogenesis results from induction of metanephric blastema by the ampullae of the ureteric buds. Blastema also gives rise to the renal stroma. Hence, in a typical Wilms' tumor, which is a primitive embryonal tumor, islands of blastema surround central epithelial tubules and are themselves surrounded by stroma. These three elements are present in most Wilms' tumors, but in varying proportions **(Fig. 10.12)**. The blastemal cells are small, primitive cells, oval or fusiform; they are closely packed; and they have scanty cytoplasm. The epithelial cells recapitulate abortive metanephrogenesis, as evidenced by formation of tubular and glomerulus-like structures with no attempts to form mature nephrons. The stromal cells are mostly spindle-shaped and have a fibroblastic appearance. In some cases, muscle, bone, and cartilage can be seen.

Aspiration Biopsy Cytology

The aspirates are richly cellular. The cells are arranged in variably sized sheets or clusters as well as in single cells. The individual blastemal cells **(Fig. 10.13)** are small,

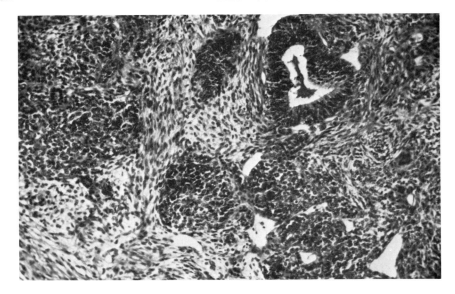

Fig. 10.12. Wilms' tumor, histologic section. Note admixture of three components: small dark blastemal cells, epithelial cells in tubular arrangement, and fusiform or elongated stromal cells. (H & E preparation; ×125).

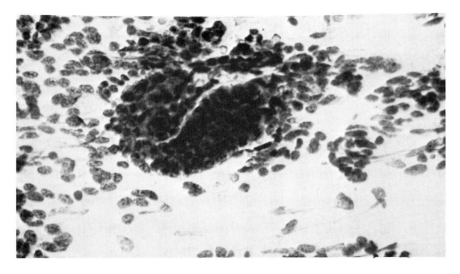

Fig. 10.13. Wilms' tumor, aspirate from a liver metastasis. Note dispersed undifferentiated blastemal cells and a solid tubular structure with well-defined border (*center of figure*). (H & E preparation; ×310).

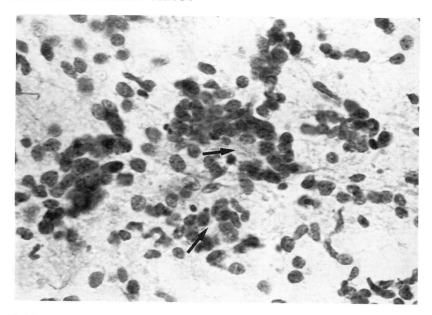

Fig. 10.14. Wilms' tumor, ABC. Note isolated, small blastemal cells and cells with epithelial differentiation. The latter is evidenced by epithelial grouping and rosetting. Arrows indicate rosette lumina. (H & E preparation; ×310). (Reproduced from Suen KC: *Atlas and Text of Aspiration Biopsy Cytology*. Baltimore, Williams & Wilkins, 1991, with permission).

round, oval, or fusiform cells, having dark-staining nuclei with fine, evenly dispersed chromatin granules and small nucleoli. Cytoplasm is scanty. The blastemal cells with epithelial differentiation are characterized by slightly larger cells with more cytoplasm. The epithelial cells are arranged in sheetlike fashion or in circular-tubular arrangements indicating tubular differentiation **(Fig. 10.13)**. The tubules have sharply defined borders. Some are solid, while others have lumina resembling rosettes[37] **(Fig. 10.14)**. The stromal component is characterized by spindle-shaped cells **(Fig. 10.15)** arranged in narrow bundles and mixed with the blastemal cells. In some cases heterologous stromal elements, such as cartilaginous tissue and striated muscle **(Fig. 10.16)**, may also be seen. In the series reported by Quijano et al,[38] the authors stressed the frequent presence of many necrotic tumor cells with nuclear pyknosis or karyorrhexis, admixed with inflammatory cells, including polymorphonuclear leukocytes, lymphocytes, and macrophages.

Diagnostic Pitfalls

Wilms' tumor may be difficult to distinguish from other small blue cell tumors of childhood. Rosettes may be seen in both Wilms' tumor and neuroblastoma and may cause confusion. Epithelial differentiation, as evidenced by tubule formations and stromal differentiation in the form of spindle cells, is characteristic of Wilms' tumor, while an eosinophilic fibrillar stroma formed by intertwining cytoplasmic processes is characteristic of neuroblastoma. However, poorly differentiated neuroblastomas may

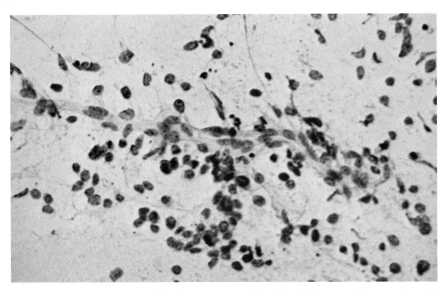

Fig. 10.15. Wilms' tumor, ABC. Note a narrow bundle of elongated mesenchymal cells, surrounded by small blastemal cells. (H & E preparation; ×310).

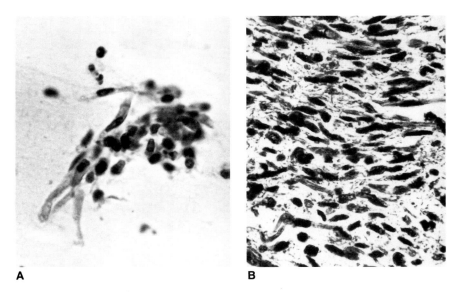

A   B

Fig. 10.16. Wilms' tumor with fetal rhabdomyomatous differentiation. **A.** ABC. Note a group of fetal striated muscle cells (strap cells). (H & E preparation; ×310). **B.** Histologic section featuring the rhabdomyomatous area of the Wilms' tumor consisting of fetal strap cells with cross-striations. (H & E preparation; ×310). (Reproduced with permission from Suen KC: *Atlas and Text of Aspiration Biopsy Cytology.* Baltimore, Williams & Wilkins, 1991).

be devoid of fibrillar matrix and cytoplasmic processes. In these cases, electron microscopic examination to demonstrate neurosecretory granules may be required to establish a definitive diagnosis.[37]

To prevent confusion with Ewing's sarcoma, lymphoma, and embryonal rhabdomyosarcoma, the cytopathologist must pay attention to the clinical and radiologic data, especially the location of the tumor, the age of the patient, and the past medical history (see Chapter 5, section under Ewing's sarcoma).

TRANSITIONAL CELL CARCINOMA AND OTHER EPITHELIAL NEOPLASMS OF THE RENAL PELVIS, URETER, AND BLADDER

Epithelial neoplasms of the renal pelvis, ureter, and urinary bladder are discussed together because of their many shared features. First, these sites are lined by transitional cell epithelium (urothelium), which gives rise to morphologically similar neoplasms. Second, as evidenced by frequent multicentricity of these tumors, cancers arising in these sites are most likely caused by the same carcinogens affecting the upper urinary tract as well as the bladder.

Primary urothelial tumors are usually diagnosed at any early, symptomatic stage by endoscopic techniques, and they are unlikely targets for percutaneous NAB. However, large recurrent tumors in the pelvis and in the retroperitoneum, metastatic urothelial carcinomas to the lungs and elsewhere as well as bulky sarcomas of the bladder are easy targets for NAB.[41-43]

Histopathology

The transitional cell epithelium gives rise to three main types of carcinoma: transitional cell, squamous cell, and adenocarcinoma. An occasional tumor may be a mixed cell type.[42] Transitional cell carcinomas are by far the most common, representing 90% of the tumors.[44] The term "transitional cell" is used to designate cells having features intermediate between those of columnar and squamous epithelia. Normal transitional cells are polygonal or columnar, with well-defined cell borders. The nuclei are regular, round to oval, with finely dispersed chromatin and tiny nucleoli. There is a moderate amount of cytoplasm, which stains pale eosinophilic with hematoxylin and eosin stain and pale green with the Papanicolaou stain. They do not show cytoplasmic keratinization as in squamous cells or mucin vacuoles as in glandular cells. When the transitional cells become malignant, the tumor may be papillary or nonpapillary and solid. Transitional cell tumors can be classified as grade I, II, or III, depending on the degree of nuclear anaplasia.

Squamous cell carcinomas constitute about 8% of urinary tract carcinomas.[44] Although these tumors may arise directly from the transitional cell epithelium, they most often arise by metaplasia from transitional cells. They are frequently associated with renal calculi and chronic inflammation.

Adenocarcinomas are the least common urinary tract carcinoma, constituting about 1–2% of the cases. Histologically, they are generally poorly differentiated glandular cancers, but many also produce mucin. Like squamous cell carcinomas, they are commonly associated with renal stones and infection.

Aspiration Biopsy Cytology

Cells derived from transitional cell carcinomas are enlarged and generally polygonal or elongated. The round nuclei may be central or eccentric; the latter may impart a plasmacytoid appearance to the cell. The cytoplasm is scanty to moderate in amount, homogeneous and eosinophilic, and shows no evidence of keratinization. The cell borders are well-defined. A cytoplasmic tail can sometimes be seen at one end of the tumor cells. Depending on the degree of differentiation, the tumor cells exhibit a wide range of atypia. Grade I transitional cell carcinoma **(Fig. 10.17)** shows cytologic features that closely resemble normal transitional cells. Cells derived from high-grade carcinomas **(Fig. 10.18)** show moderate to markedly pleomorphic cells. The nuclei are hyperchromatic with very coarse-textured chromatin, and the nucleocytoplasmic ratio is markedly increased. The nucleoli are large. However, all these malignant cytologic features are general and nonspecific. The cytopathologist will most likely not be able to classify the cell origin of the tumor unequivocally based solely on the cytologic features. In cases of recurrent or metastatic tumors, knowledge of the original histologic diagnosis is helpful for the correct classification of the tumor. More recently, Johnson and Kini[43] described the presence of spindled, pyramidal, and racquet-shaped malignant cells with eccentric nuclei and cytoplasmic features of both squamous and glandular differentiation as distinctive features of metastatic transitional cell carcinoma.

Squamous cell carcinoma of the urinary tract is usually a keratinizing squamous cancer. The malignant cells are large, irregular, and characterized by a considerable amount of eosinophilic or orangeophilic cytoplasm with sharp border. Their nuclei are irregular, are markedly hyperchromatic, and only occasionally show nucleoli. The nuclei seldom occupy as much of the total cell area as is the case with malignant transitional cells. There is considerable variability in cell size and shape **(Fig. 10.19)**.

The cytologic features of the adenocarcinomas of the urinary tract do not differ from those in other sites. The tumor cells are cuboidal to columnar, and the chromatin is generally finely granular and hyperchromatic. Some cells contain prominent single or multiple nucleoli. The cytoplasm has a lacy translucent appearance and may be vacuolated. When acinar or glandular units are formed, the tumor cells are seen arranged in a radial fashion around a central space **(Fig. 10.20)**.

URINARY TRACT SARCOMA

Bulky sarcomas are easy targets for NAB, but they are rare in the urinary system. A detailed account of the cytology of various types of sarcoma can be found in Chapter 5. Older reports often listed fibrosarcoma as the most common sarcoma afflicting the kidney. With ultrastructural studies, most of these spindle cell malignancies are now considered to be sarcomatoid renal cell carcinomas. A survey of renal sarcomas in adults was reported by Farrow et al,[45] who identified only 26 cases of sarcoma among 2,386 cases of kidney neoplasms. Leiomyosarcomas were the most common (15 cases), followed by liposarcomas (five cases), but no fibrosarcomas.

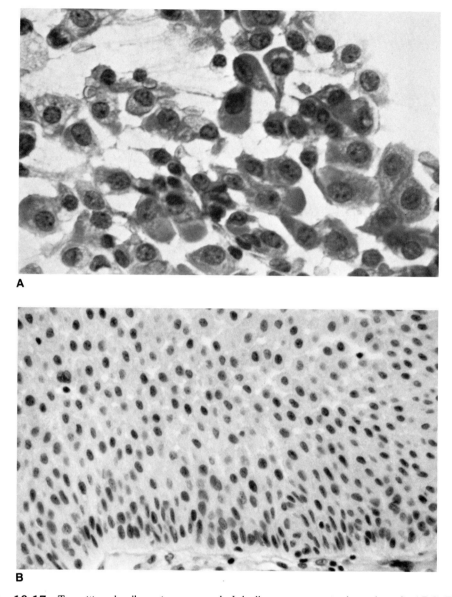

Fig. 10.17. Transitional cell carcinoma, grade I, bulky recurrence in the pelvis. **A,** ABC. The tumor cells shown here are more pleomorphic than the original grade I transitional cell carcinoma. (Papanicolaou preparation; ×500). **B.** Histologic section of the original grade I transitional cell carcinoma. (H & E preparation; ×310).

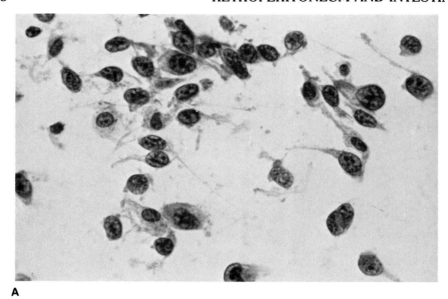

A

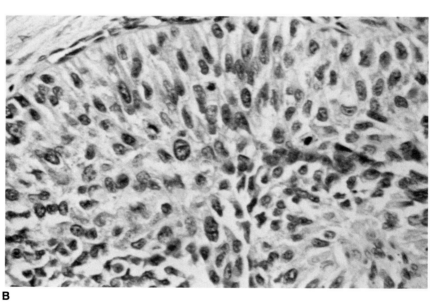

B

Fig. 10.18. Transitional cell carcinoma, grade II. **A.** ABC. Note cellular dyshesion, coarsely granular, hyperchromatic chromatin, and irregularly thickened nuclear membranes. Also note cytoplasmic elongations (tails) comparable to those seen in the histologic section. (H & E preparation; ×500). **B.** Histologic section of the previously resected, grade II transitional cell carcinoma. (H & E preparation; ×310).

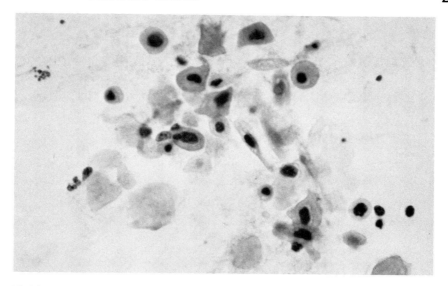

Fig. 10.19. Squamous cell carcinoma of the renal pelvis, ABC. Note opaque nuclei, dense eosinophilic cytoplasm with sharp border. The tumor cells vary widely in size and shape, and an elongated cell is present. (H & E preparation; ×310).

Embryonal Rhabdomyosarcoma

This is the most common malignant tumor of the urinary bladder in children.[46] Grossly the tumor forms a grapelike myxoid mass with a grayish-pink cut surface. The aspirates consist of variable numbers of round, hyperchromatic cells superficially resembling large lymphoid cells. However, under higher magnification, many of these round cells show irregular nuclei, prominent nucleoli, and a variable amount of eosinophilic granular cytoplasm **(Fig. 10.21).** The tinctorial eosinophilia of the cytoplasm is consis-

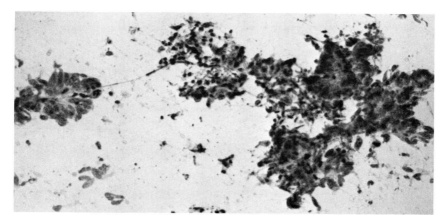

Fig. 10.20. Adenocarcinoma of the urinary bladder, ABC. Note gland formations evidenced by radial arrangement of cells around lumina. Many tumor cells are necrotic. (H & E preparation; ×250).

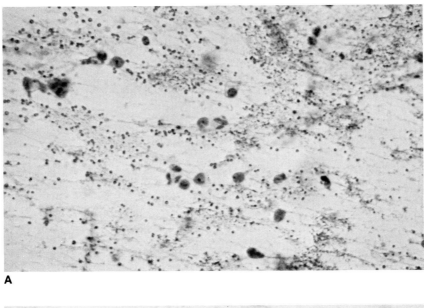

A

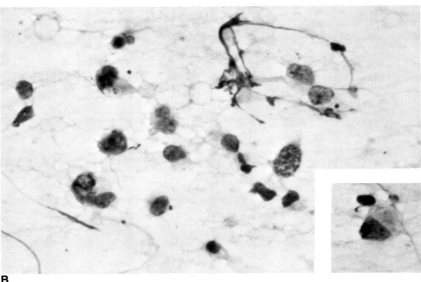

B

Fig. 10.21. Embryonal rhabdomyosarcoma. **A.** ABC. Note scattered single cells with hyperchromatic, round nuclei. (H & E preparation; ×125). **B.** ABC. High-magnification view of the tumor cells showing coarsely granular, irregularly distributed chromatin, irregular nuclear membranes, and prominent nucleoli. *Inset:* A malignant rhabdomyoblast with discernible eosinophilic cytoplasm. (H & E preparation; ×500).

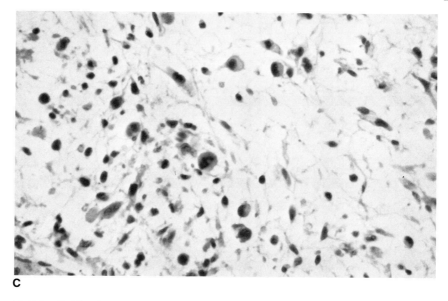

C

Fig. 10.21. C. Histologic section of embryonal rhabdomyosarcoma showing hyperchromatic tumor cells in a characteristic myxoid stroma. (H & E preparation; ×310).

tent with rhabdomyoblastic differentiation. Torres et al[47] have demonstrated the presence of myoglobin antigen in embryonal muscle cells, using the immunoperoxidase technique performed on needle aspirates.

RENAL ONCOCYTOMA

Renal oncocytoma is a benign neoplasm, derived from the intercalated cells of the collecting tubules.[48] The term "oncocytes" is used to describe the epithelial cells with abundant brightly eosinophilic and granular cytoplasm, due to the presence of numerous mitochondria in the cytoplasm. Renal oncocytomas generally are not symptomatic. The vast majority of such tumors have been discovered incidentally during evaluation for some unrelated disease or at postmortem. This important feature was originally pointed out by Klein and Valensi.[49] The low incidence of signs and symptoms reflects their benign local growth behavior.[50] The increasing use of modern abdominal imaging techniques in the investigation of a wide variety of medical complaints will undoubtedly lead to the discovery of many more asymptomatic oncocytomas in the future. The ABC of renal oncocytoma has been reported in the literature[51–54] and it has been pointed out that NAB diagnosis can reinforce the surgeon's decision for conservative partial nephrectomy.[53,55]

Histopathology

The tumor is well-circumscribed and brown-tan in color. A central stellate scar is usually seen in the larger tumors. Histologically, the tumor is composed of uniform

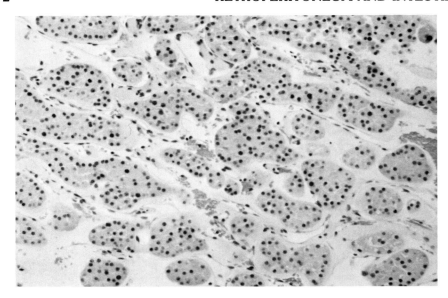

Fig. 10.22. Renal oncocytoma, histology section. Note organoid nests of oncocytic cells, separated by wide bands of mature fibrous tissue. Central lumina within the cell packets result in an alveolar pattern when seen in cross section and a tubular pattern when viewed longitudinally. This architectural arrangement of tumor cells is characteristic, yet not specific, for this tumor. (H & E preparation; ×125).

polygonal cells with abundant brightly eosinophilic, homogeneous or granular cytoplasm. The nuclei are round and uniform. The tumor cells are arranged in solid sheets, but there is a tendency towards clustering into nests and cords of cells separated by delicate fibrovascular stroma **(Fig. 10.22).** Central lumina within the cell nests give rise to an alveolar pattern when viewed in cross section and a tubular appearance when viewed longitudinally.

Lieber et al[56] reviewed 90 oncocytomas and were able to divide them into two groups, grade I and grade II, based on cytologic atypia. Four of the 28 grade II tumors resulted in metastases and death. None of the 62 patients with grade I tumors developed metastases. These authors stressed that if the term renal oncocytoma is used strictly to signify a very well-differentiated (grade I) eosinophilic granular cell renal cortical tumor then renal oncocytomas are nonaggressive tumors with a highly favorable prognosis.

Aspiration Biopsy Cytology

The ABC of renal oncocytoma shows moderate cellularity, with tumor cells lying singly or aggregated loosely in small groups or nests **(Fig. 10.23).** The cells are uniform and polygonal. Although the nuclei may be hyperchromatic, they are regular and round, with uniform distribution of the chromatin. Nucleoli may be present but are not prominent. The cytoplasm is brightly eosinophilic and the cytoplasmic border is sharply defined.

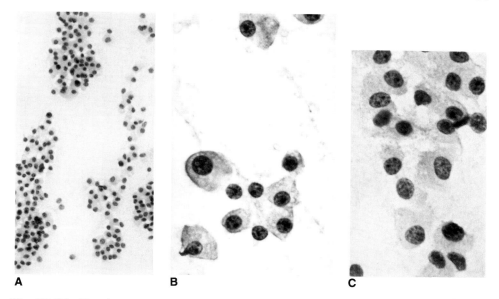

A   B   C

Fig. 10.23. Renal oncocytoma, composite ABC. **A.** Low-magnification view showing a single population of cells, arranged in nests. (H & E preparation; ×125). **B,C.** High-magnification views. The neoplastic oncocytes have polygonal shape, bland uniform nuclei, small nucleoli, and eosinophilic granular cytoplasm. (H & E preparation; B, C, ×500).

Diagnostic Pitfalls

The tumor cells of renal oncocytoma may resemble the epithelial cells of the proximal convoluted tubules. Two important features help distinguish a neoplastic aspirate from an aspirate of normal renal tissue. First, an aspirate from an oncocytoma is more cellular. Second, the cells are all of one type, i.e., oncocytes. This is in contrast to an aspirate from normal renal parenchyma, which consists typically of a mixture of proximal and distal tubular cells and renal glomeruli **(Fig. 10.1B and C).**

An occasional renal cell carcinoma may contain areas that are indistinguishable from renal oncocytoma, but examination of other parts of the tumor will show the features of renal cell carcinoma.[57] When NAB is performed, adequate multiple sampling of the lesion is therefore paramount in order to minimize the confusion between the two conditions. The presence of clear cells, a predominant papillary pattern, necrosis, mitosis, or high-grade nuclear pleomorphism rules out the diagnosis of oncocytoma.

In discussing the treatment of renal oncocytoma, Lieber et al[50,55] stated that radical (total) nephrectomy is the treatment of choice for a large solid tumor that has occupied most of the kidney if a good contralateral kidney is present, irrespective of whether the tumor is a renal cell carcinoma or a renal oncocytoma. On the other hand, if the tumor is smaller than 4 cm and has been shown by computed tomography to be well-circumscribed and confined to one pole of the kidney, partial nephrectomy is recommended. In the very elderly or very sick patient having a renal tumor with the possibility of an oncocytoma, needle biopsy of multiple areas of the lesion to demonstrate the presence solely of oncocytes provides information valuable for patient management. There are reported cases in which patients with bilateral large and unresectable renal oncocytomas proven by biopsy have been followed for many years without showing distinct progression of the tumors. Lieber[50,55] states that such observational treatment of renal oncocytomas may be entirely appropriate for the very elderly or for patients who are otherwise at very poor operative risks.

ANGIOMYOLIPOMA

Angiomyolipomas are uncommon benign tumors that are generally considered hamartomatous in nature. Before the term "angiomyolipoma" was introduced in 1951 by Morgan et al,[58] these lesions were reported as intrarenal lipomas or mixed tumors. About 50% of the cases of renal angiomyolipomas are associated with the tuberous sclerosis complex, a familial disorder consisting of gliosis of the brain, adenoma sebaceum of the face, and multiple hamartomas of the kidney, liver, and pancreas. The other 50% of renal angiomyolipomas occur independent of tuberous sclerosis. In the past, radical nephrectomy was often performed for angiomyolipomas because of the preoperative assumption that they were renal cell carcinomas. A specific preoperative diagnosis is now possible with the use of computed tomography and NAB. The characteristic low tissue density of the fat content in the lesion can be seen on computed tomography. Diagnosis of angiomyolipomas by percutaneous NAB has been reported.[3,59,60] Such a diagnosis may prompt surgical exploration of the renal mass with intraoperative frozen section biopsy.[61,62] A partial, instead of a total, nephrectomy may then be performed.[60,61,63]

Histopathology and Aspiration Biopsy Cytology

Histologically, the lesion is composed of variable proportions of mature adipose tissue, bundles of smooth muscle, fibrous connective tissue, and abnormal thick-walled blood vessels **(Fig. 10.24)**. The representation of each of these components varies from one field to another. Occasionally pleomorphic, cellular areas involving the adipose or smooth muscle elements may be present and these features do not indicate malignant behavior.

On ABC, the smears consist of fragments of mature adipose tissue admixed with irregular bundles of mesenchymal cells **(Fig. 10.25)**. The vascular component is not reliably identified. The mesenchymal cells are spindle-shaped, with faintly fibrillary cytoplasm and oval to cigar-shaped nuclei with slight pleomorphism, uniform chromatin distribution, and inconspicuous nucleoli. Immunostains for muscle-specific actin are strongly positive in the cytoplasm of these mesenchymal cells, confirming their smooth muscle origin.[60]

Diagnostic Pitfalls

The smooth muscle cells in angiomyolipoma may occasionally have an atypical morphology, mimicking a leiomyosarcoma or the sarcomatoid variant of renal cell carci-

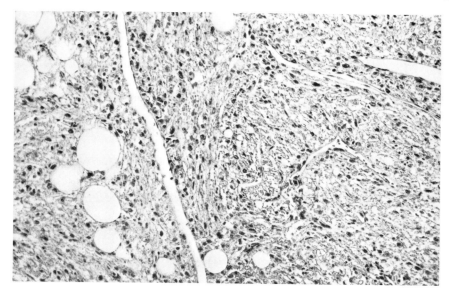

Fig. 10.24. Angiomyolipoma, histologic section. Note admixture of smooth muscle bundles, fatty tissue, and vascular spaces. (H & E preparation; ×125).

noma. Tumors that contain predominantly fatty tissue may be confused with well-differentiated liposarcoma.[64] Conversely, a false-negative report may result if the spindle and fat cells present in the aspirate are misinterpreted as being normal components derived from the perinephric fibrofatty tissue.

The presence of intimate admixtures of adipose and smooth muscle components, smooth muscle marker expression, and the lack of malignant cytologic features permit the diagnosis of angiomyolipoma to be made on NAB. Cytologic findings should always be interpreted in the light of clinical data as well as the characteristic computed tomography findings.

MESOBLASTIC NEPHROMA

The mesoblastic nephroma, also known by other names including fetal hamartoma, leiomyomatous hamartoma, and stromal hamartoma, is a congenital benign lesion and generally presents in early infancy. Only occasionally, the tumor occurs in older children and young adults. On gross examination, the tumor is a solitary mass of variable size and often resembles a leiomyoma with a tough, fibrous-appearing cut surface.

Histopathology and Needle Aspiration Cytology

Histologically the tumor is composed of fascicles of immature-appearing spindled cells resembling fibroblasts, myofibroblasts, and smooth muscle cells, with variable

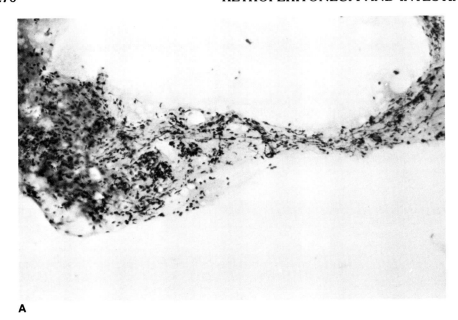

A

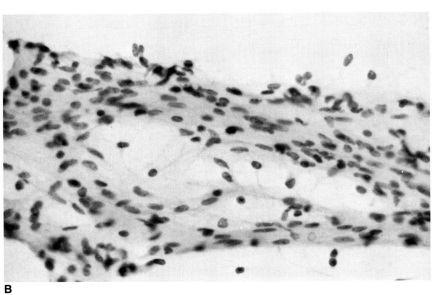

B

Fig. 10.25. Angiomyolipoma, ABC. **A.** Note a large tissue fragment composed of fat cells and spindle cells. (H & E preparation; ×125). **B.** Note spindle cells with cigar-shaped nuclei in regimented polarization, consistent with smooth muscle cells. (H & E preparation; ×310).

amounts of collagen between the cells. Mitotic activity is variable, usually it is low. When the tumor displays more mitotic activity, cellular pleomorphism, and necrosis, one must raise the suspicion that the tumor is an atypical variant, which has an aggressive behavior with a high propensity of recurrence.

Reports on the aspiration biopsy cytology of mesoblastic nephroma have been few.[65,66] In classic cases, the ABC shows variably sized sheets of spindle cells as well as dyshesive spindle cells with scanty cytoplasm and oval nuclei, some with pointed ends **(Fig. 10.26)**. Nuclear chromatin is coarse but uniformly distributed. The cells resemble closely fibroblastic or leiomyomatous cells and exhibit minimal nuclear atypia and mitosis. No epithelial, tubular, or glomeruloid differentiation is noted. Dey and associates[65] reported a case of mesoblastic nephroma in a 4-month-old child and pointed out that a correct diagnosis is possible on ABC, provided both the age and cytomorphology are taken into consideration in interpreting the smears and the aspirates are obtained from multiple sites.

Diagnostic Pitfalls

The principal lesion with which mesoblastic nephroma is likely to be confused is the nephroblastoma (Wilms' tumor) with predominantly stromal differentiation. However, the demonstration of small, dark blastemal cells, solid tubules (no lumina), or differentiated tubules with lumina permits the diagnosis of Wilms' tumor in the majority of instances. It is unusual to see the fibroma-like cells characteristic of mesoblastic nephroma occupying large areas of an aspirate from a Wilms' tumor.

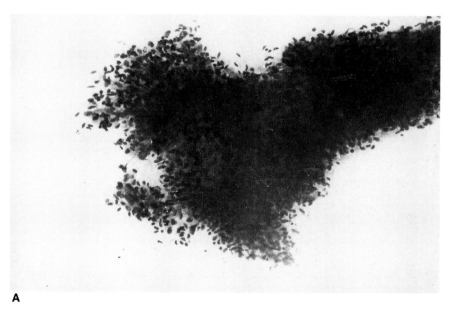

A

Fig. 10.26. Mesoblastic nephroma. **A.** ABC. Note a cohesive, thick sheet of cells and a few dyshesive spindle cells at the peripheral of the sheet. (May-Grünwald Giemsa preparation; ×110).

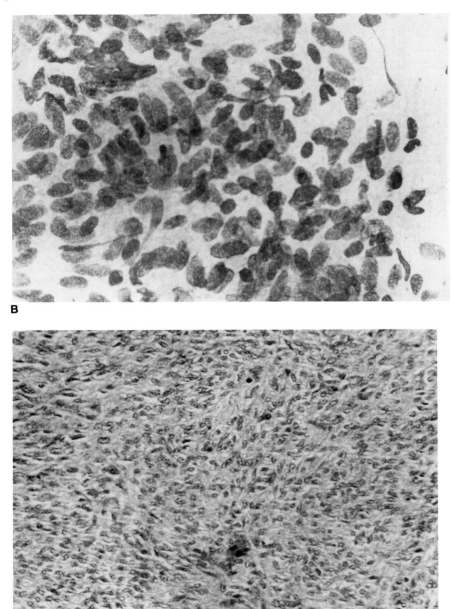

Fig. 10.26. B. ABC. Note hypercellular smear showing spindle cells with oval nuclei and uniform coarse chromatin. (May-Grünwald Giemsa preparation: ×400). **C.** Histologic section of the mesoblastic nephroma. (H & E preparation; ×110). (Reproduced from Dey P, Srinivasan R, Nijhawan R, et al: Fine needle aspiration cytology of mesoblastic nephroma. A case report. *Acta Cytol* 36:404–406, 1992, with permission).

XANTHOGRANULOMATOUS PYELONEPHRITIS

Xanthogranulomatous pyelonephritis is an uncommon unilateral chronic inflammatory disease of the kidney associated with recurrent urinary tract infections, particularly *Proteus* or pseudomonal infections. On diagnostic imaging or arteriography, the disease frequently appears as a mass lesion simulating a renal neoplasm. However, the patient often will have evidence of active chronic infection, such as fever, flank pain, and leukocytosis. Urine culture is positive for bacterial organisms in two-thirds of the patients.[67] Most patients have been treated surgically by total nephrectomy because of the preoperative uncertainty about a possible neoplasm. Sease et al[68] reported four patients who had NAB findings supportive of xanthogranulomatous pyelonephritis and ultrasound findings characteristic of the disease. A preoperative diagnosis of this inflammatory condition can spare the patient a radical nephrectomy; the disease is often localized and partial nephrectomy is the treatment of choice in most cases.

Histopathology and Needle Aspiration Biopsy

Histologically, chronic xanthogranulomatous pyelonephritis **(Fig. 10.27)** is characterized by sheets of large, lipid-laden, foamy histiocytes (xanthoma cells). There are also lymphocytes and plasma cells. Fibrosis and necrosis are common.

NAB of xanthogranulomatous pyelonephritis shows a chronic inflammatory process, composed predominantly of proliferation of foamy histiocytes with variable num-

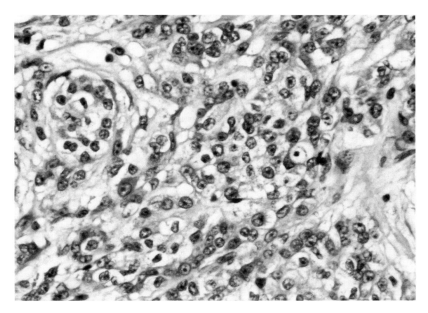

Fig. 10.27. Chronic xanthogranulomatous pyelonephritis, histologic section. Note large accumulation of histiocytes. (H & E preparation; ×310).

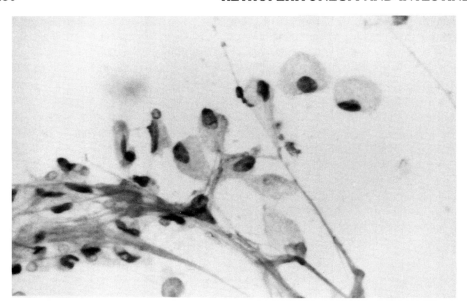

Fig. 10.28. Chronic xanthogranulomatous pyelonephritis, ABC. Note foamy histiocytes and fibroblasts. (H & E preparation; ×500). (Reproduced from Suen KC: *Atlas and Text of Aspiration Biopsy Cytology.* Baltimore, Williams & Wilkins, 1991, with permission.)

bers of lymphocytes and fibroblasts, and sometimes necrotic debris **(Fig. 10.28).** Multinucleated macrophages were noted by Nguyen.[69]

It is important to remember that foamy histiocytes may be mistaken for renal cell carcinoma of the clear cell type.

RENAL CYSTS

Benign renal cysts are common and must be differentiated from neoplastic and inflammatory processes. If the cyst is first discovered by intravenous urography, it can be further evaluated by ultrasound. On ultrasound a benign simple cyst will show a smooth, sharply defined cyst wall, absence of internal echogenicity, and acoustic enhancement beyond the posterior wall.[70] Although ultrasound is the diagnostic modality of choice for evaluation of a renal mass, alternatively computed tomography may be used. On computed tomography examination, the interiors of the benign cysts generally have a uniform attenuation value near that of water and do not change in appearance on contrast-enhanced scans. Sometimes, when ultrasound or computed tomography criteria for benign cysts are not met, a double-contrast study can be performed if one desires better definition of the inner cyst wall. Injection of contrast material may demonstrate the typical smooth wall characteristic of a simple cyst.

The use of modern imaging techniques aided by percutaneous needle aspiration has almost eliminated the need for surgical exploration of benign renal cysts. Operation is indicated only when the radiologic interpretation is equivocal, especially if a double-contrast study reveals filling defects or solid nodules protruding into the cyst cavity.[31]

Benign renal cysts yield a clear, straw-colored fluid of low fat and protein content and normal lactic acid dehydrogenase level.[31] Cytologic examination of the fluid **(Fig. 10.29)** shows a variable number of cells. The most commonly seen are the scattered histiocytes. The epithelial cells are generally attenuated and cuboidal in shape, with small bland nuclei. The epithelial cells or histiocytes or both occasionally show marked reactive atypia, mimicking malignant cells.[2,29,30,71] Koss et al[71] cautioned that as a

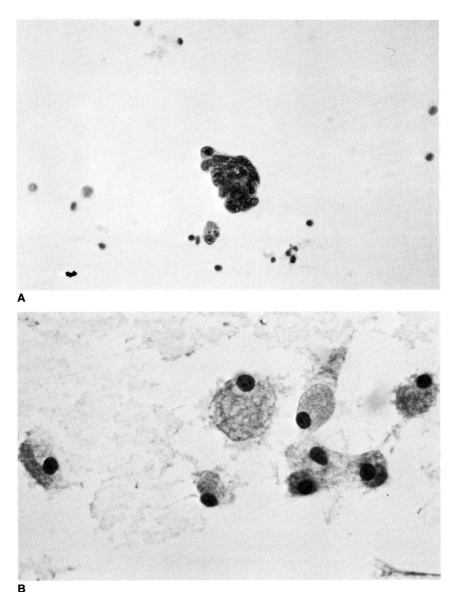

Fig. 10.29. Aspiration of renal cyst (cytocentrifuge smears). **A.** Note a small cluster of attenuated cells with bland nuclei. These cells probably represent epithelial lining cells, but they might be small histiocytes. (H & E preparation; ×310). **B.** Note scattered, large histiocytes with abundant foamy cytoplasm. (H & E preparation; ×500).

TABLE 10.4. Criteria for Diagnosis of Benign Renal Cysts by Needle Puncture

1.	Ultrasound shows a regular, smooth inner wall. Alternatively, injection of contrast material shows a typical smooth walled cyst completely filling the mass seen on prior intravenous pyelogram.
2.	Aspiration of clear, straw-colored fluid.
3.	No cytologic abnormalities (absence of atypical or malignant cells in the aspirate).
4.	No biochemical abnormalities (benign cysts have low fat and protein content and normal lactic dehydrogenase activity. Fluid from a cystic cancerous lesion contains fat, considerable protein, and low lactic dehydrogenase activity).

general rule the diagnosis of cancer should not be made from cyst fluid except on the basis of massive cytologic evidence. Steg[31] outlined the criteria for the diagnosis of a benign cyst **(Table 10.4).** In a study of 1,342 renal cysts, he reported that no case was found in which the diagnostic criteria of benign cyst were satisfied and the lesion was not benign.

NEOPLASMS METASTATIC TO THE KIDNEY

The most common sites of primary cancers that metastasize to the kidney are: lung, colon, opposite kidney, and melanomas from various body sites.[72] The clinical presentation may mimic renal cell carcinoma, with hematuria, pyrexia and a palpable mass. The differential diagnosis is helped by knowing that the patient has been treated for a primary cancer arising elsewhere. A metastatic carcinoma in the kidney is generally far advanced when diagnosed; therefore, with few exceptions, extensive investigation and radical treatment are generally not indicated. The cytologic features of various metastatic tumors are discussed in detail in Chapter 6.

ACCURACY OF NEEDLE ASPIRATION BIOPSY

Pilotti et al[6] analyzed the results of 132 cases of NAB of renal masses and reported that the sensitivity, specificity, and predictive values for positive results were, respectively, 93%, 96%, and 93.5%, with one false-positive diagnosis in a case of multilocular cystic nephroma. Cristallini et al[8] studied 72 kidney masses by NABs and achieved an overall accuracy rate of 93.05%. Shah and Kini[13] reviewed 92 cases and the diagnostic errors included four false-negatives (three unsatisfactory, one misinterpreted as negative) and one false-positive. Cajulis et al[14] found a high (80–92%) concordance between nuclear grading in NAB material and histologic specimens and advocated the use of NAB for tumor grading.

Although, based on the available data in the literature, most authors indicate that NAB can be effectively applied to the diagnosis of renal masses, this opinion is not shared by all investigators. Torp-Pedersen and associates[7] recently recorded seven false-positive cytologic reports in 49 noncancer cases. Of these seven cases, five did not have any neoplasm; one had an angiomyolipoma; and in another a dysplastic kidney was diagnosed by arteriography. No reasons were given to explain why the false-positive results had occurred in the five "normal" kidneys, but these authors indicated that the false-positive rate was too high for NAB to be clinically useful in their hands.

REFERENCES

1. Franzen S, Brehmer-Andersson E: Cytologic diagnosis of renal cell carcinoma. In Kuss R, Murphy GP, Khoury S, et al (eds): *Renal Tumors.* New York, Alan R Liss, 1981, pp 425–432.

2. Helm CW, Burwood RJ, Harrison NW, et al: Aspiration cytology of solid renal tumors. *Br J Urol* 55:249–253, 1983.

3. Glenthoj A, Partoft S: Ultrasound-guided percutaneous aspiration of renal angiomyolipoma. *Acta Cytol* 28:265–268, 1984.

4. Juul N, Torp-Pedersen S, Gronvall S, et al: Ultrasonically guided fine needle aspiration biopsy of renal masses. *J Urol* 133:579–581, 1985.

5. Luciani L, Scappini P, Pusiol T, et al: The role of aspiration cytology in the management of ureteral obstruction in patients with known cancer. *Cancer* 59:1936–1946, 1987.

6. Pilotti S, Rilke F, Alasio L, et al: The role of fine needle aspiration in the assessment of renal masses. *Acta Cytol* 32:1–10, 1988.

7. Torp-Pederson S, Juul N, Larsen T, et al: US-guided fine needle biopsy of solid renal masses—comparison of histology and cytology. *Scand J Urol Nephrol* 137(Suppl):41–43, 1991.

8. Cristallini EG, Paganelli C, Bolis GB: Role of fine-needle aspiration biopsy in the assessment of renal masses. *Diagn Pathol* 7:32–35, 1991.

9. Stewart BH, Pasalis JK: Aspiration and cytology in the evaluation of renal mass lesions. *Cleveland Clin Quart* 43:1–6, 1976.

10. Murphy WM, Zambroni BR, Emerson LD, et al: Aspiration biopsy of the kidney. Simultaneous collection of cytologic and histologic specimens. *Cancer* 56:200–205, 1985.

11. Nguyen GK: Percutaneous fine-needle aspiration biopsy cytology of the kidney and adrenal. *Pathol Annu* 22(part 1):163–191, 1987.

12. Vassiliades VG, Bernardino ME: Percutaneous renal and adrenal biopsies. *Cardiovasc Intervent Radiol* 14:50–54, 1991.

13. Shah AR, Kini SR: Efficacy of fine needle aspiration of solid tumors involving the kidney (abstract). *Acta Cytol* 35:595, 1991.

14. Cajulis RS, Katz RL, Dekmezian R, et al: Fine needle aspiration biopsy of renal cell carcinoma. Cytologic parameters and their concordance with histologic and flow cytometric data. *Acta Cytol* 37:367–372, 1993.

15. Nunez D Jr, Yrizarry JM, Nadji M, et al: Renal cell carcinoma complicating long-term dialysis: Computed tomography-guided aspiration cytology. *CT* 10:61–66, 1986.

16. Ishikawa I, Kovacs G: High incidence of papillary renal cell tumors in patients on chronic hemodialysis. *Histopathol* 22:135–139, 1993.

17. Bray G, Pendergrass TW, Schaller RT Jr, et al: Preoperative chemotherapy in the treat-

ment of Wilms' tumor diagnosed with the aid of fine needle aspiration biopsy. *Am J Pediatr Hematol Oncol* 8:75–78, 1986.

18. Luciani L, Scappini P, Pusiol T, et al: The role of aspiration cytology in the management of ureteral obstruction in patients with known cancer. *Cancer* 59:1936–1946, 1987.

19. Freiman DB, Ring EJ, Oleaga JA, et al: Thin needle biopsy in the diagnosis of ureteral obstruction with malignancy. *Cancer* 42:714–716, 1978.

20. Bradham RR, Wanamaker CC, Pratt-Thomas HR: Renal cell carcinoma metastases 25 years after nephrectomy. *JAMA* 223:921–922, 1973.

21. Linsk JA, Franzen S: Aspiration cytology of metastatic hypernephroma. *Acta Cytol* 28:250–260, 1984.

22. Lasser A, Rothman JG, Calamia VJ: Renal cell carcinoma metastatic to the thyroid. *Acta Cytol* 29:856–858, 1985.

23. Nguyen GK: Fine needle aspiration biopsy cytology of metastatic renal cell carcinoma. *Acta Cytol* 32:409–414, 1988.

24. Skinner DG, Colvin RB, Vermillion CD, et al: Diagnosis and management of renal cell carcinoma. A clinical and pathologic study of 309 cases. *Cancer* 28:1165–1177, 1971.

25. Schreeb von T, Franzen S, Ljungquist A: Renal adenocarcinoma: Evaluation of malignancy on a cytologic basis. A comparative cytologic and histologic study. *Scand J Urol Nephrol* 1:265–269, 1967.

26. Nurmi M, Tyrkko J, Puntala P, et al: Reliability of aspiration biopsy cytology in the grading of renal adenocarcinoma. *Scand J Urol Nephrol* 18:155–156, 1984.

27. Zajicek J: *Aspiration Biopsy Cytology, Part 2: Cytology of Infradiaphragmatic Organs.* Basel, Karger, 1979, pp 1–36.

28. Syrjanen K, Hjelt L: Grading of human renal adenocarcinoma. *Scand J Urol Nephrol* 12:49–55, 1978.

29. Plowden KM, Erozan YS, Frost JK: Cellular atypia associated with benign lesions of the kidney as seen in fine needle aspirates. *Acta Cytol* 28:648, 1984.

30. Reddy VB, Gattuso P, Abraham KP, et al: Computed tomography-guided fine needle aspiration biopsy of deep-seated lesions. A four-year experience. *Acta Cytol* 35:753–756, 1991.

31. Steg A: Does percutaneous puncture still have a role to play in the diagnosis of renal tumors? In Kuss R, Murphy GP, Khoury S, et al (eds): *Renal Tumors.* New York, Alan R Liss, 1981, pp 417–423.

32. Tolamo TS, Shonnard JW: Small renal adenocarcinoma with metastases. *J Urol* 124:132–134, 1980.

33. Cass AS: Large renal adenoma. *J Urol* 124:281–282, 1980.

34. Mostofi FK, Davis CJ: Pathology of urologic cancer. In Javadpou N (ed): *Principles and Management of Urologic Cancer,* ed 2. Baltimore, Williams & Wilkins, 1983, p 65.

35. Bennington JL: Cancer of the kidney—etiology, epidemiology and pathology. *Cancer* 32:1017–1029, 1973.

36. Drut R, Pollono D: Anaplastic Wilms' tumor. Initial diagnosis by fine needle aspiration. *Acta Cytol* 31:774–776, 1987.

37. Akhtar M, Ali AM, Sackey K, et al: Aspiration cytology of Wilms' tumor: Correlation of cytologic and histologic features. *Diagn Cytopathol* 5:269–274, 1989.

38. Quijano G, Drut R: Cytologic characteristics of Wilms' tumors in fine needle aspirates. A study of ten cases. *Acta Cytol* 33:263–266, 1989.

39. Howell LP, Russell LA, Howard PH, et al: The cytology of pediatric masses: A differential diagnostic approach. *Diagn Cytopathol* 8:107–115, 1992.

40. De Kraker J, Lemerle J, Voute PA, et al: Wilms' tumor with pulmonary metastases at diagnosis. *J Clin Oncol* 8:1187–1190, 1990.

41. Weithman AM, Morrison G, Hurt MA: Metastatic transitional-cell carcinoma to the mandible. A case report. *Diagn Cytopathol* 4:156–158, 1988.

42. Hayes MMM, Jones EC, Verma AK, et al: Transitional cell carcinoma of the renal pelvis metastatic to the metacarpal. *Acta Cytol* 36:946–950, 1992.

43. Johnson TL, Kini SR: Cytologic features of metastatic transitional cell carcinoma. *Diagn Cytopathol* 9:270–278, 1993.

44. Bennington JL, Beckwith JB: *Tumors of the Kidney, Renal Pelvis, and Ureter. Atlas of Tumor Pathology.* Fascicle 12, Second Series. Washington, DC, Armed Forces Institute of Pathology, 1975, pp 243–310.

45. Farrow GM, Harrison EG Jr, Utz DC, et al: Sarcomas and sarcomatoid and mixed malignant tumors of the kidney in adults. *Cancer* 22:545–550, 1968.

46. Dehner LP: Pathology of the urinary bladder in children. In Young RH (ed): *Pathology of the Urinary Bladder.* New York, Churchill Livingstone, 1989, pp 179–211.

47. Torres V, Ferrer R: Cytology of fine needle aspiration biopsy of primary breast rhabdomyosarcoma in an adolescent girl. *Acta Cytol* 29:430–434, 1985.

48. Zerban H, Nogueira E, Riedasch G, et al: Renal oncocytoma: Origin from the collecting duct. *Virchow Arch* 52:375–387, 1987.

49. Klein MJ, Valensi QJ: Proximal tubular adenomas of kidney with so called oncocytic features. A clinicopathological study of 13 cases of a rarely reported neoplasm. *Cancer* 38:906–914, 1976.

50. Lieber MM: Renal oncocytoma. *Urol Clin North Am* 20:355–359, 1993.

51. Rodriquez CA, Buskop A, Johnson J, et al: Renal oncocytoma. Preoperative diagnosis by aspiration biopsy. *Acta Cytol* 24:355–359, 1980.

52. Nguyen GK, Amy RW, Tsang S: Fine needle aspiration biopsy cytology of renal oncocytoma. *Acta Cytol* 29:33–36, 1985.

53. Alanen KA, Tyrkko JES, Nurmi MJ: Aspiration biopsy cytology of renal oncocytoma. *Acta Cytol* 29:859–862, 1985.

54. Cochand-Priollet B, Rothschild E, Chagnon S, et al: Renal oncocytoma diagnosed by fine-needle aspiration cytology. *Br J Urol* 61:534–535, 1988.

55. Lieber MM, Tsukamoto T: Renal oncocytoma. In deKernion JB, Pavone-Macaluso (eds): *Tumors of the Kidney.* Baltimore, Williams & Wilkins, 1986, pp 257–273.

56. Lieber MM, Tomera KM, Farrow GM: Renal oncocytoma. *J Urol* 125:481–485, 1981.

57. Barnes CA, Beckman EN: Renal oncocytoma and its congeners. *Am J Clin Pathol* 79:312–318, 1983.

58. Morgan GS, Straumfjord JY, Hall EF: Angiomyolipoma of the kidney. *J Urol* 65:525–527, 1951.

59. Nguyen GK: Aspiration biopsy cytology of renal angiomyolipoma. *Acta Cytol* 28:261–264, 1984.

60. Pueblitz S, Paulson J, Edmonds P, et al: The cytologic features of renal angiomyolipoma (abstract). *Am J Clin Pathol* 94:510, 1990.

61. Williams G: Angiomyolipoma. In DeKernion JB, Pavone-Macaluso M (eds): *Tumors of the Kidney.* Baltimore, Williams & Wilkins, 1986, pp 320–330.

62. Kaneti J, Kruguak K, Hirsh M, et al: Rupture of renal angiomyolipoma: Conservative surgery. *J Urol* 129:810–811, 1983.

63. Barrilero AE: Renal angiomyoliopma: A study of 13 cases. *J Urol* 117:547–552, 1977.

64. Hruban RH, Bhagavdan BS, Epstein JL: Massive retroperitoneal angiomyolipoma: A lesion that may be confused with well differentiated liposarcoma. *Am J Clin Pathol* 92:805–808, 1989.

65. Dey P, Srinivasan R, Nijhawan R, et al: Fine needle aspiration cytology of mesoblastic nephroma. A case report. *Acta Cytol* 36:404–406, 1992.

66. Drut R: Cytologic characteristics of congenital mesoblastic nephroma in fine-needle aspiration cytology. A case report. *Diagn Cytopathol* 8:374–376, 1992.

67. Oosterhof GON, Delaeere KPJ: Xanthogranulomatous pyelonephritis: A review with 2 case reports. *Urol Int* 41:180–186, 1986.

68. Sease WC, Elyaderani MK, Belis JA: Ultrasonography and needle aspiration in diagnosis of xanthogranulomatous pyelonephritis. *Urology* 24:231–235, 1987.

69. Nguyen GK: Percutaneous fine-needle aspiration cytology of the kidney and adrenal. *Pathol Annu* 22 (Part 1):115–134, 1987.

70. Letourneau JG, Elyaderani MK: Percutaneous biopsy of kidneys and adrenals and drainage of nephric and perinephric fluid collections. In Letourneau JG, Elyaderani MK, Castaneda-Zuniga WR (eds): *Percutaneous Biopsy, Aspiration and Drainage.* Chicago, Year Book, 1987, pp 79–103.

71. Koss LG, Woyke S, Olszewski W: *Aspiration Biopsy. Cytologic Interpretation and Histologic Bases.* New York, Igaku-Shoin, 1992, p 593.

72. Silva FG, Childers JH: Adult renal diseases. In Sternberg SS (ed): *Diagnostic Surgical Pathology.* New York, Raven Press, 1989, p 1323.

Index

A

Abdominal imaging, 27–37
  adrenals, *see* Adrenals
  computed tomography, 29, 31–33
  fluoroscopy, 29–30
  gastrointestinal tract, 35–36
  intestine, 169–197
  kidney, *see* Kidney
  localization of mass, 28–34
  magnetic resonance imaging, 29, 34
  modalities, comparison, 29
  palpation, mass, 28–30
Abscess, retroperitoneum, 126
Acquired immunodeficiency syndrome, lymphomas associated with, 70
Adenocarcinoma
  intestine, 176–178
  malignant mesothelioma, peritoneal, distinguishing, 210
  retroperitoneum, 137–144
  stomach, 171–176
Adjuvant diagnostic techniques, 11
Adrenals, 213–246
  adrenocortical adenoma, 217–221
  adrenocortical carcinoma, 221–227
    renal cell carcinoma, distinguishing features, 227, 260
  adrenocortical nodules, 217–221
  anatomy, 213–214
  cyst, 239
  diagnostic accuracy, 242–243
  embryology, 213–214
  ganglioneuroblastoma, 237–238
  ganglioneuroma, 237–238
  imaging, 36
  incidentally discovered mass, role of needle aspiration biopsy, 241–242
  metastases to adrenal gland, 239–241
  myelolipoma, 239
  neuroblastoma, 234–237
  normal cytology, 215–216
  pheochromocytoma, 227–234
  tumors, overview of, 214–215
Adrenocortical adenoma, 217–221
Adrenocortical carcinoma, 221–227
  renal cell carcinoma, distinguishing features, 227
Adrenocortical nodules, 217–221
AIDS, *see* Acquired immunodeficiency syndrome
Alpha-fetoprotein, immunologic marker, 13, 156
Anaplastic carcinoma, small cell, retroperitoneum, 145–146, 222
Anaplastic large cell lymphoma, 69–70
Anatomy
  adrenals, 213–214
  intestine, 169–170
  peritoneal mesothelioma, 199–200
  retroperitoneum, 39–40
  stomach, 169–170
Angiomyolipoma, kidney, 274–275
Antibody
  for differentiating carcinoma, sarcoma, lymphoma, 12
  to leukocyte common antigen, immunocytochemistry, retroperitoneum, lymphoproliferative disorder, 53
Anti-kappa antibodies, lymphoproliferative disorder, 53
Anti-lambda antibodies, lymphoproliferative disorder, 53
Approach to interpretation, multiparameter, 10–24
  electron microscopy, 17–22
  clinical applications, 19–22
  flow cytometry, 14–17
  clinical applications, 15–17
    DNA ploidy/cell proliferation study, 15–16
    immunophenotyping, 16–17
  immunocytochemistry, 10–14
  clinical applications, 12–14
  molecular genetic study, 22–24
Architectural pattern, in needle aspiration biopsy, 7, 9
Aspiration
  biopsy cytology
    results, retroperitoneum, 79–80

Aspiration (*contd.*)
   retroperitoneum
      metastatic tumor, 137–163
      normal and reactive cells, 43–45
   technique, 2–3
Attributes, for cytopathologist, 4
Atypical immunoreactions, in some neoplasms, 14

B

Background material, noncellular, in needle aspiration biopsy, 8–9
Bladder, transitional cell carcinoma, 265–266
British Columbia Cancer Agency, fine needle aspiration biopsy, 2
Burkitt's lymphoma, 63, 66

C

Carazzi's hematoxylin, preparation of, 4
Carbowax solution, 2
Carcinoembryonic antigen, immunologic marker, 13
Carcinoid tumor, intestine, 184–189
   diagnostic pitfalls, 186–189
   pathology, 185–186
Carcinosarcoma, retroperitoneum, 150
Castleman's disease, retroperitoneum, 74
CEA, *see* Carcinoembryonic antigen
Cell kinetics analysis, DNA content, lymphoproliferative disorder, 56–57
Chordoma, retroperitoneum, 113
Choriocarcinoma, retroperitoneum, 156, 161
Chromogranin, immunologic marker, 13
Chromosome, translocations, 11, 24, 62, 66, 110
Colon, lymphoma, 182
Complications, of needle aspiration biopsy, retroperitoneum, 43
Computed tomography, abdominal imaging, 29, 31–33
Consultation, importance of, 6
Core needle biopsy, *see* Cutting needle biopsy
Cutting needle biopsy, fine needle aspiration biopsy, versus, 42–43
Cyst
   adrenal, 239
   renal, 280–282
   retroperitoneum, 124
Cytokeratin, immunologic marker, 13
Cytologic patterns, summary of, 9
Cytometry
   flow, technique of, for successful needle aspiration biopsy, 5
   image, technique of, for successful needle aspiration biopsy, 5
Cytopathologist, attributes of, 4

D

Desmin, immunologic marker, 13, 87
Diagnostic criteria, knowledge of, for successful needle aspiration biopsy, 5
Differential diagnosis, knowledge of, for successful needle aspiration biopsy, 5
DNA content/cell kinetics analysis, lymphoproliferative disorder, 56–57

DNA ploidy/cell proliferation study, flow cytometry, 15–16

E

Electron microscopy
   adjuvant diagnostic technique, 11
   multiparameter approach to interpretation, 17–22
      clinical applications, 19–22
   retroperitoneum, sarcoma, 87–88
   technique of, for successful needle aspiration biopsy, 5
Embryology
   adrenals, 213–214
   kidney, 247–248
   peritoneal mesothelioma, 199–200
   retroperitoneum, 39–40
   stomach, 169–170
Embryonal carcinoma, retroperitoneum, 156
Eosin staining procedure, 4
Epithelioid leiomyosarcoma, retroperitoneum, 113
Epithelial membrane antigen, immunologic marker, 13, 208, 225
Epithelioid variant, of smooth muscle tumor, intestine, 190, 193–194
Ewing's sarcoma, 108–110, 116–117

F

False-positive/negative report, reasons for, 9–10
Fibrosarcoma, retroperitoneum, 97
Fibrosis, idiopathic retroperitoneal fibrosis, retroperitoneum, 124–125
Fixation, 3
   for specimen quality, for successful needle aspiration biopsy, 5
Flow cytometry
   adjuvant diagnostic technique, 11
   multiparameter approach to interpretation, 14–17
      clinical applications, 15–17
      immunophenotyping, 16–17
   retroperitoneum, lymphoproliferative disorder, 55–57
      applications, lymph node pathology, 56
      histogram, interpretation as abnormal, criteria, 56
   technique of, for successful needle aspiration biopsy, 5
Fluoroscopy, abdominal imaging, 29–30

G

Ganglioneuroblastoma, adrenals, 237–238
Ganglioneuroma, adrenals, 237–238
Gastrointestinal lymphoma, 181–184
Gastrointestinal tract, imaging, 35–36
Genetics, molecular
   multiparameter approach to intepretation, 22–24
   technique of, for successful needle aspiration biopsy, 5
Genotypic study, molecular, lymphoproliferative disorder, 57–59

Germ cell tumor, retroperitoneum, 135–167
Giant follicular hyperplasia, retroperitoneum, 74
Gynecologic tumor, retroperitoneum, 150–155

H
Hematoma, retroperitoneum, 124–126
Hematoxylin
    Carazzi's, preparation of, 4
    procedure, rapid, 4
Histology, knowledge of, for successful needle aspiration biopsy, 5
HMB45, immunologic marker, 13, 152
Hodgkin's disease, 71–72
    retroperitoneum, interpretive pitfalls, 77

I
Idiopathic retroperitoneal fibrosis, retroperitoneum, 124–125
Image cytometry, technique of, for successful needle aspiration biopsy, 5
Immunocytochemistry
    adjuvant diagnostic technique, 11
    retroperitoneum
        lymphoproliferative disorder, 53–55
        sarcoma, 87–88
    technique of, for successful needle aspiration biopsy, 5
Immunologic marker analysis, retroperitoneum, lymphoproliferative disorder, 55
Immunophenotyping, flow cytometry, 15–16
Immunoreaction, atypical, in some neoplasms, 14
Intestine
    adenocarcinoma, 176–178
    anatomy, 169–170
    carcinoid tumor, 184–189
        diagnostic pitfalls, 186–189
        pathology, 185–186
    endoscopic biopsy, versus needle aspiration biopsy, 170–171
    gastrointestinal lymphoma, 181–184
    imaging, 169–197
    pseudomyxoma peritonei, 178–181
    small, lymphoma, 182
    smooth muscle tumor, 189–195

K
Kappa light chain, immunologic marker, 13
Kidney, 247–265, 271–286
    angiomyolipoma, 274–275
    embryology, 247–248
    imaging, 36
    mesoblastic nephroma, 275–278
    needle aspiration biopsy, role of, 248
    needle biopsy, accuracy of, 282–283
    neoplasm, metastatic, 282
    nephroblastoma, 261–265
    normal cytology/histology, 248–250
    renal cell carcinoma, 251–261
    renal cyst, 280–282
    renal oncocytoma, 271–274

transitional cell carcinoma, 265–266
Wilms' tumor, 261–265
xanthogranulomatous pyelonephritis, 279–280
Ki-1 lymphoma, 69–70

L
Lambda light chain, immunologic marker, 13
Leiomyoma, retroperitoneum, 124
Leiomyosarcoma, retroperitoneum, 90–94
Leukocyte common antigen, immunologic marker, 13
Leu-M-1, immunologic marker, 13
Leu-M1 antibody, retroperitoneum, lymphoproliferative disorder, 53
Lipoma, retroperitoneum, 120–124
Liposarcoma, low-grade, retroperitoneum, 94–97
    well-differentiated, 94–97
Localization of mass, abdominal, 28–34
Low-grade liposarcoma, retroperitoneum, well-differentiated, 94–97
Lymphadenitis
    acute, retroperitoneum, 73
    chronic, retroperitoneum, 73–74
Lymphoblastic lymphoma, retroperitoneum, 66
Lymphocyte subsets, immunologic marker, 13
Lymphoid hyperplasia
    reactive, retroperitoneum, 73–75
Lymphoma, antibody, for differentiating from carcinoma, sarcoma, 12
Lymphoproliferative disorder, retroperitoneum, 49–84
    acquired immunodeficiency syndrome, lymphomas associated with, 70
    ancillary diagnostic procedures, 52–59
    antibody to leukocyte common antigen, immunocytochemistry, 53
    anti-kappa antibodies, 53
    anti-lambda antibodies, 53
    aspiration biopsy cytology results, 79–80
    Burkitt's lymphoma, 63, 66
    cytology interpretation, clinical data relevant to, 51
    DNA content/cell kinetics analysis, 56–57
    fine needle biopsy, role of, 51–52
    flow cytometry, 55–57
        applications, lymph node pathology, 56
        histogram, interpretation as abnormal, criteria, 56
        immunologic marker analysis, 55
    giant follicular hyperplasia, 74
    Hodgkin's disease, 71–72
    immunocytochemistry, 53–55
    interpretive pitfalls, 75–79
        histologic type, 75–76
        Hodgkin's disease, 77
        lymphoma, versus nonlymphoid neoplasm, 77, 79
        sclerosis, 76–77
    Leu-M1 antibody, 53
    lymphadenitis
        acute, 73
        chronic, 73–74
    lymphoblastic lymphoma, 66
    lymphoid hyperplasia, 73–74

Lymphoproliferative disorder, retroperitoneum (*contd.*)
    malignant lymphoma, 50–51
      classification, 50–51
    molecular genotypic study, 57–59
    non-Hodgkin's, working formulation for, 50
    non-Hodgkin's lymphoma, 59–70
      malignant lymphoma, 59–61
        large cell
          cleaved and noncleaved, 63
          immunoblastic, 63
        mixed small/large cell, 63
        small cleaved cell, 62
        small noncleaved cell, 63, 66
      small lymphocytic, 59–61
    nonlymphoid markers, 53–55
    reactive lymphoid hyperplasia, 73–75
    tuberculous lymphadenitis, 75

M

Magnetic resonance imaging, abdominal imaging, 29, 34
Malignant lymphoma, retroperitoneum, lymphoproliferative disorder, 50–51
    classification, 50–51
Malignant melanoma, retroperitoneum, 146–150
Markers, immunologic, common, 13
Melanoma, malignant, 146–150
Mesoblastic nephroma, 275–278
Mesothelioma, malignant, adenocarcinoma, peritoneal, distinguishing, 210
Metastatic tumor, retroperitoneum, 135–167
Molecular genetics
    adjuvant diagnostic technique, 11
    multiparameter approach to interpretation, 22–24
    retroperitoneum, lymphoproliferative disorder, 57–59
    technique of, for successful needle aspiration biopsy, 5
Morphology, cell, knowledge of, for successful needle aspiration biopsy, 5
Multiparameter approach to interpretation, 10–24
    electron microscopy, 17–22
      clinical applications, 19–22
    flow cytometry, 14–17
      clinical applications, 15–17
        DNA ploidy/cell proliferation study, 15–16
        immunophenotyping, 16–17
    immunocytochemistry, 10–14
      clinical applications, 12–14
    molecular genetic study, 22–24
Muscle-specific actin, immunologic marker, 13
Myelolipoma, adrenals, 239
Myoglobin, immunologic marker, 13, 87
Myxoid liposarcoma, retroperitoneum, 94

N

Needle aspiration specimen, assessment, overview, 6–9
    architectural pattern, 7, 9
    cellularity of smear, 6–7
    morphology of individual cells, 7–8
    noncellular background material, 8–9
Nephroma, mesoblastic, 275–278

Nerve sheath tumor, peripheral, retroperitoneum, malignant, 97
Neuroblastoma, adrenals, 234–237
Noncellular background material, in needle aspiration biopsy, 8–9
Non-Hodgkin's lymphoma, 50
    retroperitoneum, 59–70
      lymphoproliferative disorder, small lymphocytic, 59–61
      malignant lymphoma, 59–61
        large cell
          cleaved and noncleaved, 63
          immunoblastic, 63
        mixed small/large cell, 63
        small cleaved cell, 62
        small noncleaved cell, 63, 66
Nonlymphoid markers, retroperitoneum, lymphoproliferative disorder, 53–55

O

Oncocytoma, renal, 271–274

P

Palpation, mass, abdominal imaging, 28–30
Papillary carcinoma, retroperitoneum, 144–145
Paraganglioma, retroperitoneum, 110, 114
Pathology, surgical, knowledge of, for successful needle aspiration biopsy, 5
Pattern
    cytologic, summary of, 9
    recognition, knowledge of, for successful needle aspiration biopsy, 5
Peripheral nerve sheath tumor, retroperitoneum, malignant, 97
Peritoneal mesothelioma
    anatomy, 199–200
    benign, peritoneal mesothelioma, 201
    embryology, 199–200
    imaging, 199–212
    malignant, peritoneal mesothelioma, 201–211
    normal cytology, 200
Pheochromocytoma, adrenals, 227–234
Pleomorphic sarcoma, retroperitoneum, 97–108
    diagnostic problems, 115–116
    malignant fibrous histiocytoma, 97–101
    pleomorphic rhabdomyosarcoma, 106–108
Polygonal cell sarcoma, retroperitoneum, 110–113
    diagnostic problems, 119
Pontifex, Hugh, M.D., fine needle aspiration biopsy, British Columbia Cancer Agency, 2
Prerequisites, for successful needle aspiration biopsy, 5
Prostate-specific antigen, immunologic marker, 13
Pseudomyxoma peritonei, 178–181
Pyelonephritis, xanthogranulomatous, 279–280

R

Radiologist, consultation with, 6
Rapid hematoxylin, procedure, 4

Reactive lymphoid hyperplasia, retroperitoneum, 73–75

Reading, immediate, for specimen quality, for successful needle aspiration biopsy, 5

Rectum, lymphoma, 182

Renal
  cell carcinoma, 251–261
    adrenocortical carcinoma, distinguishing features, 227
  cyst, 280–282
  disorders, see also Kidney
  oncocytoma, 271–274

Rhabdomyosarcoma, embryonal, retroperitoneum, 108–109

Rhabdomyosarcoma, pleomorphic, retroperitoneum, 102, 107

Round cell sarcoma, 108–110

S

Saccomanno's Carbowax solution, 2

Sampling, adequacy of, for specimen quality, for successful needle aspiration biopsy, 5

Sarcoma
  antibody, for differentiating from carcinoma, lymphoma, 12
  retroperitoneum, 85–119
    classification, 86–88
    diagnostic problems, 113–119
      pleomorphic sarcoma, 115–116
      polygonal cell sarcoma, 119
      small round cell sarcoma, 116–119
      spindle cell, 113, 115
    electron microscopy, 87–88
    Ewing's sarcoma, 108–110
    immunocytochemistry, 87–88
    needle aspiration cytology, 88–90
    pathology, 86–88
    pleomorphic, 97–108
      malignant fibrous histiocytoma, 97–101
      rhabdomyosarcoma, 97–101
    round cell, 108–110
    spindle cell, 90–97
      leiomyosarcoma, 90–94
      liposarcoma
        low-grade, 94–97
        low-grade, myxoid, 94
        low-grade, well-differentiated, 94–97
      peripheral nerve sheath tumor, malignant, 97
    spindle cell sarcoma, 90–97
  urinary tract, 266–271

Schwannoma, retroperitoneum, 119–120

Sclerosis, lymphoma, interpretive pitfalls, 76–77

Seminoma, retroperitoneum, 156

Small cell anaplastic carcinoma, retroperitoneum, 145–146

Small round cell sarcoma, retroperitoneum, diagnostic problems, 116–119

Smooth muscle tumor, intestine, 189–195
  epithelioid variant, 190, 193–194

Soft tissue tumor, retroperitoneum, 85–133

Solution, Carbowax, as fixative, 2

S100 protein, immunologic marker, 13, 97, 152

Specimen, quality of, 5–6

Spindle cell sarcoma
  liposarcoma, low-grade, well-differentiated, 94–97
  retroperitoneum, 90–97
    diagnosis problems, 113, 115
    fibrosarcoma, 97
    leiomyosarcoma, 90–94
    liposarcoma, low-grade, myxoid, 94
    peripheral nerve sheath tumor, malignant, 97

Squamous cell carcinoma, 137

Staining, 3
  for specimen quality, for successful needle aspiration biopsy, 5

Stomach
  adenocarcinoma, 171–176
  anatomy, 169–170
  embryology, 169–170
  endoscopic biopsy, versus needle aspiration biopsy, 170–171
  imaging, 169–197
  lymphoma, 181–182

Suen, Kenneth C., development of fine needle aspiration biopsy, 2

Surgical pathology, knowledge of, for successful needle aspiration biopsy, 5

T

T-cell lymphoma, retroperitoneum, 66, 68–69

Team approach
  abdominal imaging, 34–35
  importance of, 6

Technique, of aspiration, 2–3

Teratoma, retroperitoneum, 161

Transitional cell carcinoma, 265–266

Tuberculoma, retroperitoneum, 126–127

Tuberculous lymphadenitis, retroperitoneum, 75

U

Ultrasound, abdominal imaging, 29–31

Ultrastructural diagnosis of tumors, 19

Ureter, transitional cell carcinoma, 265–266

Urinary tract, 265–271
  sarcoma, 266–271

V

Vimentin, immunologic marker, 13

W

Wilms' tumor, 261–265; see Nephroblastoma

X

Xanthogranulomatous pyelonephritis, 279–280

Y

Yolk sac tumor, retroperitoneum, 156